Computational Methods and Algorithms for Medicine and Optimized Clinical Practice

Kwok Tai Chui
City University of Hong Kong, Hong Kong

Miltiadis D. Lytras
Deree - The American College of Greece, Greece

A volume in the Advances in Medical Technologies and Clinical Practice (AMTCP) Book Series

IGI Global
DISSEMINATOR OF KNOWLEDGE

Published in the United States of America by
IGI Global
Medical Information Science Reference (an imprint of IGI Global)
701 E. Chocolate Avenue
Hershey PA, USA 17033
Tel: 717-533-8845
Fax: 717-533-8661
E-mail: cust@igi-global.com
Web site: http://www.igi-global.com

Library of Congress Cataloging-in-Publication Data

Names: Chui, Kwok Tai, editor. | Lytras, Miltiadis D., 1973- editor.
Title: Computational methods and algorithms for medicine and optimized clinical practice / Kwok Tai Chui and Miltiadis D. Lytras, editors.
Description: Hershey PA : Medical Information Science Reference, [2019] | Includes bibliographical references.
Identifiers: LCCN 2018050068| ISBN 9781522582441 (hardcover) | ISBN 9781522582458 (ebook)
Subjects: | MESH: Computing Methodologies | Clinical Medicine--methods | Algorithms
Classification: LCC R855.3 | NLM W 26.5 | DDC 610.285--dc23 LC record available at https://lccn.loc.gov/2018050068

This book is published in the IGI Global book series Advances in Medical Technologies and Clinical Practice (AMTCP) (ISSN: 2327-9354; eISSN: 2327-9370)

British Cataloguing in Publication Data
A Cataloguing in Publication record for this book is available from the British Library.

Advances in Medical Technologies and Clinical Practice (AMTCP) Book Series

ISSN:2327-9354
EISSN:2327-9370

MISSION

Medical technological innovation continues to provide avenues of research for faster and safer diagnosis and treatments for patients. Practitioners must stay up to date with these latest advancements to provide the best care for nursing and clinical practices.

The **Advances in Medical Technologies and Clinical Practice (AMTCP) Book Series** brings together the most recent research on the latest technology used in areas of nursing informatics, clinical technology, biomedicine, diagnostic technologies, and more. Researchers, students, and practitioners in this field will benefit from this fundamental coverage on the use of technology in clinical practices.

COVERAGE

- Medical Informatics
- Diagnostic Technologies
- Nutrition
- Clinical Nutrition
- Nursing Informatics
- Clinical Studies
- Patient-Centered Care
- Clinical High-Performance Computing
- Telemedicine
- Biomedical Applications

The Advances in Medical Technologies and Clinical Practice (AMTCP) Book Series (ISSN 2327-9354) is published by IGI Global, 701 E. Chocolate Avenue, Hershey, PA 17033-1240, USA, www.igi-global.com. This series is composed of titles available for purchase individually; each title is edited to be contextually exclusive from any other title within the series. For pricing and ordering information please visit http://www.igi-global.com/book-series/advances-medical-technologies-clinical-practice/73682. Postmaster: Send all address changes to above address.

Titles in this Series

For a list of additional titles in this series, please visit:
https://www.igi-global.com/book-series/advances-medical-technologies-clinical-practice/73682

Computer Applications in Drug Discovery and Development
A. Puratchikody (Anna University, India) S. Lakshmana Prabu (Anna University, India) and A. Umamaheswari (Anna University, India)
Medical Information Science Reference • ©2019 • 332pp • H/C (ISBN: 9781522573265) • US $255.00

Computational Techniques for Dental Image Analysis
K. Kamalanand (Anna University, India) B. Thayumanavan (Sathyabama University Dental College and Hospital, India) and P. Mannar Jawahar (Anna University, India)
Medical Information Science Reference • ©2019 • 334pp • H/C (ISBN: 9781522562436) • US $225.00

Emerging Trends in the Diagnosis and Intervention of Neurodevelopmental Disorders
Sanjeev Kumar Gupta (All India Institute of Speech and Hearing, India) Srinivasan Venkatesan (All India Institute of Speech and Hearing, India) S.P. Goswami (All India Institute of Speech and Hearing, India) and Rajeev Kumar (Indian Institute of Technology Kharagpur, India)
Medical Information Science Reference • ©2019 • 394pp • H/C (ISBN: 9781522570042) • US $265.00

Histopathological Image Analysis in Medical Decision Making
Nilanjan Dey (Techno India College of Technology, India) Amira S. Ashour (Tanta University, Egypt) Harihar Kalia (Seemantha Engineering College, India) R.T. Goswami (Techno India College of Technology, India) and Himansu Das (KIIT University, India)
Medical Information Science Reference • ©2019 • 340pp • H/C (ISBN: 9781522563167) • US $265.00

Healing Through the Arts for Non-Clinical Practitioners
Jenny Bopp (Westtown School, USA) Amy M. Grebe (Zinnia Consulting and Design, USA) and Joanna Hope Denny (Pellisippi State Community College, USA)
Medical Information Science Reference • ©2019 • 309pp • H/C (ISBN: 9781522559818) • US $255.00

Medical Image Processing for Improved Clinical Diagnosis
A. Swarnambiga (Indian Institute of Technology Madras, India)
Medical Information Science Reference • ©2019 • 313pp • H/C (ISBN: 9781522558767) • US $245.00

For an entire list of titles in this series, please visit:
https://www.igi-global.com/book-series/advances-medical-technologies-clinical-practice/73682

IGI Global
DISSEMINATOR OF KNOWLEDGE

701 East Chocolate Avenue, Hershey, PA 17033, USA
Tel: 717-533-8845 x100 • Fax: 717-533-8661
E-Mail: cust@igi-global.com • www.igi-global.com

Table of Contents

Detailed Table of Contents

speech and memory lateralization. First, the imaging modality data is excluded and just clinical, electrographic and neuropsychological data are investigated. Afterward, the imaging data are investigated and a comparison between the prediction results of the two types of data is done. In the case of using non-imaging multimodal data, 56% and using imaging features, about 71% of correct outcome prediction was obtained.

Healthcare reform and health information technology (HIT) are transforming physicians' roles in delivering healthcare. New technologies present physicians with exciting new opportunities and challenges to enhance medical practice, reduce costs, and improve patient experiences, as well as opportunities to develop new competencies and standards of professionalism. The Dreyfus model for skills acquisition may provide a helpful framework. Within the competency context, understanding and leveraging drivers of and the barriers to HIT adoption can promote a learning culture that may more readily assimilate new HIT. Involving physicians in designing and implementing HIT systems could result in increasing physician satisfaction. Supportive staffing and technical assistance may aid physicians in successfully implementing the systems without increasing workload or decreasing professional satisfaction. Understanding the needs of 21st century physicians related to HIT solutions should greatly increase the successful integration of HIT into the 21st century healthcare workplace.

Predicting patient turnover within health services is beneficial for resource planning. In this chapter, patient turnover is viewed as a form of customer churn. As such, the authors examine whether free-form notes are useful for solving the classification problem typically associated with customer churn. The authors show that classifiers which incorporate free-form notes, using natural language processing techniques, are up to 11% more accurate than classifiers that are solely developed using structured data. In addition, the authors show that free-form notes aggregated for each account perform better than treating each note separately. It is suggested that hospitals and chronic disease management clinics can use structured data and free-form notes from electronic health records to predict which patients are likely to cease receiving care from their facilities. Classification tools for predicting patient churn are of interest to hospital administrators; such information can aid in resource planning and facilitates smoother handoffs between care providers.

Developing an efficient algorithm for traversing large ontologies is a key challenge for many semantic-based applications. This chapter introduces an approach, spreading activation over ontology (SAOO), to explore the relationship between two human diseases using an ontology-based spreading activation approach. SAOO comprises two phases: semantic matching and diseases relatedness detection. In the semantic matching phase, user-submitted diseases are semantically identified in the ontology graph using the proposed matching algorithm. Semantic matching conducts more analysis in the matching process, which comprises term normalization; phrase analysis, and word sense disambiguation. In the diseases relatedness detection phase, the URIs of these diseases are passed to the relatedness detector to detect the relationship connecting them. SAOO improves healthcare systems by considering semantic domain knowledge and a set of SWRL rules to infer diseases relatedness. We present a use case that outlines how SAOO can be used to explore relationships between vaccines in the vaccine ontology.

The complexity of clinical decision-making is immensely increasing with the advent of big data with a clinical relevance. Clinical decision systems represent useful e-health tools applicable to various tasks within the clinical decision-making process. This chapter is devoted to basic principles of clinical decision support systems and their benefits for healthcare and patient safety. Big data is crucial input for clinical decision support systems and is helpful in the task to find the diagnosis, prognosis, and therapy. Statistical challenges of analyzing big data in psychiatry are overviewed, with a particular interest for psychiatry. Various barriers preventing telemedicine

Preface

The famous saying "Wealth is Health" means a well-managed, modern clinical practice is vital to our healthy life. In earlier days, life was not so on the go. People were living simple and having fewer challenges as compared with these days, however medicine and clinical practices were underdeveloped. When it comes to today's technological era, we would like to emphasise that the busy workload that people having leads to sub-health and being more prone to disease.

Healthcare industry starts increasing their trust of computation algorithms for medicine and clinical practices as the way out of global healthcare challenges: (1) an ageing population (Søreide & Wijnhoven, 2016); (2) inadequacies of medical personnel (Liu, Goryakin, Maeda, Bruckner, & Scheffler, 2017); and (3) increasing healthcare expenditure (Baltagi, Lagravinese, Moscone, & Tosetti, 2017).

Have you noticed computing tools which have been utilized in healthcare applications? Magnetic resonance imaging (MRI), computed tomography (CT), positron emission tomography (PET) scans, and electronic health record sharing systems (eHRSS) are typical examples. These features have received positive feedback from both medical workers and users. What are the main obstacles in extensive deployment of computational algorithms for medicine? The top concern comes to major people mind is that technology may eliminate jobs. Nevertheless, authors believe that this is true in all areas, as sometimes it changes them, sometimes beyond recognition. It is a trend to have smart healthcare as a global vision. Particularly, the direction is to relieve medical doctors of routine work so that they can have more time to carry out surgery, which is difficult to achieve via automation.

ORGANIZATION OF THE BOOK

We are glad to deliver this editing volume with the support and contribution from international experts. This book is a manifestation of some of the most interesting aspects of theoretical and applied research covering complementary facets of the computational methods and algorithms for medicine and optimized clinical practice:

- Assessment of human cognitive abilities via digital technologies and smart devices
- Information and communication technology in the health sector
- Heart rate monitoring for preventing mental disease
- Localization related epilepsy using clinical, neuropsychologies and imaging data
- Implications of information technology for physician practice and professionalism
- Predicting customer churn using free-form call center notes
- Ontology-based spreading activation approach for disease relationship analysis
- Clinical decision support for mental health
- Glycemic monitoring and prediction with response improvement via Psyllium

This book covers the discussion on the computational methods and algorithms for medicine as well as optimized clinical practice via 9 chapters. The summary of each chapter is given.

Chapter 1 discusses various devices and technologies to assess neuropsychology. The smart devices computer, tablet and smartphones could be virtual reality enabled. It takes advantage of testing situations, is less labor intensive, more cost-efficient, and increases real-world experience and allows freedom from examiner biases and judgement. Unfortunately, the disadvantages are technical glitches and data loss, the affordability of digital technology, and human interaction versus automation. The author has shared the adoption of smart devices and technologies for healthcare in India.

The second chapter is about the satisfaction of Nigerian medical personnel when using information and communication technology (ICT). A survey taken by 106 participants, shows the extent of use of ICT, tasks and activities carried out with ICT, and the year of adoption of ICT. The results have indicated that female staff tend to use ICT more when compared to male staff. Examined by age, the age group of 26-35 years old contribute 50% of the respondents. Considering the data by title, doctors, nurses, pharmacists and physiotherapists contribute 75% of the respondents who use ICT functions. The reflection from health workers on ICT in healthcare is it could increase the efficiency in medical diagnoses, improve the doctor-patient rapport, increase the number of publications, create more exposure to scrutiny from patients, facilitate remote consultation, improve diagnoses and treatment, allow for easy collaboration among physicians and allow access to relevant medical training.

In Chapter 3, authors aimed at developing stress support system using smart finger plethysmogram measurement which visualizes the heart rate of body based on stress and heart rate interrelation. This chapter has summarized three phases for preventing mental illness based on preventive medicine: (1) primary prophylaxis by getting rid of the stressor; (2) secondary prophylaxis by early detection and early medical examination; and (3) tertiary prophylaxis by recurrence prevention treatment. Future development, maintenance and improvement of comprehensive daily health are ahead of this research. By generalizing the measurement of the state of mind, attention to ethics and safety are required.

Multimodal attributes analytics in localization-related epilepsy was carried out in Chapter 4 examining the effect on the selection of patients for surgery. It is noted that imaging modality data was neglected to avoid invasion and only neuropsychological, electrographic and clinical data was selected. The texture features extracted from magnetic resonance imaging (MRI) data related to the left and right hippocampus have a great potential to predict the surgical outcome. Various algorithms are implemented with different combinations of feature selection, clustering, and Engle classification approaches are used in order to estimate the status of localization-related epilepsy patients after surgery.

Chapter 5 presents physicians with new chances and challenges to improve patient experience, reduce costs, enhance the medical practice, as well as bring new opportunities to develop new competencies and standards of professionalism. Involving physicians in designing and implementing health information systems could result in leveraging physician satisfaction. Technical staffing and supportive assistance may aid physicians in successfully implementing the systems without increasing workload or lowering professional satisfaction.

Chapter 6 relates to the identification of some popular algorithms, as well as text mining techniques for modelling churn with semi-structured data. The key limitation was related to customer service notes which were used as opposed to actual patient notes from an electronic health record. In the future, the experiment should be repeated in order to evaluate whether the findings and conclusion hold true whenever anonymized patient data are available.

Spreading activation over ontologies was applied in the detection of two types of human diseases in Chapter 7. The methodology was divided into two parts, named semantic matching and diseases relatedness detection. Generally, the advantages of the proposed algorithm are to ease the process of finding the root of a disease which might be related to another disease that causes this disease. It can be used to find the relationship between any two instances in the biomedical ontologies such as diseases and vaccines. Various future works were recommended, for instance: (1) to find the relatedness between more than two diseases using multiple-goal search algorithms and provide the relatedness graph between them not only a simple path; and (2) a set of relationships is returned to the user which is a subset of the power set of the input diseases.

Clinical decision support is desired to relieve the workload of medical workers due to insufficient numbers of medical personnel worldwide and to reduce the medical expenditures. Chapter 8 discusses a clinical decision support system and its benefits using big data technology. Specifically, the authors were focused on diagnostics and therapy, as well as psychiatry. A reliable and tailor-made artificial intelligence technique such as classification and clustering of patient data is a key application.

At last, a review was made towards glycemic monitoring and prediction with response improvement via psyllium. Diabetes is one of the series epidemic diseases in the world. Over 400 million people in the world are living with diabetes. Many patients have to rely on medication in their lifetimes to control diabetes. Therefore, interventions that help glycemic control are worth discussing and investigating. It was suggested that psyllium might possibly give glycemic response improvement, and is greater among type 2 diabetes mellitus patients.

Kwok Tai Chui
City University of Hong Kong, Hong Kong

Miltiadis D. Lytras
Deree – The American College of Greece, Greece

REFERENCES

Baltagi, B. H., Lagravinese, R., Moscone, F., & Tosetti, E. (2017). Health care expenditure and income: A global perspective. *Health Economics*, *26*(7), 863–874. doi:10.1002/hec.3424 PMID:27679983

Liu, J. X., Goryakin, Y., Maeda, A., Bruckner, T., & Scheffler, R. (2017). Global health workforce labor market projections for 2030. *Human Resources for Health*, *15*(1). doi:10.118612960-017-0187-2

Søreide, K., & Wijnhoven, B. P. L. (2016). Surgery for an ageing population. *British Journal of Surgery*, *103*(2), e7–e9. doi:10.1002/bjs.10071 PMID:26771471

Chapter 1
Feasibility of Using Smart Devices and Digital Technologies in the Assessment of Human Cognitive Abilities:
Perspective for India

Aparna Sahu
Turiyan Psyneuronics Pvt. Ltd, India

ABSTRACT

The chapter covers topics concerning the use of smart devices such as smartphones, tablet devices, computer-based testing, and digital technology such as virtual reality, for the use of neuropsychological assessments. Several research results show promise for the use of the aforementioned technologies for the benefit of assessments for discriminating between patients and normal controls, and the increasing comfort levels of participants. Key advantages and disadvantages to using these technologies and future directions in terms of adopting newer technologies are discussed in the light of current developments. A specific emphasis is also laid on countries such as India that is ready to adopt such technologies in the healthcare sector.

DOI: 10.4018/978-1-5225-8244-1.ch001

INTRODUCTION

Psychology has come a long way since its inception as a scientific discipline. Empirical testing, evidence-based research, and ecological validity of assessments for neurological and psychiatric conditions are now the hallmark of the field.

This review chapter is specifically based on neuropsychological /neurocognitive assessment tools that are used to supplement diagnosis of neurological conditions. Furthermore, the key feature of the chapter is to check for the feasibility of integrating new developments with a specific emphasis on smart devices, and digital reality with assessments, and their use on neurological patients in India.

Neuropsychological assessments are "means of measuring in a quantitative, standardized fashion the most complex aspects of human behavior—attention, perception, memory, speech and language, building and drawing, reasoning, problem solving, judgment, planning, and emotional processing" (p.60, Lezak, Howieson, Bigler, & Tranel, 2012). Neuropsychological assessments till date use paper-pencil versions. Assessment tests for various cognitive functioning are known to have strong psychometric properties, and are known to be highly reliable (test scores are consistent over time) and valid (test measures what it is meant to measure). However, since the last two decades or so, researchers and clinicians have experimented with integrating technological advances with cognitive assessments. These have included,

1. Web-based assessments and computer-based assessments, which are typically conducted on the computer either as an installed application on the system or in the online modality,
2. Tablet-device based assessments that normally involve carrying out the assessment on a tablet device where data gets stored and/or being transferred to the cloud into an online database, and
3. Digital reality technology, which simulates reality in different ways (Cook, Cotteleer, & Holdowsky, 2018).

The chapter concentrates on the use of smart devices and digital reality for cognitive assessments. In keeping with this intention, the chapter is broadly divided into the following sub-sections:

1. Use of computer and smart devices and digital reality for cognitive assessments,
2. Benefits, and concerns about integrating smart devices and digital reality with neuropsychological assessments, and
3. Scope of integrating technology in the cognitive healthcare sector in India

COMPUTER BASED ASSESSMENTS, SMART DEVICES AND DIGITAL REALITY FOR COGNITIVE ASSESSMENTS

Generically, smart devices are interactive electronic gadgets that can connect to other devices via wireless protocols such as Bluetooth, WI-FI, LI-FI, and 3G-5G. Smart devices include smart phones, tablet devices, smart watches, smart bands, and smart speakers. These devices have artificial intelligence networks at the backend, and may be said to be characterized with a level of intuition as programmed by the makers of these devices.

However, the American Academy of Clinical Psychology and the American Academy of Neuropsychology consider computer based and smart devices under the umbrella term of Computerized Neuropsychological Assessment Devices (CNAD) for administering, scoring, and even interpreting test results pertaining to behaviour and neurological conditions (Bauer et al., 2012). Within the CNADs, there are variations that would either include or exclude an examiner, typically a clinical psychologist or a neuropsychologist who is trained in administering, and interpreting test results (Bauer et al., 2012). For instance, few computerized batteries are used for assessing neuropsychological functioning that comprise important domains such as attention, memory, language, speed of processing; these are compromised and are influence by the neurological conditions such as epilepsy and even the use of anti-epileptic medications. Data obtained from these batteries are automatically scored, and may be interpreted by a trained clinician (Witt, Alpherts, & Helmstaedter, 2013).

Several CNADs can be self-administrative in nature and hence do not require expertise to interpret the data. Most often these would be used for research or clinical trials. For instance, the computerized composite for preclinical Alzheimer's disease (C3-PAD), created by Rentz et al. (2016), is a tablet-device based testing of cognitive functioning with reportedly strong reliability and validity indices for older participants enrolled in clinical trials. Another self-administered test designed for cognitive assessment for dementia, iPad version (CADi) created by Onoda et al. (2013) is used for assessing cognition with the advantage of assessing large groups of elderly, thus reducing administration and data collection times. Self-administered CNADs may also be used as initial screeners for potential cognitive deficits for neurological deficits following brain concussion during sport activities (e.g., Collie, et al., 2003); additionally, self-administered computerized cognitive assessment batteries have been used in detecting mild cognitive impairment a condition characterised by confusion, disorientation, and abnormal cognitive functioning prior to a complete onset of dementia (Petersen, 2016; Tornatore, Hill, Laboff, & McGann, 2005).

The past two decades have witnessed a major addition in the area of digital technology and this essentially includes virtual reality (VR), augmented reality

(AR), and mixed reality (MR). Most studies have so far used VR technology and have shown its benefit in the assessment arena.

VR technology allows for interaction and immersion in an environment that is artificially created to replicate the real world; essentially, VR is a digitally created environment that replaces one's real-world environment (Cook, Cotteleer, & Holdowsky, 2018). With greater advancement over time, VR technology affords individuals with not just a three-dimensional environment, but also integrates tactile stimulation, making the experience all the more real. Given such a stimulating environment, individuals who experience VR, are also at the liberty to walk or turn around in the space he/she is viewing the environment. This happens because of the add-on hardware such as the head-mounted displays, and the eye tracking systems that integrate the data from the individual and allows the computer to adapt, generate-regenerate images in correspondence to the manner in which the individual is exploring the VR environment (Schultheis, Himelstein, & Rizzo, 2002).

VR technology has been in use for assessing neuropsychological functioning since the last two decades, which is suggestive of the point that technologies were available and were being tested for use in the clinical world. For instance, Pugnetti et al. (1998) used the VR environment for assessing memory processing, specifically for incidental memory (a memory processing characterised by remembering information from one's day-to-day happenings from one's life), and spatial memory, and found strong sensitivity for its use for both normal controls and cognitively impaired patient groups. Additionally, VR technology has also been used to assess other cognitive functions such as executive functioning, a cognitive parameter that represents higher-order processing that influences goal-directed behaviour, and adapting to complex, novel and uncertain situations (Hughes, 2013). Studies have shown robust findings in terms of accurately detecting executive dysfunction and/or normal executive functioning in patients and normal controls, respectively (Elkind et al., 2001; Pugnetti et al., 1998).

In more recent times, VR technology has increasingly been used in research and clinical setups to assess for specific types of memory processing such as allocentric and egocentric memories in neurological conditions such as mild cognitive impairment (Weniger et al., 2011), prospective memory or completion of task set for at a future time point, e.g., remembering to post a letter, or switch off the oven after some minutes (e.g., Knight & Titov, 2009), or simply assessing daily cognitive functioning in real setups such as shopping at a grocery store (e.g., Parsons, McPherson, & Interrante, 2013). In fact, a recent meta-analytic review has shown that using VR technology in the area of assessment is a sensitive measure to use and has more benefits than the traditional paper-pencil test (Negut, Matu, Sava & David, 2016).

Psychometric Characteristics of Smart Device and Digital Technology Based Assessments

An essential piece of information to be considered when incorporating such advances is whether these are able to demonstrate strong psychometric properties, an expectation that is held for psychological or cognitive tests for use on human subjects. A psychological test is a standardized way to measure a specific psychological construct, which are represented by scores. Furthermore, tests have norms or standards by which one's scores can be compared to judge, predict, interpret how similar or different their test performances are (Gregory, 2015). In keeping with these standards, researchers have shown that smart devices are significantly comparable to the gold standard of an established psychometrically sound cognitive/ psychological test.

Computerized neuropsychological tests have been deemed to be sensitive measures and are comparable to paper-pencil tests for measuring and reporting sensitively about cognitive functioning in the elderly (e.g., Collerton et al., 2007), for conducting memory tests and showing potential for detecting mild cognitive impairments and dementia (e.g, Chan, Kwong, Wong, Kwok, & Tsoi, 2018), and in detecting cognitive deficits in traumatic brain injury (Arrieux, Cole, & Ahrens, 2017). Similarly, tablet-based tests also showed robust psychometric properties and sensitivity in comparison to paper-pencil testing, and has been successful in discriminating cognitive performance between healthy controls and patients of Alzheimer's (Onoda & Yamaguchi, 2014). Researchers have also shown the comparable performances between a computerized and an ipad based cognitive assessment for the elderly (e.g., Meilke et al., 2015). Specifically, these researchers also found that there were some accuracy-based differences with the mouse producing quicker responses for a specific learning task over touchscreen on the tablet device; however, on a subjective level of reporting, participants preferred the tablet device over the computer for the assessment.

VR has also demonstrated its strengths in terms of establishing strong ecological validity. This type of validity consists of two components, a) an emphasis is placed on whether data collection methods are reflective of real-life tasks, and b) do test results reflect and predict one's cognition and behaviour in the real world (Franzen & Wilhem, 1996). VR environments have been used for studying spatial memory in mild cognitive impairment patients (Weniger, Ruhleder, Lange, Wolf, & Irle, 2011), predetermining a dementia diagnosis (Tarnanas, et al., 2013), and assessing executive functioning in post-stroke patients (Raspelli et al., 2011). Furthermore, VR environments have demonstrated a very high ecological validity in terms of representing real-life scenario and the manifestation of cognitive behaviour. In order to study how soldiers can adapt and show superior cognitive functioning such as being alert, assessing threat levels, problem-solving, coordinating psychomotor performance, researchers were able to assess these in the backdrop of a VR military scene (Parsons, Courtney, Arizmendi, & Dawson, 2011).

ADVANTAGES AND DISADVANTAGES ABOUT INTEGRATING SMART DEVICES AND DIGITAL REALITY WITH NEUROPSYCHOLOGICAL ASSESSMENTS

Advantages

1. **Rigor of Testing Situations:** Cognitive tests have most often emanated from experimental testing, which are later adapted for use in the clinical set up. Hence, some tests are heavily dependent on response times and correctness of responses. In this regard, smart devices are shown to be reliable in reporting these parameters with much rigor. For instance, a controlled environment which allows for increased precision in recording responses is deemed important in assessing visual processing of information; this ability is affected in certain neurological and psychological conditions, and even in normal aging (e.g., Duncan et al 1999; Finke et al., 2013; Finkel et al., 2007). Foerster et al. (2016) used the oculus rift for VR application and found it to be a highly reliable measure in testing for visual processing. One of the key aspects about tests of visual attention is that in addition to measuring the required parameters (correct responses, reaction times), such environments are characterised by heightened control for light, sound, foreground, and background stimuli.
2. **Less Labor Intensive:** One of the most acknowledged characteristics of automation in smart devices and other technologies is their ability to carry out assessing and scoring the input data. From an administration perspective, some tests can be heavily labor intensive. For instance, the cognitive ability of planning is affected in some neurological conditions; one way of measuring the planning ability is to administer cognitive tasks such as Tower of London test, and Wisconsin card sorting test. From a real-world perspective, Shallice and Burgess (1991) developed the multiple errands test (MET), which measures similar functions in a grocery store set up, where patients are assessed on their planning ability within a time frame. While the MET is a robust test to detect planning deficits, it is also known to be heavily dependent on the requirement of personnel for conducting the test in such a realistic way. However, adapting the same task in a VR based grocery store environment has demonstrated its

feasibility as well as success in reducing the requirement for increased personnel involvement (Raspelli et al., 2011) and has been implemented for assessing patients with neurological conditions, such as Parkinson's disease (Serino et al., 2014)

Furthermore, paper-pencil based neuropsychological assessments are known to be quite labor demanding as behavioural responses are required to be converted into scores, which are then compared to standardized norms to detect whether the obtained scores are in the normal or compromised ranges. By merely automating this process, clinicians can instead spend more quality time in interpreting the data and working out the next steps for the benefit of their patients. On a related note, and as mentioned previously, standardized norms are an important requirement before a test can be deemed as established. Collection of norms on a large-scale basis followed by scoring the data and creating specific norms based on statistical analyses, are possible using smart devices.

3. **Cost-Efficiency:** In a day and age where the environment we live in is getting heavily compromised due to climate change and with limited availability and/or incurring increased cost of resources (e.g., paper), using smart devices would be a significant and a much-needed replacement for paper-pencil versions.
4. **Increased Real-World Experience:** Tests created on smart devices and cognitive functions which are tested in the VR environment, are increasingly more representative of the real-world, and participants are more likely to relate with and identify with the testing situation, hence taking care of their innate biases about the usefulness of such testing. Furthermore, such technologies can afford the integration of more hardware to gather more relevant data, such as eye tracking devices (e.g., Rosa et al., 2015), galvanic skin response and heart rate measuring devices (e.g., Parsons et al., 2011), and even electroencephalograms for cerebral data derived from event-related potentials (e.g., Lin et al., 2007).
5. **Freedom From Examiner Biases and Judgement:** Most testing takes place on a one-on-one basis with a neuropsychological rater/examiner, who is witness to a participant's performance. Consequently, participants may experience discomfort, or may get defensive when they are unable to perform by their standards, which may further affect their performances on other tests. With self-administered smart device-based tests and / or tests within a VR environment, participants are less likely to feel self-conscious, and are more likely to be immersed in the testing situation.

Disadvantages

1. **Technical Glitches and Data Loss:** One of the constant fears of using and integrating technology with behavioural studies has been the possibility of a technical problem with the device, which could lead to data loss. In some cases, operating system updates on a smart device can also deem the previously installed application as outdated (most often, applications made on open source programs such as python, may not be necessarily updated or receive a patch fix by the creators due to the lack of funding).
2. **Affordability of Digital Technology:** While smart devices have now become cost friendly, perhaps migrating to tablet and computer-based testing might not necessarily be a problem. However, at the moment, digital technology is yet not affordable. As a result, integrating these with the psychology world is going to take some time. Perhaps in due time, this technology would become affordable, however given VR testing is meant for one person at a time, standardizing tests with the VR environment could not only be expensive but also a time-consuming process.
3. **Automation vs. Human Interaction:** One of the concerns for using automation is that interpretation of scores is simply at a superficial level and would not necessarily contribute towards patient care. While automation has its benefits, they are without doubt, tools for use for patient care. Clinicians are strongly required to be the point of contact as they play a key role in interpreting neuropsychological data and planning the future course in terms of remediation plans, for better patient management.

SCOPE OF INTEGRATING TECHNOLOGY IN THE COGNITIVE HEALTHCARE SECTOR FOR INDIA

It is crucial to study consumer attitudes and receptiveness of such technologies as these factors play important roles in assessing the feasibility of using these for neurological and psychiatric conditions.

India, like most other countries has successfully adopted such technologies once markets were flooded with affordable smart devices. A caveat to be considered while reading this sub-section; almost all studies discussing the use of smart devices consider smart phones as the point of reference; hence, this device will be used as a representative for people's attitudes towards adopting and adapting to smart technologies.

The influence and acceptance of smart devices has been pervasive in India. This is clearly witnessed based on current and predictive forecast of smart phone usage, which was at 199.08 million users in 2015, to a projected estimate of 442.5 million users by 2022 (Statista, 2018). A study by Watkins, Kitner, and Mehta (2012) showed the increased use of smart phones for communication in the urban sector, whereas rural areas did show a slowed acceptance of the technology due to reduced digital literacy and income. In order to deal with the slowed acceptance on the rural front, government initiatives to enable more education, exposure, and affordable technologies have managed in making individuals from these sectors, open to using such technologies (Ranade, Londhe, & Mishra, 2015).

Smartphone use has also shown its mark across generations. Needless to say, the young age group, specifically adolescents, has demonstrated quick adaptation of such technologies (Davey & Davey, 2014) for varied uses including educational reasons (e.g., Gavali, Khismatrao, Gavali, & Patil, 2017). However, the elderly individuals have also taken to smartphone use in a positive light, where such gadgets are used for communication over phone and participating in interactions over social media, and using applications for photographs and even health-monitoring (William & Murugesh, 2016).

In summary, the process of recognizing, and accepting smart devices (cell phones) in day-to-day life is on its way to becoming a common device in the lives of people. Increased exposure to such technologies would increase familiarity, hence, using such technologies may be a feasible option at the level of assessments.

India certainly has great chances of levelling herself to the western world in terms of adopting such technologies in the healthcare sector. While there have already been advances in some medical areas such as neurosurgery, physiotherapy, speech therapy, there is now great promise of seeing developments in the neuropsychological sector in the coming years.

Future Directions

A few upcoming start-up companies in India are already working towards creating and testing web applications and smart device applications for assessment purposes. However, two specific areas that are going to need increased attention in the coming years are, data management protocols, and the integration of Internet of things (IoT) in patient assessment.

Data management protocols will need to take into consideration how data are collected, stored, and managed by specific personnel in the field. A conceptual framework for tablet device based testing by Sahu (2017) is based on data gathering on the smart device and/or transferred to an online database, and an analysed report with scores can be generated. However, a detailed review by Bauer et al. (2012) addresses some additional aspects of the CNAD and issues as far as device use and management are concerned. Some of the areas that need an in-depth understanding for users of smart devices include, the variety of CNADs available for neuropsychological assessments, personnel and their expertise that needs involvement when administering tests on CNADs, technical information related to hardware, software that needs to be provided by CNAD developers, psychometric properties of test that are used for CNADs, awareness about the devices for the end-user, and privacy of data obtained and security of patients'/participants' identifying information, medical information.

One of the most talked about developments in recent times is about the Internet of Things (IoT), and this is going to change the face of neuropsychological assessment in a few decades. In recent times, IoT has already begun taking into consideration digital footprints of individuals who are in touch with the relevant IoT technology. In fact, there are already trials and speculations underway on how IoT is impacting the healthcare industry, where an individual's behaviour is tracked in real-time using sensors on patients and these data help in guiding healthcare professionals in diagnosing, and prescribing treatment plans (Chui et al., 2010). One way in which IoT may be used to track a person's cognitive performance in real time and within a real environment is by assessing how the individual interacts with their surroundings and devices connected to the internet (assuming several systems are kept on non-automatic level of functioning). This would reflect one's optimal functioning in the cognitive arena. For example, imagine a morning scenario where as it happens in daily life, a person wakes up in the morning, and needs to begin the day keeping the coffee for brewing, complete toilet chores while the coffee is getting ready, toast the bread while preparing fruit smoothie in the blender, and pack lunch while ordering some groceries over the phone. All these steps would constitute planning, a part of executive functioning. However, the key point to consider would be that all devices would be part of the IoT system;, the point of interest then from the point of view of neuropsychology would be to see how and when some of the behavioural deviations happen (e.g., forgetting some aspect of the routine) and if these could be considered early signs for the onset of a neurological condition.

To conclude, the world of neuropsychological assessments has already shown signs of being benefitted from the use of smart devices for patient diagnosis and cognitive tracking. Furthermore, digital technology, specifically VR has been used successfully in assessing cognitive functions in a simulated environment which has a strong real-life relevance. The future for the union between technology and neuropsychology certainly seems do-able and exciting as more developments in the technology world are here to change the face of cognitive assessments.

REFERENCES

Arrieux, J. P., Cole, W. R., & Ahrens, A. P. (2017). A review of the validity of computerized neurocognitive assessment tools in mild traumatic brain injury assessment. *Concussion*, *2*(1). doi:10.2217/cnc-2016-0021 PMID:30202572

Baucr, R. M., Ivcrson, G. I., Ccrnich, A. N., Binder, L. M., Ruff, R. M., & Naugle, R. I. (2012). Computerized Neuropsychological Assessment Devices: Joint Position Paper of the American Academy of Clinical Neuropsychology and the National Academy of Neuropsychology. *Archives of Clinical Neuropsychology*, *27*(3), 362–373. doi:10.1093/arclin/acs027 PMID:22382386

Chan, J. Y. C., Kwong, J. S. W., Wong, A., Kwok, T. C. Y., & Tsoi, K. K. F. (2018). Comparison of Computerized and Paper-and-Pencil Memory Tests in Detection of Mild Cognitive Impairment and Dementia: A Systematic Review and Meta-analysis of Diagnostic Studies. *Journal of the American Medical Directors Association*, *19*(9), 748–756. doi:10.1016/j.jamda.2018.05.010 PMID:29921507

Chui, M., Löffler, M., & Roberts, R. (2010). The internet of things. *The McKinsey Quarterly*, *2*, 1–9.

Collerton, J., Barrass, K., Bond, J., Eccles, M., Jagger, C., James, O., ... Kirkwood, T. (2007). The Newcastle 85+ study: biological, clinical and psychosocial factors associated with healthy ageing: Study protocol. *BMC Geriatrics*, *7*(1), 14. doi:10.1186/1471-2318-7-14 PMID:17594470

Collie, A., Maruff, P., Makdissi, M., McCrory, P., McStephen, M., & Darby, D. (2003). CogSport: Reliability and correlation with conventional cognitive tests used in postconcussion medical evaluations. *Clinical Journal of Sport Medicine*, *13*(1), 28–32. doi:10.1097/00042752-200301000-00006 PMID:12544161

Cook, A., Cotteleer, M., & Holdowsky, J. (2018). *Digital reality – A technical primer*. Deloitte Insights.

Davey, S., & Davey, A. (2014). Assessment of smartphone addiction in Indian adolescents: A mixed method study by systematic review and metaanalysis approach. *International Journal of Preventive Medicine*, *5*(12), 1500–1511. PMID:25709785

Duncan, J., Bundesen, C., Olson, A., Humphreys, G., Chavda, S., & Shibuya, H. (1999). Systematic analysis of deficits in visual attention. *Journal of Experimental Psychology. General*, *128*(4), 450–478. doi:10.1037/0096-3445.128.4.450 PMID:10650583

Elkind, J. S., Rubin, E., Rosenthal, S., Skoff, B., & Prather, P. (2001). A simulated reality scenario compared with the computerized Wisconsin card sorting test: An analysis of preliminary results. *Cyberpsychology & Behavior*, *4*(4), 489–496. doi:10.1089/109493101750527042 PMID:11708728

Finke, K., Myers, N., Bublak, P., & Sorg, C. (2013). A biased competition account of attention and memory in Alzheimer's disease. *Philosophical Transactions of the Royal Society of London. Series B, Biological Sciences*, *368*(1628), 1–11. doi:10.1098/rstb.2013.0062 PMID:24018724

Finkel, D., Reynolds, C. A., McArdle, J. J., & Pedersen, N. L. (2007). Age changes in processing speed as a leading indicator of cognitive aging. *Psychology and Aging*, *22*(3), 558–568. doi:10.1037/0882-7974.22.3.558 PMID:17874954

Foerster, R. M., Poth, C. H., Behler, C., Botsch, M., & Schneider, W. X. (2016). Using the virtual reality device Oculus rift for neuropsychological assessment of visual processing capabilities. *Scientific Reports*, *6*(1), 37016. doi:10.1038rep37016 PMID:27869220

Franzen, M. D., & Wilhelm, K. L. (1996). Conceptual foundations of ecological validity in neuropsychological assessment. In R.J. Sbordone & C.J. Long (Eds.), Ecological validity of neuropsychological testing (pp. 91-112). Delray Beach, FL: Gr Press/St Lucie Press, Inc.

Gavali, M. Y., Khismatrao, D. S., Gavali, Y. V., & Patil, K. B. (2017). Smartphone, the new learning aid amongst medical students. *Journal of Clinical and Diagnostic Research*, *11*(5), JC05–JC08. doi:10.7860/JCDR/2017/20948.9826 PMID:28658804

Gregory, R. J. (2015). *Psychological testing: History, principles, and applications* (7th ed.). Boston: Allyn and Bacon.

Hughes, C. (2013). Executive function: development, individual differences, and clinical insights. In J. L. R. Rubenstein & P. Rakic (Eds.), *Neural Circuit Development and Function in the Brain, - Comprehensive Developmental Neuroscience* (pp. 429–445). Amsterdam: Academic Press. doi:10.1016/B978-0-12-397267-5.00062-5

Knight, R., & Titov, N. (2009). Use of Virtual Reality Tasks to Assess Prospective Memory: Applicability and Evidence. *Brain Impairment*, *10*(1), 3–13. doi:10.1375/brim.10.1.3

Lezak, M. D., Howieson, D. B., Bigler, E. D., & Tranel, D. (2012). *Neuropsychological assessment* (5th ed.). New York, NY: Oxford University Press.

Lin, C., Chung, I., Ko, L., Chen, Y., Liang, S., & Duann, J. (2007). EEG-based assessment of driver cognitive responses in a dynamic virtual reality driving environment. *IEEE Transactions on Biomedical Engineering, 54*(7), 1349–1352. doi:10.1109/TBME.2007.891164 PMID:17605367

Meilke, M. M., Machulda, M. M., Hagen, C. E., Edwards, K. K., Roberts, R. O., Pankratz, V. S., ... Petersen, R. C. (2015). Performance of the CogState computerized battery in the Mayo clinic study on aging. *Alzheimer's & Dementia, 11*(11), 1367–1376. doi:10.1016/j.jalz.2015.01.008 PMID:25858683

Neguț, A., Matu, S., Sava, F. A., & David, D. (2016). Virtual reality measures in neuropsychological assessment: A meta-analytic review. *The Clinical Neuropsychologist, 30*(2), 165–184. doi:10.1080/13854046.2016.1144793 PMID:26923937

Onoda, K., Hamano, T., Nabika, Y., Aoyama, A., Takayoshi, H., Nakagawa, T., ... Yamaguchi, S. (2013). Validation of new mass screening tool for cognitive impairment: Cognitive assessment for dementia, iPad version. *Clinical Interventions in Aging, 8*, 353–360. doi:10.2147/CIA.S42342 PMID:23569368

Onoda, K., & Yamaguchi, S. (2014). Revision of the cognitive assessment for dementia, iPad version (CADi2). *PLoS ONE, 9*(10), e109931. doi:.pone.0109931 doi:10.1371/journal

Parsons, T. D. (2015). Ecological Validity in Virtual Reality-Based Neuropsychological Assessment. In M. Khosrow-Pour, D.B.A. (Ed.), Encyclopedia of Information Science and Technology (3rd ed., pp. 1006-1015). Hershey, PA: IGI Global. doi:10.4018/978-1-4666-5888-2.ch095

Parsons, T. D., Courtney, C. G., Arizmendi, B., & Dawson, M. (2011). Virtual reality stroop task for neurocognitive assessment. *Studies in Health Technology and Informatics, 163*, 433–439. PMID:21335835

Parsons, T. D., McPherson, S., & Interrante, V. (2013). Enhancing neurocognitive assessment using immersive virtual reality. In *2013 1st Workshop on Virtual and Augmented Assistive Technology, VAAT 2013; Co-located with the 2013 Virtual Reality Conference - Proceedings* (pp. 27-34). IEEE Computer Society. 10.1109/VAAT.2013.6786190

Petersen, R. C. (2016). Mild cognitive impairment. Continuum, 22(2), 404 – 418.

Pugnetti, L., Mendozzi, L., Attree, E. A., Barbieri, E., Brooks, B. M., Cazzullo, C. L., ... Rose, F. D. (1998). Probing memory and executive functions with virtual reality: Past and present studies. *Cyberpsychology & Behavior, 1*(2), 151–161. doi:10.1089/cpb.1998.1.151

Ranade, P., Londhe, S., & Mishra, A. (2015). Smart villages through information technology – need for emerging India. *International Journal of Information Technology, 3*(7), 1–7.

Raspelli, S., Pallavicini, F., Carelli, L., Morganti, F., Poletti, B., & ... Riva, G. (2011). Validation of a neuro virtual reality –based version of the multiple errands test for the assessment of executive functions. *Studies in Health Technology and Informatics, 167*, 92–97. PMID:21685648

Rentz, D. M. (2016). Validating Use of Technology for Cognitive Test Assessment. *EBioMedicine, 11*, 23–24. doi:10.1016/j.ebiom.2016.08.002 PMID:27498366

Rosa, P. J., Gamito, P., Oliveira, J., Morais, D., Pavlovic, M., & Smyth, O. (2015). Show me your eyes! The combined use of eye tracking and virtual reality applications for cognitive assessment. In *Proceedings of the 3rd 2015 Workshop on ICTs for improving Patients Rehabilitation Research Techniques (REHAB '15)* (pp. 135-138). New York, NY: ACM. 10.1145/2838944.2838977

Sahu, A. (2017). Feasibility of using tablet-based cognitive screening tools in India: A short review. *International Journal of Computers in Clinical Practice, 2*(1), 34–44. doi:10.4018/IJCCP.2017010103

Schultheis, M., Himelstein, J., & Rizzo, A. A. (2002). Virtual reality and neuropsychology: Upgrading the current tools. *The Journal of Head Trauma Rehabilitation, 17*(5), 378–394. doi:10.1097/00001199-200210000-00002 PMID:12802250

Serino, S., Pedroli, E., Cipresso, P., Pallavicini, F., Albani, G., ... Riva, G. (2014). The role of virtual reality in neuropsychology: The virtual multiple errands test (VMET) for the assessment of executive functions in Parkinson's disease. *Intelligent Systems. The Reference Librarian, 68*, 257–274. doi:10.1007/978-3-642-54816-1_14

Shallice, T., & Burgess, P. (1991). Deficits in strategy application following frontal lobe damage in man. *Brain, 114*(2), 727–741. doi:10.1093/brain/114.2.727 PMID:2043945

Statista. (2018). Forecast of mobile phone users in India. Retrieved from https://www.statista.com/statistics/274658/forecast-of-mobile-phone-users-in-india/

Tarnanas, I., Schlee, W., Tsolaki, M., Müri, R., Mosimann, U., & Nef, T. (2013). Ecological validity of virtual reality daily living activities screening for early dementia: longitudinal study. *JMIR Serious Games, 1*(1), 1-14.

Tornatore, J. B., Hill, E., Laboff, J. A., & McGann, M. E. (2005). Self-administered screening for mild cognitive impairment: Initial validation of a computerized test battery. *The Journal of Neuropsychiatry and Clinical Neurosciences, 17*(1), 98–105. doi:10.1176/jnp.17.1.98 PMID:15746489

Watkins, J., Kitner, K. R., & Mehta, D. (2012). Mobile and smartphone use in urban and rural India. *Journal of Media & Cultural Studies, 26*(5), 685–697. doi:10.1080/10304312.2012.706458

Weniger, G., Ruhleder, M., Lange, C., Wolf, S., & Irle, E. (2011). Egocentric and allocentric memory as assessed by virtual reality in individuals with amnestic mild cognitive impairments. *Neuropsychologia, 49*(3), 518–527. doi:10.1016/j.neuropsychologia.2010.12.031 PMID:21185847

William, J. A., & Murugesh, R. (2016). Cognitive modeling in human computer interaction: Understanding technology usage in elderly people. In *2016 IEEE International Conference on Advances in Computer Applications (ICACA)* (pp. 115-120). 10.1109/ICACA.2016.7887934

Witt, J.-A., Alpherts, W., & Helmstaedter, C. (2013). Computerized neuropsychological testing in epilepsy: Overview of available tools. *Seizure, 22*(6), 416–423. doi:10.1016/j.seizure.2013.04.004 PMID:23628168

Chapter 2
An Empirical Study of Information and Communications Technology (ICT) in the Nigerian Health Sector

Jeremiah Ademola Balogun
Obafemi Awolowo University, Nigeria

Ngozi Chidozie Egejuru
Hallmark University, Nigeria

Peter Adebayo Idowu
https://orcid.org/0000-0002-3883-3310
Obafemi Awolowo University, Nigeria

Temilade Aderounmu
Obafemi Awolowo University Teaching Hospital Complex (OAUTHC), Nigeria

ABSTRACT

This study focuses on the assessment of different ICT tools used by Nigerian health workers. Structured questionnaires were used to collect information from 106 respondents. The questionnaire consists of 5 sections, namely: demographics, extent of use of ICT, tasks and activities carried out with ICT, the year of adoption of ICT. Descriptive statistics tools were used for data summarization and visualization. The results showed that the ICT devices were more commonly used among females than male medical personnel which were most common among the age group of 26-30 years and were nurses and doctors with less than 5 years' experience. The earliest ICT tool adopted was the PC in 1994 followed by mobile phones and search engines in 1996 and the projector in 2001. A majority of the health workers used ICT for administrative functions followed by research and personal work. ICT majorly impacted ICT by promoting collaboration among physicians, quicker medical diagnoses of diseases, increased efficiency and facilitated remote consultation, diagnoses and treatment.

DOI: 10.4018/978-1-5225-8244-1.ch002

INTRODUCTION

It is no longer news that Information and Communication Technology (ICT) is arguably the most rapidly growing segment of the world ecosystem (Toyo, 2016). The development in the sector permeates every human activity: social, economic, cultural, religious, political or health care (Idowu et al., 2008). The huge networking possibilities afforded by ICT has significantly transformed the health care systems in the world; dispersing health care information with comparative ease, bringing patients closers to caregivers, making access to the best health care technology and expertise available to the remotest parts of the world (Akadiri et al., 2009). ICT has been integrated into business operation and management for decades. Investments in ICT have become crucial organizational strategies for survival and competitive advantage (Melville et al., 2004). One of the most common questions when utilizing ICT in business operation is when the business is considered to be successful at using ICT or what determines the stage of success (Ekene, 2014).

ICTs with their gathering, processing and retrieval abilities can simplify the numerous information and communication needs required for such collaboration. Shittu et al. (2008), list the information and communication requirements of the health institution to include information and research tasks, interacting and gathering information daily from several patients, cross-checking patients' histories, discussing with colleagues to examine and share experiences as well as updating knowledge on diseases and drugs (Udousoro, 2014). Networking was the ground-breaking digital innovation which altogether modified the landscape for the use of ICTs (Kundi et al., 2013). Computer is no more the central feature of computer-based systems rather it is just a node on the network. Internet is one of the convenient and cheapest sources that save time for searching information by the healthcare professionals. This is supported by (Mittman and Cain, 1999) they found that availability of online health care information save time, efforts and make the access easier. As according to Griffiths et al. (2006) one of the most common functions of internet is that it provides all sorts of health-related information through use of different websites.

According to Idowu et al. (2006), the last 20 years has witnessed incredible swift and dynamic execution of information technology (IT) which has turned the world into a global village. Nations have also enjoyed an unparalleled increase in productivity as well as sustainable economic growth and development due to this evolving trend. However, this laudable development has not been evenly spread. In particular, the health sector was relatively slower than other industries in the adoption and use of information technology based solutions for its services where the use of computers, mobile phones, multimedia projectors, video conferencing, audio conferencing and internet for the improvement of individual and collective effort on the job productivity of workers in the health care system is not commonly recognized (Idowu et al., 2003).

Innovation in healthcare is crucial for improving patient outcomes. However, this potential can only be fully realized when innovation is effectively spread, adopted and used. The incorporation of IT in the health sector plays the following roles (Idowu et al., 2006; Srivastava, 2005): ICT enables remote consultation, diagnosis and treatment through telemedicine. This is increasingly being used in developing countries to transmit patient's information to medical practitioners and specialists who then advice on treatments to be given; the connectivity via the Internet and satellites promotes collaboration among physicians by enabling the sharing of knowledge regarding new methods of treatment and case-specific consultation for expert opinion thereby ensuring more effective treatment; ICT supports research in healthcare by enabling a network of libraries and other information agencies, transmission of field information for remote analysis by research institutes, and exchanging ideas on similar research fields between researchers from different institutes; and the Internet can be used for the surveillance of epidemics and outbreaks in order to plan mass vaccination campaigns. The benefits of IT in the healthcare sector are very numerous. Among the various benefits of IT in the healthcare sector includes: efficient and effective sharing of health-related information and skills; easy information dissemination for disease treatment and control; reduced costs and inconvenience of patients' transfer; disease surveillance information and interventions accessible by all; and databases of health management information systems for efficient planning and policy formulation.

Despite the growing proliferation of ICT into the Nigerian Health sector, there is a still a number of limitations facing the adoption of ICT in Nigeria. One of the major problems facing the adoption of ICT is the epileptic supply of power in Nigeria by the Power Holding Company of Nigeria (PHCN) whereas ICT tools require electricity in order to function and be used for any purpose as required by the user instead the power situation in Nigeria has caused a lot of damage to research computer laboratory equipment. In addition Internet connectivity also suffered massive downtime owing to epileptic power thus leading to the purchase of diesel electricity generating plants as alternate power supply which on the long run leads to more expenses covering the purchase of diesel and the maintenance of the generating plants (Adebayo and Edward, 2014).

In Nigeria, ICT tools like the mobile phones, personal computers and the Internet are becoming ubiquitous by workers of the Nigerian tertiary hospitals (Afolayon and Oyekunle, 2014; Adeyemi and Ayegboyin, 2004). Furthermore, there is a growing number of ICT tools users in the Nigerian health sector as many more people are adopting ICT in their personal life and also their research activities especially with the use of the Google search engine for searching for related materials and collaborative groups where fellow practitioners are met in order to share insights and breakthrough more easily and speedily. It is of importance that the present state of the identification, adoption and the usage pattern of different ICT tools be identified especially in the health sector of Nigeria so as to stress the importance of the adoption of ICT for the ease and efficiency of the medical practice by tertiary health workers using ICT. Hence, an empirical study of the various ICT tools used are discussed alongside their distribution, availability and functionality using descriptive statistics tools like frequency distribution tables for the summarization of distribution and bar charts for the visualization of the distribution.

RELATED WORKS

A number of studies have been made in the area of the adoption and the use of ICT in various sectors of the economy, namely: education, business, finance, health etc. Among those identified in the review of literature are a number of related works which are discussed in the following paragraphs.

Idowu et al. (2017), proposed an ICT infusion model for the Nigerian transport sector. The study was aimed at identifying the various ICT devices that were adopted and used in the transport sector following which a polynomial model was used to formulate the infusion model for the identified ICT devices adopted in the transport sector of Nigeria. Structured questionnaires were used to collect information regarding the use of the ICT devices used in the Nigerian transport sector identified from 100 staffs selected from six (6) different transport companies in southwestern Nigeria. The different ICT devices identified were: smartphones, SMS, e-mails, company website, bulk SMS, ticket reservations, vehicle trackers, POS systems and 2-way radio. The results of the study showed that majority of respondents were married male drivers of Ibo ethnicity within ages of 31 – 40 years which was 57% of the respondents selected. The results of the study also showed that the earliest ICT tools adopted were: SMS, e-mails, bulk SMS, company websites, ticket reservations and vehicle trackers in 2001 while smartphones, POS and 2-way radios were adopted by 2006.

Okundaye (2016), presented a study on the adoption of ICT in the Nigerian small and medium enterprises (SMEs). The study explored how SME leaders in Lagos, Nigeria, adopted information and communication technology (ICT) as a business strategy to increase profitability and compete globally. Data was collected from 5 SME leaders from 4 SMEs which had successfully integrated ICT into their business. The data was analyzed following which the technology acceptance model (TAM) was adopted. The study revealed that the adoption of ICT by SMEs will create a social change by creating jobs thus alleviating poverty and promoting socio-economic development by adopting ICT.

Wilson et al. (2014), presented an analysis of University of Education, Winneba students' use of Information and Communication Technology. The study described the ability of students' in using a wide range of ICT devices to support their personal learning. The study used a self-answering questionnaire and focus-group-discussions (FGD) to collect data from students. A total of thousand five hundred (N = 1500) students were selected using stratified sampling. The data from the questionnaires were analysed using SPSS software to identify and compare students' ICT use and ability. The findings revealed that a good number of the students had access to ICT tools and devices, and were competent in using a wide range of ICT tools and devices both for the context of academic and non-academic use. It was evident in the data that most students used this technology on a frequent basis.

Shabi et al. (2011) determined the extent, purpose, determinants and the impact of the utilization of internet medical databases among medical practioners in Osun state. A descriptive cross-sectional survey of 540 randomly selected physicians at two tertiary institutions in Osun State, Nigeria. Questionnaires was distributed to 444 physicians located in the two selected locations. The results showed that 53.8% used Internet resources at least once in 2 weeks, while 12.2% used the resources every day. 40.4% say that the Internet resources has positively impacted clinical practice while 65.5% said it has impacted research output. The study concluded that there has been considerable increase in the extent and quality of utilizaion of online medical databases which has a positive impact on clinical practices and research output of the physicians.

Olatokun and Adeboyejo (2009), investigated reproductive health workers' (RHW) use of ICTs, the effects of ICTs on their job functions alongside the challenges limiting full exploitation of ICTs. The study adopted a descriptive survey design. Stratified sampling technique was used to select a sample of 360 RHWs of the University College Hospital, Nigeria. A questionnaire obtained the data, and frequencies and percentage distributions were the analytical techniques adopted. Findings revealed that RHWs indicated extensive use of ICTs in their job functions. Faster access to relevant medical information, easy exchange of information with colleagues, and increased efficiency were the major impacts of ICT usage on their activities. The information accessed through ICTs was primarily educational, health, and research. Findings equally revealed that the major challenges in ICT use were erratic power supply and inadequate access to ICT facilities. Based on the findings, recommendations were made towards enhancing better utilization of ICTs by RHWs.

Asanganasi et al. (2008), performed a survey of the use of computers among medical doctors in Nigerian tertiary hospitals. The study used questionnaires to evaluate information on the level of computer and Internet use among doctors located in the University College Hospital (UCH), Ibadan. The study population consisted of 600 interns and resident doctors undergoing traomomg at UCH in various specialties using a 24-item questionnaire. 87% of doctors could use statistical software but 37.9% could not use word processing software while about 51.7% of them had their own personal computers. The study revealed that there was a strong association between those who owned their pseronal computers with the longer duration of practice, postgraduate qualification, word procesing skills and browsing the Internet at home alongside publishing more papers.

Ajuwon (2006), investigated the use of internet for health information by physicians for patient care in a teahcing hosptal in Ibadan, Nigeria. The study used standardized questionnaire to elicit information from 172 physicians at the University College Hospital (UCH), Ibadan, Nigeria consisting of 31 items while Epi-Info software was use for analysis. The results showed that the mean age of users was 31.95 years with 98% of users virtually making use of the Internet while 76% used the cyber-cafes. The most commonly used service was the e-mail comprising of 64% of repondents. 90% had obtained patient acre-related information from the Internet from which 76.2% had accessed a database with the most frequently accessed database being MADLINE/PubMed. The study identified the barriers to the use of Internet as being poor availablity of broadband (fast conection speed) Internet access, lack of infromation searching skills, costs of access and information overload.

MATERIALS AND METHODS

This study made use of structured questionnaire for the purpose of eliciting information about the types of ICT components used, how many people used the resources and for how long the IT devices had been in use among the respondents considered for the study. The study considered respondents selected from four (4) teaching hospitals located in south-western part of Nigeria, namely: Bowen University Teaching Hospital (BUTH), Ogbomoso; Ladoke Akintola University Technology Teaching Hospital (LAUTH), Ogbomoso; Olabisi Onabanjo University Teaching Hospital (OOUTH), Sagamu and Obafemi Awolowo University Teaching Hospital Complex (OAUTHC), Ile-Ife. Thus, two (2) hospitals from Oyo state and one (1) each from Ogun and Osun state respectively were considered for this study.

The instrument of data collection was used to collect information from the respondents of the study, such data included: demographic information, Information and Communications Technology (ICT) components used at each sites alongside the impact of the ICT components. Following the collection of data from the respondents, the data was analyzed using standard descriptive statistics tools: tables for data presentation and graphs for data presentation. The IT infusion model was formulated using polynomial functions needed to represent sequences and series of data – representing the total number of people who use each ICT for each period of time between the periods of infusion till 2015. The infusion model for ICT was presented for each ICT component identified given a base year.

The study population for this study was identified as the members of staffs (male and female) of Teaching Hospitals located in four (4) hospitals identified in the earlier section which comprises of the following: medical doctors, nurses, pharmacists, medical laboratory scientists, orderly, attendants, consultants; and physiotherapists. The study also considered respondents within the age group of 26 years and above with 160 respondents – 40 selected from each tertiary institutions selected for this study.

This study incorporated the use of descriptive statistical techniques for the purpose of analyzing the data collected for this study from the respondents. The descriptive statistics methods used helped in the simplification of large amount of data in a much sensible way by the provision of summary using both numerical and graphical tools using frequency tables and charts respectively.

RESULTS AND DISCUSSIONS

Based on the findings of this study, the ICT tools investigated among the 106 respondents chosen for this study were: multimedia projectors, mobile phones, personal computers, e-mail, the Web, video and audio conferencing and search engines. Following the results of the demographic information of the respondents in order to identify those that make use of these ICT tools within the Nigerian teaching hospitals, it was observed that there were more female users (51.9% of respondents) than there were male users (40.6%) of ICT tools working in Nigerian teaching hospitals as shown in Table 1. The results also showed that users within the age interval of 26 – 35 (28.3% for the interval 26-30 and 22.6% of respondents for the interval 31-35) are more likely to use ICT tools compared to other tertiary hospital users as shown in Table 2.

Doctors (30.2% of respondents) were the most likely to use ICT tools followed by nurses (28.3% of respondents) and pharmacists (17.0% of respondents) among all respondents which may be associated with the demand of their job functionalities in the tertiary hospitals as shown in Table 3. The results further showed that most

Table 1. Gender of respondents that use ICT tools

Gender	Total	%
Male	43	40.57
Female	55	51.89
Missing	8	7.55
Total	106	100.00

Table 2. Age group distribution of respondents using ICT tools

Age-Group	Total	%
26-30	30	28.30
31-35	24	22.64
36-40	10	9.43
41-45	8	7.55
46-50	14	13.21
51 and above	16	15.09
Missing	4	3.77
Total	106	100.00

Table 3. Distribution of the Job category of users of ICT tools

Category	Total	%
Nurse	30	28.30
Doctor	32	30.19
Pharmacist	18	16.98
SLT	4	3.77
Attendant	4	3.77
Physiotherapist	12	11.32
Consultant	5	4.72
Orderly	1	0.94
Missing	0	0.00
Total	106	100.00

common users of ICT tools constitute of respondents with 0 – 5 years of work experience (34.9% of respondents) and the number of users reduced as due to an increase in the number of years of work experience as shown in Table 4. Hence, women and doctors or nurses alongside respondents within the age group of 26 – 35 years are most likely to use ICT tools in Nigerian tertiary hospitals. Regarding the availability and functionality of ICT tools in tertiary institutions it was observed that personal computers, mobile phones, multimedia projectors, search engines and e-mails are available and functional to a majority of users representing an average of 70.0% of respondents while video and audio conferencing services are not available to a smaller proportion of users representing an average of 40.0% of respondents as shown in Figure 1.

With respect to the use of ICT tools among users, the results showed that Video and audio conferencing services have never been used by a majority of users representing 54.0% and 55.0% of respondents although a majority of users representing 62.3% and 45.3% of respondents use mobile phones and personal computer very often while an average of 23.6% of respondents use projectors, e-mails, the Web and search engines often as shown in Figure 2. Based on the type of activities carried out by respondents, results showed that 65.0% of respondents did not use ICT tools for staff record purposes, collaboration, skill acquisition and health care delivery while a majority representing 85.0% of respondents do not use ICT tools for the purpose of administrative tasks as shown in Figure 3. Also, 65.0% of respondents representing a majority of users used ICT tools for research, PowerPoint presentation

Table 4. Distribution of work experience of users of ICT tools

Experience	Total	%
0-5	37	34.91
6-10	20	18.87
11-15	13	12.26
16-20	9	8.49
21-25	14	13.21
26-30	9	8.49
31 and above	4	3.77
Missing	0	0.00
Total	106	100.00

Figure 1. ICT tools' availability and functionality among users

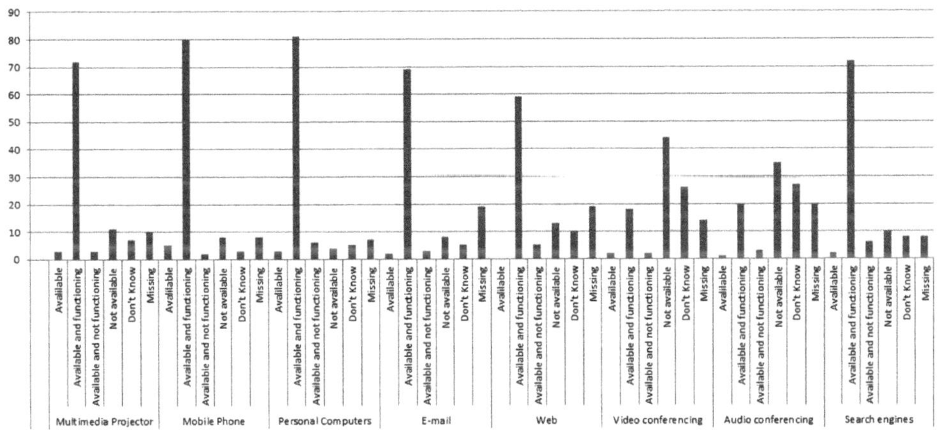

Figure 2. Frequency of use of ICT tools among users

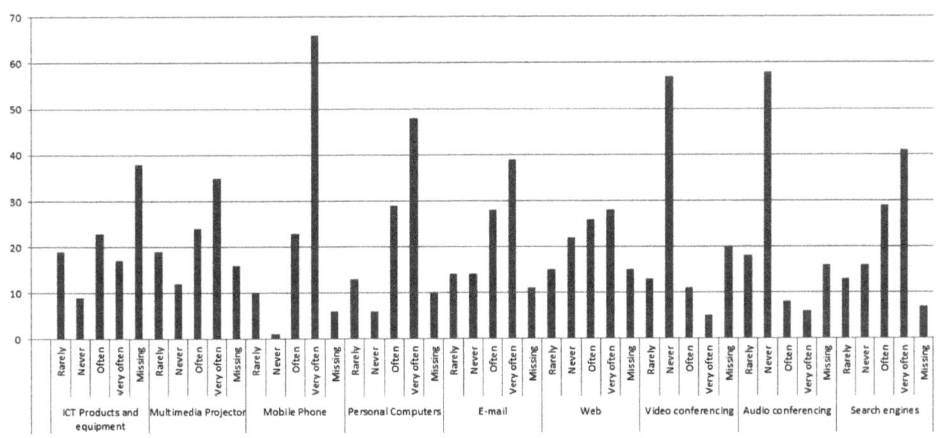

and personal work as shown in Figure 4. The significant proportion of users who use ICT tools for power point presentations can be associated with the proportion of respondents who use projectors in tertiary institutions.

The results of the impact of ICT tools on job productivity and functionality showed that a majority representing 32.0% of respondents believed that the impact of ICT was very good for increased efficiency, 34.0% of respondents believed that the impact of ICT was good for quicker medical diagnoses, 28.0% of respondents believed that the impact of ICT was very good for better doctor-patient rapport, 29.0% of respondents believed that the impact of ICT was good for increased number

Figure 3. Tasks and activities carried out using ICT tools among users

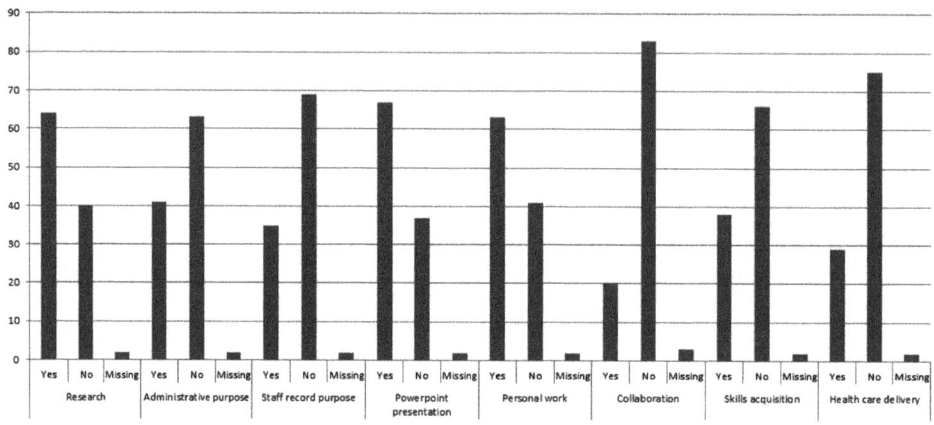

Figure 4. Health-related activities carried out using ICT tools among users

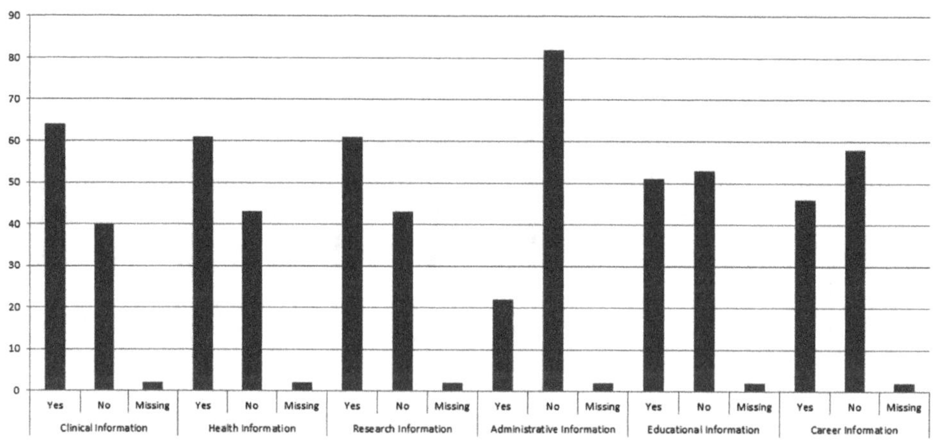

of publication, 30.0% of respondents believed that the impact of ICT was good for facilitating remote consultation, diagnoses and treatment, 36.0% of respondents believed that the impact of ICT was good for easy collaboration among physicians while 29.0% of respondents believed that the impact of ICT was very good for access to relevant training as shown in Figure 5. Thus most of the respondents believed ICT tools promoted collaboration among physicians, quicker medical diagnoses of diseases, increased efficiency and facilitated remote consultation, diagnoses and treatment.

Figure 5. Distribution of the impact of ICT tools on job productivity and functionality of respondents

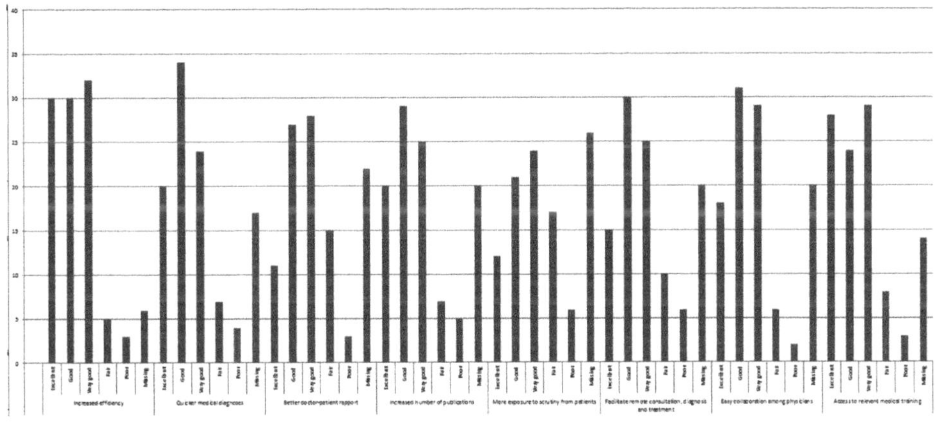

Based on the results of this study, a number of observations were made about the distribution of ICT among health workers in Nigerian tertiary hospitals which include the following. ICT tools were more commonly used among female workers than among male workers with a very small marginal difference and more commonly used among respondents between the age group of 26 – 35 years of age. Doctors and nurses with at most 10 years working experience were identified to be among the respondents who use ICT tools among the respondents selected for this study. Also, among the identified ICT tools selected for this study, the multi-media projector, mobile phones, personal computers, e-mails, the Web and search engines were identified to be available and functioning by at least 60% of health workers selected for this study.

Among the ICT tools identified to be used by the health workers selected for this study, the mobile phones, personal computers, e-mails and search engines were used most often by majority of the respondents while the audio and video conferences were most rarely used by majority of Nigerian health workers in tertiary hospitals. Also, majority of respondents used ICT tools for the purpose of research, presentations and collaboration with fellow health workers located at other remote locations while the health-related activities most commonly performed with ICT were clinical, health information, health research and educational information by at least 60% of health workers.

CONCLUSION

This study presented an empirical study into the infusion of ICT in the Nigerian tertiary hospitals by healthcare workers in South-western Nigeria. It is obvious that the health professionals in the selected study area are aware of the usefulness of ICTs to the medical profession; however, volumes of ICTs are low. The health professionals are handicapped because there are some core ICT enabled services like video and audio conferencing that are not available for use which further affected the adoption and use of such services among Nigerian health workers. Even though the health professionals can afford to provide for themselves other ICT enabled services like Internet and search engines; the provision of ICT equipment and services by hospitals is very fundamental to achieving the desired impact of ICTs in the health sector.

It can then be inferred that Information and communication technology adds to the job productivity of workers in the health care system as well as to positive growth of the health care delivery system in Nigeria universities teaching hospitals. As regard the use of ICT tools, the results showed that respondents are more likely to make use of ICT products and equipment, multimedia projectors, mobile phones, personal computers, e-mail, Web and search engines very often and/or often while respondents are more likely to never and/or rarely use video and audio conferencing services in the discharge of their respective duties in the office.

Finally, the result showed that health workers felt the impact of ICT tools on their jobs for the following: increasing the efficiency, quicker medical diagnoses, doctor-patient rapport, increased number of publications, creating more exposure to scrutiny from patients, facilitating remote consultation, diagnoses and treatment, easy collaboration among physicians and accessing relevant medical training.

REFERENCES

Adebayo, K., & Edward, O. (2014). Issues on E-health Adoption in Nigeria. *International Journal of Modern Education and Computer Science*, *6*(9), 36–46. doi:10.5815/ijmecs.2014.09.06

Adeyemi, A., & Ayegboyin, M. (2004). A study on the use of information systems to prevent HIV/AIDS in Lagos state, Nigeria. *Paper presented at 3rd Virtual Congress in Internet Informedica: Information and Communication Technologies in Healthcare Development.*

Afolayan, A., & Oyekunle, S. (2014). Availability, Accessibility and Frequency of Use of ICT Tools by Health Professionals in Ilorin Metropolis. *Covenant Journal of Informatics and Communication Technology*, *2*(1), 1–15.

Ajuwon, G. (2006). Use of the Internet for health information by physicians for patient care in a teaching hospital in Ibadan, Nigeria. *Biomedical Digital Libraries*, *3*(12), 1–9. PMID:17163991

Akadiri, O.A., Olusanya, A.A., & Omitola, O.O. (2009). Impact of Improved Telecommunication Services on Health Care Delivery in Nigerian Teaching Hospitals – A Survey of Opinions. *Journal of Information Technology Impact*, *9*(3), 125–134.

Asanganasi, I. A. (2008, January). Computer use among doctors in Africa: Survey of trainees in a Nigerian teaching hospital. *Journal of Health Informatics in Developing Countries*, *2*(1), 10–14.

Ekene, E. A. (2014). ICT adoption in logistics operations: An emerging trend for sustainable development and human capacity building in South-Eastern Nigeria. *Journal of Emerging Trends in Engineering and Applied Sciences*, *5*(7), 24–28.

Griffiths, F., Lindenmeyer, A., Powell, J., Lowe, P., & Thorogood, M. (2006). Why are health care interventions delivered over the internet? A systematic review of the published literature. *Journal of Medical Internet Research*, *8*(2), 10–17. doi:10.2196/jmir.8.2.e10 PMID:16867965

Idowu, P., Cornford, D., & Bastin, L. (2008). Health informatics development in Nigeria. *Journal of Health Informatics in Developing Countries*, *2*(1), 15–23.

Idowu, P. A., Adagunodo, E. R., & Adedoyin, R. (2006). Information technology infusion model for health sector in a developing country: Nigeria as a case. *Technology and Health Care*, *14*, 69–77. PMID:16720950

Idowu, P. A., Eyitope, O., & Idowu, B. (2003). Information and Communications Technology in Nigeria - The Health Sector Experience. *Journal of Information Technology Impact*, *3*(2), 69–73.

Idowu, P. A., Oyetunji, M. O., Oladeji, F. A., & Balogun, J. A. (2017). An ICT Infusion Model for Nigerian Transport Sector. *Computing, Information Systems. Development Informatics and Allied Research Journal*, *8*(1), 103–120.

Kundi, G. M., Shah, B., Qureshi, A., Nawaz, A., Miankhel, A. K., Chishti, K. A., & Qureshi, N. A. (2013). Infrastructural Barriers to e-Health Implementation in Developing Countries. *European Journal of Sustainable Development*, *2*(1), 163–170.

Melville, N. K., Kraemer, & Gurbaxani. (2004). Review: Information technology and organizational performance: An integartive model of IT business value. *Management Information Systems Quarterly*, *28*(2), 283–322. doi:10.2307/25148636

Mittman, R., & Cain, M. (1999). *The Future of the Internet in Health Care: Five Year Forecast*. California Healthcare Foundation.

Okundaye, K. E. (2016). Adoption of Information and Communication Technology in Nigerian Small – to – Medium size Enterprises [PhD Thesis]. College of Management and Technology. Walden University, USA.

Olatokun, W. M., & Adeboyejo, O. C. (2009). Information and Communication Technology use by Reproductive Health Workers in Nigeria: State of the art, issues and challenges. *Human Technology*, *5*(2), 181–207. doi:10.17011/ht/urn.200911234470

Shabi, I. S., Shabi, O. M., Akewukereke, M. A., & Udofia, E. P. (2011). Physicians utilisation of internet medical databases at the tertiary health institutions in Soun state, south west Nigeria. *Health Information and Libraries Journal*, *28*(4), 313–320. doi:10.1111/j.1471-1842.2011.00962.x PMID:22051130

Shittu, A., Ajayi, A., and Garba, S. (2008). Information and Communication Technologies (ICT) Knowledge and Utilization for Healthcare Delivery among Zaria Medical Doctors. *The Nigerian Journal of Communication, 6*(1 & 2), 28-43.

Srivastava, A. (2005). *Accelerating Delivery of Health Services*. New Delhi: UN World Food Programme.

Toyo, O. D. (2016). Information and Communication Technology (ICT): A catalyst for promoting primary healthcare delivery services in rural communities in Nigeria. *International Journal of Sustainable Development, 11*(1), 49-57. Retrieved from www.africarsearchcorps.com

Udousoro, N.W. (2014). Use and gratification of ICTs by Health Care Personnel in Nigerian South-South Tertiary Hospitals. *Asian Journal of Social Sciences and Humanities, 3*(4), 226-235.

Wilson, K. B., Tete-Mensah, I., & Boateng, K.A. (2014). Information and Communication Technology Use in Higher Education: Perspectives from Students. *European Scientific Journal, 10*(19), 161–171.

Chapter 3
Consideration of Stress Coping Support System for Prevention of Mental Disease Using Smart Heart Rate Monitor

Hidehiko Hayashi
Hokusei Gakuen University, Japan

Akinori Minazuki
Kushiro Public University, Japan

ABSTRACT

In recent years, there has been a significant increase in the number of patients suffering from mood disorders in Japan, reaching 1.041 million in 2008. In 2014, the number of patients reached 1.116 million, the highest number recorded in the past. In modern society with the fourth industrial revolution, with its multitude of stressors that we encounter on a daily life, a characteristic of mental disorders is that there is a risk to increase them at the unconscious level, and even if the patient were to detect the condition, they are difficult to treat. Therefore, in everyday life, it is desirable to always measure the stress and detect the early signature before they get worse. Thus, this study aims to develop stress coping support system using smart finger plethysmogram measurement, visualizing the internal signals through the heart rate which is affected by stress.

DOI: 10.4018/978-1-5225-8244-1.ch003

INTRODUCTION

In recent years, as a term like the Fourth Industrial Revolution (4IR) (Schwab, 2016; Schwab, 2018) represents, social changes that create new values by utilizing Information Technology (IT, such as computers, the Internet, smart phones, social media, mobile devices, wearable devices, and so on) or digital technologies (DX, such as AI, IoT, Robotics and so on) are progressing in all industries. Digitization of the medical field is progressing. Developing human sensing technology which is detect human condition and behavior are also remarkable progress. Technology development to estimate human stress conditions in everyday life has also progressed.

In modern society with 4IR, the survey of patients in Japan by the Ministry of Health, Labor and Welfare (MHLW, 2018) revealed the total number of estimated patients with mood disorders included depressions climbed to more than 111.6 million people in 2014: number of people with mood disorders was 0.433milion in 1996 (Figure 1). This disease, called "modern-day illness", is largely the result physical stress and psychological stress (Lazarus and Folkman, 1984; Kawakami and Haratani, 1999; Stansfeld et al., 1999). In modern society, we have a broad range of stressors which load to depression; therefore, we are at an increased risk for this illness. However, there are many potential patients despite being affected by a disease. Depression can be defined subjectively or objectively; thus, patients with depression to accept or be aware of their disease. Although a diagnostic test which examines stress level has been invented, it is difficult to help conscious about

Figure 1. Increase of depressed patients within mood disorders

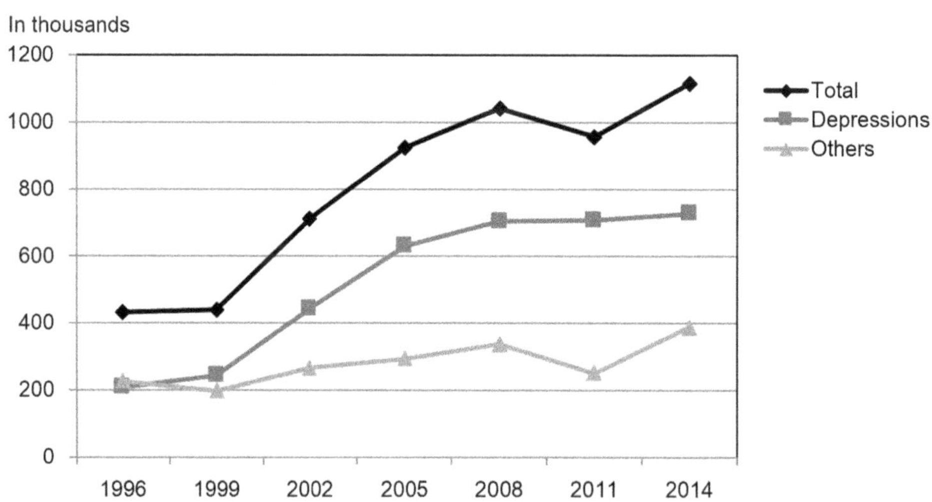

their disease. The reason is that the test is easily affected arbitrary and subjective elements (Aasman et al., 1987; Haas, 1979; Radloff, 1977). There are three phases of prevention of mental illness based on preventive medicine.

1. Primary prophylaxis by getting rid of the stressor.
2. Secondary prophylaxis by early detection and early medical examination.
3. Tertiary prophylaxis by recurrence prevention treatment.

SYSTEM OUTLINE

This study proposes a system using "visual studio net flame work, "The C# Programming Language" and Arduino (Arudino, 2005), A.P.Sheild (Koress, 2010) for open source hard ware (Figure 2, Figure 3).

A.P.Sheild is an expansion board for Arduino compatible computers using photo sensors which make it possible to change an electric currency by catching infrared light emitted from the expansion board. We detect a change of blood flow by using finger photo sensors to measure finger plethysmogram (Fujimoto et al, 2004; Fujimoto et al, 2005) as shown in Figure 4. This system can be used by connecting

Figure 2. Arudino

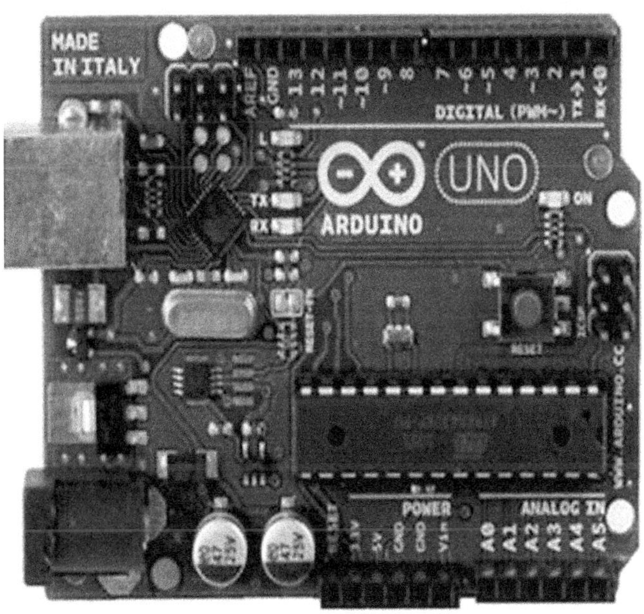

Figure 3. Arduino and A.P.Sheild

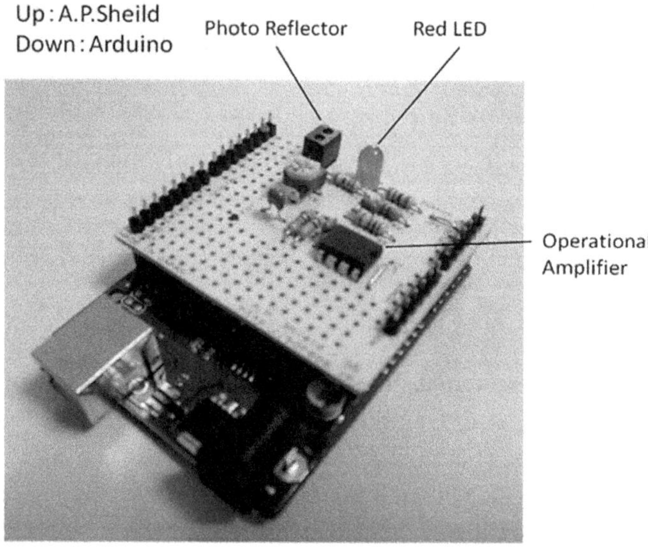

Figure 4. Example of using development system

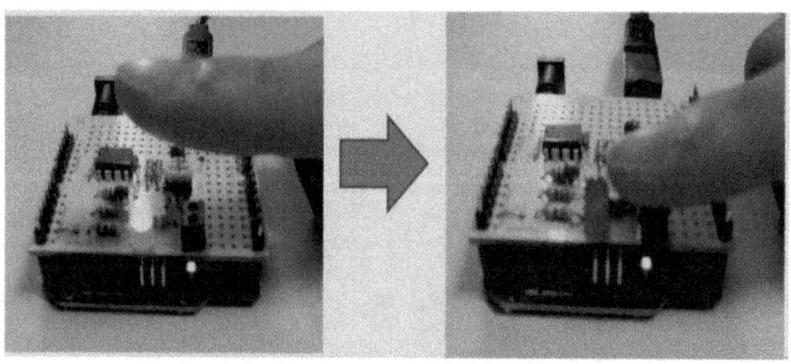

a personal computer and Arduino attached to A.P.Sheild with a USB cable. This system makes it possible to measure and visualize stress level easily, such as like taking one's temperature, measuring one's weight, or measuring blood pressure to self-assess the risk of disease as developing a prototype. The system we invented aims for measuring of stress level as a means of management in the home such as measuring weight, blood pressure and body temperature.

In addition, by providing feedbacking of results and putting the data in chronological order, this system would help patients with become more aware of the causes of their stress. Moreover, this system prevents people from being potential patients by giving an objective quantitative assessment makes measuring one's stress level using this system is as easy as taking one's temperature.

STRESS MEASUREMENT

Internal organs such as the heart are function under the influence of the automatic nervous system. The autonomic nerve is divided into the sympathetic nerve, which responds to physical stimulation or psychological stimulation and the parasympathetic nerve which responds during rest. The sympathetic nerve becomes predominant when humans experience stress and then the finger plethysmogram will be affected. The heart interval (R-R Interval: RRI) has fluctuations, and this is called heart rate variability (HRV). There is previous studies that HRV is related stress (Collins et al., 2005; Glei et al., 2007; Hanson et al., 2001; Hintsanen et al., 2007; McEwen and Lasley, 2003; Meijman and Mulder, 1998; Riese et al., 2004; Vrijkotte et al., 2000; Zanstra et al., 2006), and especially work stress measurement models (Karasek, 1979; Siegrist et al., 2004). The range of HRV can be derived by frequency analyzing a time series. Three main frequency components are identified for the R-R Interval time series (Sayers 1973; Tabe et al, 1996; Shimono et al, 1998; Minamitani et al, 1999; Takatsu et al, 2000; Hamanaka et al, 2006).

1. **Very Low Frequency – VLF:** Mainly affected by sympathetic nerve activity in part and has a frequency component of 0.00-0.05Hz.
2. **Low Frequency – LF:** Affected by sympathetic nerve activity and parasympathetic nerve activity and has a frequency component of 0.05-0.15Hz.
3. **High Frequency:** Affected by only parasympathetic nerve activity and has frequency component of 0.15-0.40Hz.

The ratio between Low Frequency and High Frequency (LF/HF) is regarded as a measure describing a balance of automatic nerves. We believe that higher the numerical number, the higher the stress. Since R-R interval corresponds approximately to P-P interval, because of the ease of measurement and low cost, this system uses pulse interval to derive stress instead of finger plethysmogram (Figure 5, Figure 6).

Figure 5. Process of Stress Management on Stress Coping Support System

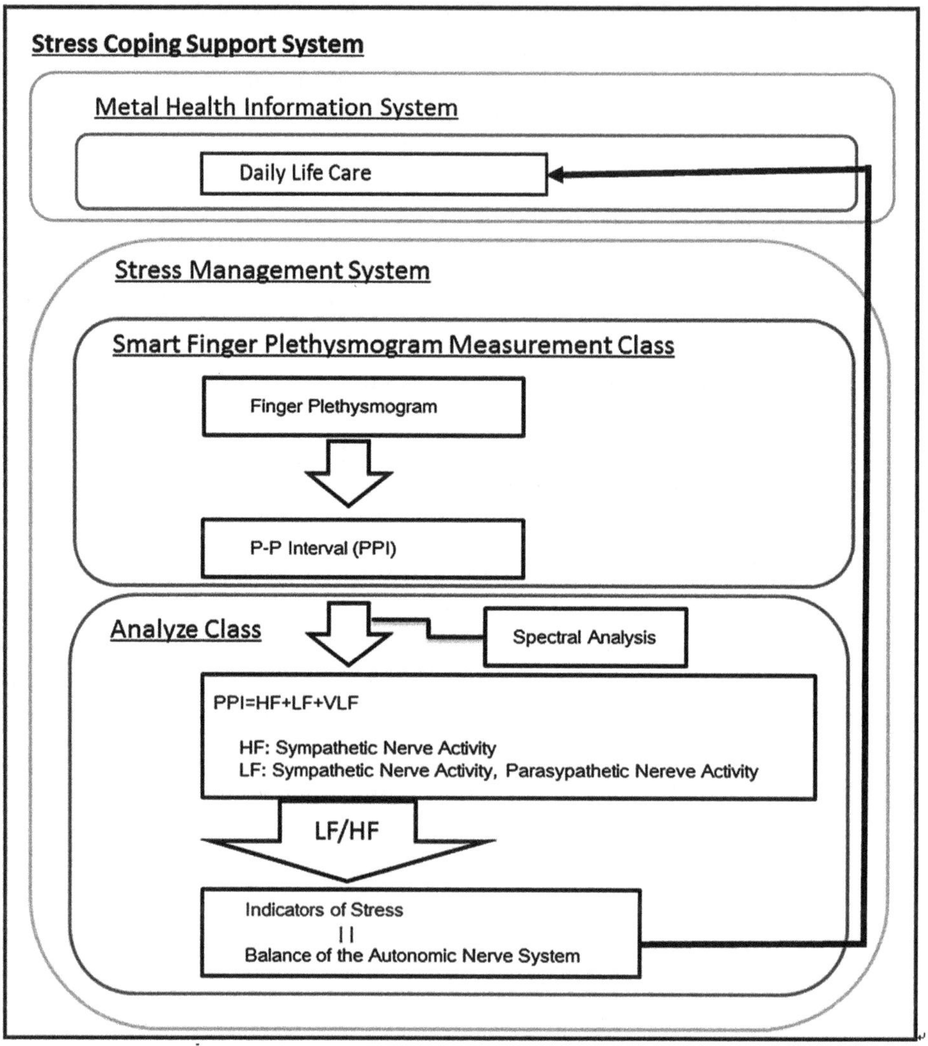

EXPERIMENTAL METHOD

In order to validate the functionality of the system developed by this study, 13 college students were selected, and a stress test was administered to them to measure their stress levels as students. From the results, 1 student was selected from each of the following categories: Students with high, medium and low levels. These 3 students were chosen as subjects, and as experiment 1, both stress tests and this

Figure 6. Visualization of stress measurement

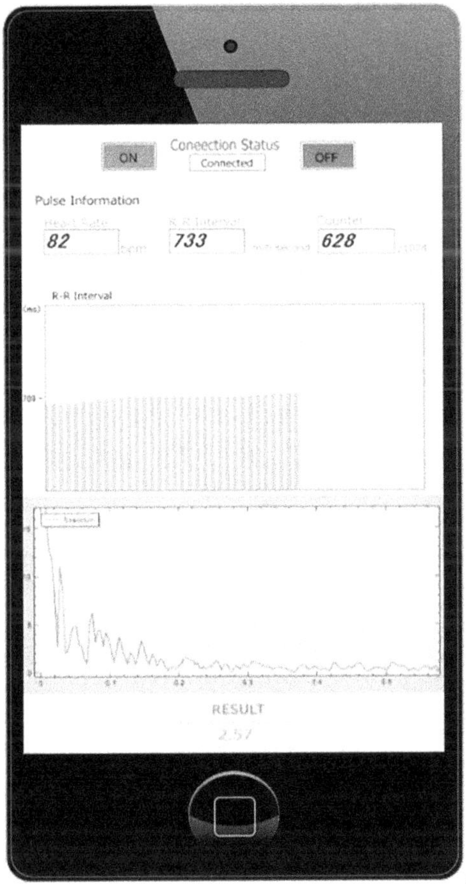

system were managed to measure the difference between them. As experiment 2, in order to evaluate the influence due to the time zone to be measured, experiments were conducted to measure time zones in the morning, daytime and night. For use in everyday life, a usage period of about 2 weeks was set.

Experimental results have found that individual differences in stress may be characterized, for example, at the time of start and end of stress. We also found that consideration of measurement conditions due to time zone differences between daytime and nighttime will be the subject of consideration.

EXPERIMENTAL RESULTS

The results of this study showed that it is the influence of individual difference of stress measurement. In Experiment 1, the authors found the possibility that the start point and the end point receiving stress are individually different. Also, the results of this study reveal a gap between the evaluation by this system and the results of stress testing. This gap is due to the subjective judgments being made, and we believe that this gap can be closed by using this system as it is able to eliminate subjective ratings of stress. However, the precision of machines can bring about noise in the readings, which could give rise to a margin of error, and we believe that comparison to other systems needs to be made in order to improve the accuracy of this system.

Also, in Experiment 2, it was confirmed whether there is a characteristic due to the time zone to be measured. The result was that the morning was most relaxed and the night was the most stressful time (Table 1). In addition, the variation was the largest in the morning relaxing time zone. In this way, the authors found that there is a possibility of a difference in influence due to the time zone.

CONSIDERATION AND DISCUSSION

In this study, using statistical data, we show the possibility that mental health problems is increasing, and one of the causes is described as the possibility that it is effect of stress.The problem of stress is an interdisciplinary theme that spans many academic fields such as psychology, sociology, basic medicine, industrial medicine and so on. In contemporary complex society, there are interests in stress theme in many research areas. It can be considered that digitalization and globalization of the world is a social background. Digitization has made the speed at which information can be obtained much faster. Globalization faces a variety of issues related to cross-cultural communication. Due to these factors, contemporary society can consider that the stress society is accelerating. The increase in the mental health problem may be

Table 1. Mean, S.D., and CV of LF/HF under condition of morning, daytime, and night

	Morning	Daytime	Night
Mean	1.44	0.64	0.59
S.D.	1.13	0.33	0.43
CV (%)	78	51	72

caused by such an increase in stress. However, verification in the social environment based on the scientific basis is not sufficient until now. This is probably because there was no tool that can conveniently and conveniently measure stress. Therefore, we are developing a system that can measure stress personally in daily life.

In the developed system, it is a heart rate monitor that estimates stress by touching the system with your finger. The authors developed an algorithm to detect stress. By implementing for smartphone application, stress measurement can be easily carried out. Experimental results have found that individual differences in stress may be characterized, for example, at the time of start and end of stress. We also found that consideration of measurement conditions due to time zone differences between daytime and nighttime will be the subject of consideration. In this way, there is a possibility that individual differences are large, so it is expected that further experimental data will be gathered from now on. However, unlike animal experiments, experiments targeting humans have more constraints on ethics. Therefore, experiments that consider such ethics and safety are required in the future. It is also important to develop mental health education programs. It is also necessary to provide educational programs according to individual circumstances, including stress measurement, with reference to previous research (Davis, Eshelman and McKay 2000). In developing educational programs, it is recommended that programs be developed with the assumption that stress cannot be reduced to zero but can be reduced. In other words, stress management education is necessary that can deal with and manage stress appropriately. Chronic addition of excessive stress has various adverse effects on the mind and body, so it is necessary to cope with stress properly and maintain health. Such a way to cope with stress is called stress coping. In other words, stress coping is a technique and ability to face well with stress when feeling stress in everyday life. Stress can be reduced as much as possible by dealing strategically and appropriately with stress.

There are two main types of stress coping concepts. One is problem focus coping. This method is a direct action to a stressor (a source of stress). It is an example that always carries a coat whenever the air-conditioner feels cold. By wearing a coat, it is a method of removing direct stressors like coldness due to air conditioning. Since this method is direct, high effect can be expected as coping with stress. However, it may take time and expenses to eliminate the cause of stress, and in many cases, it may be difficult to realize. Another way to do that is to have emotional focus coping. This is a way to make positive how to recognize stress. Problem focus coping functions on the stressor itself, but emotional focusing coping is a way to change thinking and feeling about stress. For example, if the interpersonal relationship is a stressor, it is a way to change your way of thinking and feeling about it.

Stress coping has been studied in various fields. By subject, there are studies targeting professionals such as athletes who utilize special skills, nurses, care workers, physical therapists, Yogo teachers (school nurse teachers) etc. There is also stress research on adolescence. High school students, college students and others are stressed with concerns about the future and carrier selection. It is research to prevent these stresses from becoming excessive. In addition, as part of work environment and employee health management in the workplace, there is research on stress management. Other studies focusing on characteristics and feelings of individuals, research on stress of collapse of love relationship. Some studies focused on stress in the state of mind of positive life events such as stress of childbirth and stress of marriage.

For example, athletes have various competitive stresses, and there are studies targeting athletes. An example in which the stress of competition appears in the most typical form is a symptom called burnout. Athletic Burnout Inventory (ABI) and Athlete Burnout Questionnaire (ABQ) are studies (Tanaka and Sugiyama 2015) as an assessment scale of burnout in order for athletes to avoid this symptom. This ABI research has been prepared for university student athletes, so that they cannot be burned out so that they can evaluate their degree and condition from the following four aspects. One is an emotional exhaustion feeling for the competition. This refers to a state of psychological exhaustion through competitive activities. Secondly, it is a decline in personal fulfillment. This refers to the reduction of competence in the competition group. The third is lack of communication with teammates. This refers to deterioration of interpersonal relationship. The fourth is the confusion of self-introduction into the competition. This refers to a reduction in self-engagement in the competition. In order for the athlete to check the stress condition, we can utilize the system proposed in this research as evaluation of such burnout. Detecting the state before burnout and performing stress coping makes it possible to prevent burnout. In addition, since this system can be conveniently used in everyday life, by taking advantage of its characteristics, it will be useful for physical and mental health and management by measuring stress in everyday life. Maintaining physical and mental health often emphasizes large stresses that affect life. However, there is a study that accumulation of minor stresses experienced in daily life also affects physical and mental health. That is, the importance of measuring stress in daily life is suggested.

Also, some models of stress coping have been proposed. In particular, in the field of cognitive psychology, there is research on a theoretical model (Lazalus et al. (1984)). The stress coping model by Lazarus is that the psychological adaptation varies depending on how various stressors experienced in daily life are taken as cognitive behavior and coping and how to deal with it. In these studies, for example, there is a study on the relationship between self-compression and stress coping (Neff, 2016; Muris and Petrocchi, 2017; Sirois et al., 2015; Strauss et al., 2016). Self-compaction is a method that can be gentle to both yourself and others, and it has three elements. One is kindness to yourself. That is to be kind to myself as well as being kind to others. This has the effect of increasing self-esteem. The second is common humanity. This is a perception that people are not perfect, sometimes they fail. In other words, it is the idea that failure is inevitable in life. The third is mindfulness. This is to concentrate on things before my eyes without being concerned with thinking and feelings (Neff, 2016). It is said that four effects can be realized by having these three elements. The effect is that procrastination is cured, it is not perfectionism, it can be gentle to others or to yourself, the satisfaction of life rises.

Also, there is a possibility that delays in cognitive stress may complicate implementing appropriate stress coping. If we can utilize stress measurement information from this system, it will be possible to give clues to problems concerning these stress perceptions. The system proposed in this research is expected to contribute to various fields because it can measure easily as compared with the method of measuring with pasting electrodes.

Particularly, dealing with stress is a serious problem depending on job type and work content. It is also an important social problem, and attention is rising in Japan as a part of reforming how to work. Also, it is important to maintain a better working environment not only in Japan but also throughout the world. Therefore, research that deals with the effects of excessive stress on society will also contribute to sustainable development goals (SDGs). SDGs are the goals of sustainable social development set by the United Nations, aiming at achievement in 2030. SDGs are action plan for man, the earth and prosperity. It also aims to integrate world peace for more freedom. 17 targets and 169 targets are defined. The goals are broad and interdependent, yet each has a separate list of targets to achieve. Among them, the goal that everyone can lead a healthy life, and the goal to achieve a good workplace are set. Research on stress measurement will contribute to achieving several goals. It is important to continue these research and to accumulate the latest knowledge. We would like to contribute to society applicable to stress.

Evolution of humanity has a history of properly coping with stress. In the future beyond the 4th industrial revolution, not only in the humanities and social sciences but also in the natural sciences, the academic field that emphasizes human mind is expanded, like stress measurement for mental health in this research. At that time, this rescarch will bc proved to be one of the pioneering research.

CONCLUSION

In this study, we developed a system that can measure stress individually in everyday life. In particular, we showed that we could develop algorithms for measurement. The system developed by thus study measures weight, blood pressure, temperature and other measurements that can be easily taken at home as part of one's' routine health care at home. In addition to measuring stress levels, the results of the measurements can be taken to form a time series data, which can be used to support one's personal risk management. Furthermore, by evaluating stress levels from an objective perspective, one is able to see the gap compared with stress levels which were evaluated subjectively, and it can serve as a bridge to a specialist consultation. Therefore, by using this system, we believe that we are able to prevent the emergence of potential patients.

Future Development, maintenance and improvement of comprehensive daily health is ahead of this research. By generalizing the measurement of state of mind, attention to ethics and safety will be required. We plan to study them comprehensively, including handling of personal data. Since the A.P.Sheild generates noise when we use this system because A.P.Sheild is not made for medical use. Therefore, when developing as medical use, we need high-precision medical devices such as sensitive pulse beat sensors, and to formulate a comprehensive system which connects with other institutions and to adapt standards in line with guidelines of organizations that aim to handle health management. experiments that consider such ethics and safety are required in the future.

REFERENCES

Aasman, J., Mulder, J., & Mulder, L. J. M. (1987). Operator effort and the measurement of heartrate variability. *Human Factors*, *29*(2), 161–170. doi:10.1177/001872088702900204 PMID:3610181

Arudino. (2005). Arudino. http://www.arduino.cc/

Fujita, E., Ogura, Y., Ochiai, N., Miao, T., Shimizu, T., Kamei, T., . . . Kaneko, S. (2004). Development of simplified appraisal method of fatigue on sitting for extended periods by the data of finger plethysmogram. Japan Ergonomics Society, 40(5), 254-263.

Fujita, E., Ogura, Y., Ochiai, N., Yasuda, E., Doi, S., Murata, K., . . . Kaneko, S. (2005). Development of the measurement method of the prediction of sleep by finger plethysmogram data. Japan Ergonomics Society, 41(4), 203-212.

Glei, D. A., Goldman, N., Chuang, Y. L., & Weinstein, M. (2007). Do chronic stressors lead to physiological dysregulation? Testing the theory of allostatic load. *Psychosomatic Medicine*, *69*(8), 769–776. doi:10.1097/PSY.0b013e318157cba6 PMID:17942833

Haas, R. W. (1979). Reducing stress and depression with exercise. *Bulletin - American Protestant Hospital Association*, *43*, 24–25. PMID:10246574

Hamanaka, Y., Nomura, R., Nakazono, Y., & Mizusawa, J. (2006). Development and Evaluation of stress measuring mouse. *IEICE*, *106*(253), 69–72.

Hanson, E. K., Godaert, G. L., Maas, C. J., & Meijman, T. F. (2001). Vagal cardiac control throughout the day: The relative importance of effort-reward imbalance and within day measurements of mood, demand and satisfaction. *Biological Psychology*, *56*(1), 23–44. doi:10.1016/S0301-0511(01)00066-7 PMID:11240313

Hintsanen, M., Elovainio, M., Puttonen, S., Kivimäki, M., Koskinen, T., Raitakari, O. T., & Keltinkangas-Järvinen, L. (2007). Effort-reward imbalance, heart rate and heart rate variability: The cardiovascular risk in young Finns study. *International Journal of Behavioral Medicine*, *14*(4), 202–212. doi:10.1007/BF03002994 PMID:18001235

Karasek, R. (1979). Job demands, job decision latitude, and mental strain: Implications for job redesign. *Administrative Science Quarterly*, *24*(2), 285–305. doi:10.2307/2392498

Kawakami, N., & Haratani, T. (1999). Epidemiology of job stress and health in Japan: Review of current evidence and future direction. *Industrial Health*, *37*(2), 174–186. doi:10.2486/indhealth.37.174 PMID:10319566

KORESS. (2010). A.P.Sheild 05: Arduino corresponding Heart Rate sensor (Pulse sensor) shield. Retrieved from http://koress.jp/2010/05/arduinoap_shield.html

Lazarus, R. S., & Folkman, S. (1984). *Stress, appraisal, and coping*. New York: Springer Publishing.

McEwen, B., & Lasley, E. N. (2003). Allostatic load: When protection gives way to damage. *Advances in Mind-Body Medicine*, *19*, 28–33. PMID:12825411

Meijman, T. F., & Mulder, G. (1998). Psychological aspects of workload. In P. J. D. Drenth, H. Thierry, & C. J. de Wolff (Eds.), *New handbook of work and organizational psychology.2 Work Psychology* (pp. 5–33). Hove, UK: Psychology Press.

MHLW. (2018). Patients survey. Retrieved from http://www.mhlw.go.jp/toukei/list/10-20.html

Minamitani, H., Hayashi, S., & Nagata, T. (1999). Heart rate variability related with mental stress and cumulative fatigue: Assessment of the autonomic nervous functions by using neural networks. *IEICE*, *98*(672), 115–122.

Muris, P., & Petrocchi, N. (2017). Protection or vulnerability? A meta-analysis of the relations between the positive and negative components of self-compassion and psychopathology. *Clinical Psychology & Psychotherapy*, *24*(2), 373–383. doi:10.1002/cpp.2005 PMID:26891943

Neff, K. D. (2016). Does self-compassion entail reduced self-judgment, isolation, and over-identification? A Response to Muris, Otgaar, and Petrocchi (2016). *Mindfulness*, *7*(3), 791–797. doi:10.100712671-016-0531-y

Radloff, L. S. (1977). The CES-D Scale: A Self-Report Depression Scale for Research in the General Population. *Applied Psychological Measurement*, *1*(3), 385–401. doi:10.1177/014662167700100306

Riese, H., Van Doornen, L. J., Houtman, I. L., & De Geus, E. J. (2004). Job strain in relation to ambulatory blood pressure, heart rate, and heart rate variability among female nurses. *Scandinavian Journal of Work, Environment & Health*, *30*(6), 477–485. doi:10.5271jweh.837 PMID:15635758

Sayers, B. M. (1973). Analysis of heart rate variability. *Ergonomics*, *16*(1), 17–32. doi:10.1080/00140137308924479 PMID:4702060

Schwab, K. (2016). The Fourth Industrial Revolution. World Economic Forum, Geneva, Switzerland.

Schwab, K., & Davis, N. (2018). Shaping the Fourth Industrial Revolution. World Economic Forum, Geneva, Switzerland.

Shimono, F., Ohsuga, M., & Terashita, H. (1998). Method for assessment of mental stress during high-tension and monotonous tasks using heart rate. respiration and blood pressure. Japan Ergonomics Society, 34(3), 107-115.

Siegrist, J., Peter, R., Junge, A., Cremer, P., & Seidel, D. (1990). Low status control, high effort at work and ischemic heart disease: Prospective evidence from bluecollar men. *Social Science & Medicine*, *31*(10), 1127–1134. doi:10.1016/0277-9536(90)90234-J PMID:2274801

Sirois, F. M., Molnar, D. S., & Hirsch, J. K. (2015). Self-compassion, stress, and coping in the context of chronic illness. *Self and Identity*, *3*(3), 334–347. doi:10.1080/15298868.2014.996249

Stansfeld, S. A., Fuhrer, R., Shipley, M. J., & Marmot, M. G. (1999). Work characteristics predict psychiatric disorder: Prospective results from the Whitehall II study. *Occupational and Environmental Medicine*, *56*(5), 302–307. doi:10.1136/oem.56.5.302 PMID:10472303

Strauss, C., Lever Taylor, B., Gu, J., Kuyken, W., Baer, R., Jones, F., & Cavanagh, K. (2016). What is compassion and how can we measure it? A review of definitions and measures. *Clinical Psychology Review*, *47*, 15–27. doi:10.1016/j.cpr.2016.05.004 PMID:27267346

Tabe, N., Tkara, T., & Hoshino, K. (1996). Pupillary diameter and heart rate under active and passive stress. *IEICE*, *96*(116), 75–79.

Takatsu, H., Murnakata, M., Ozeki, O., Yokoyama, K., Watanabe, Y., & Takata, K. (2000). An Evaluation of the Quantitative Relationship between the Subjective Stress Value and Heart Rate Variability. *The trans. of the Institute of Electrical Engineers of Japan*, *120*(1), 104-110.

Tanaka, T., & Sugiyama, Y. (2015). Improvement effect of positive affect on aggravation of burnout tendency in university athletes: Focusing on negative affect. *Japan J. Phys. Educ. Hlth. Sport Sci.*, *60*(2), 479–488. doi:10.5432/jjpehss.15016

Vrijkotte, T. G., van Doornen, L. J., & de Geus, E. J. (2000). Effects of work stress on ambulatory blood pressure, heart rate, and heart rate variability. *Hypertension*, *35*(4), 880–886. doi:10.1161/01.HYP.35.4.880 PMID:10775555

Zanstra, Y. J., Schellekens, J. M., Schaap, C., & Kooistra, L. (2006). Vagal and sympathetic activity in burnouts during a mentally demanding workday. *Psychosomatic Medicine*, *68*(4), 583–590. doi:10.1097/01.psy.0000228012.38884.49 PMID:16868268

Chapter 4
Algorithmic Analysis of Clinical, Neuropsychological, and Imaging Data in Localization-Related Epilepsy

Masoud Latifinavid
University of Turkish Aeronautical Association, Turkey

Kost Elisevich
Spectrum Health System, USA

Hamid Soltanian-Zadeh
Henry Ford Health System, USA

ABSTRACT

The current study examines algorithmic approaches for analysis of multimodal attributes in localization-related epilepsy (LRE), specifically, their impact on the selection of patients for surgical consideration. Invasive electrographic data is excluded here to concentrate upon the localized anatomical landmarks and identified/initialized brain structures in volumetric MR images as well as initial clinical presentation and the varied elements of the seizure history, ictal semiology, risk and seizure-precipitating factors and physical findings in addition to several features of the neuropsychological profile including various parameters of cognition and both speech and memory lateralization. First, the imaging modality data is excluded and just clinical, electrographic and neuropsychological data are investigated. Afterward, the imaging data are investigated and a comparison between the prediction results of the two types of data is done. In the case of using non-imaging multimodal data, 56% and using imaging features, about 71% of correct outcome prediction was obtained.

DOI: 10.4018/978-1-5225-8244-1.ch004

INTRODUCTION

In the United States alone, there are approximately 250,000 medically refractory (i.e., interactable) epileptic patients (Elisevich et al., 1996). Previous studies on predictors of postoperative seizure freedom using multivariable analysis differ in both methodology and results, some including invasive tests or image modality data (Armon, Radtke, Friedman, & Dawson, 1996; Berg, Walczak, Hirsch, & Spencer, 1998; Clusmann et al., 2002; Hennessy et al., 2001; Janszky et al., 2005; Janszky et al., 2006; Jeha et al., 2006; Spencer et al., 2005; Tonini et al., 2004; Yun et al., 2006).

Uijl et al. (Uijl et al., 2008) proposed a model for prognosis after temporal lobe epilepsy surgery using a combination of predictors. The results of this study showed 85% seizure-freedom among patients with a high probability of seizure freedom, and 40% seizure-freedom among patients with a high risk of not becoming seizure-free. In another study, Antel et al. (Antel et al., 2002) predicted surgical outcome in temporal lobe epilepsy patients using MRI and MRSI. In the Antel study, 75% of patients predicted accurately to fall in Engel class 1 after surgery on the basis of imaging alone. In the present study, we have developed a new algorithm based solely upon clinical, electrographic and neuropsychological data to predict surgical outcome. The main purpose of the study is to examine standard non-imaging evaluations as means of prognostication without relying on extraoperative electrocorticography (eECoG) or the many different imaging techniques used in these investigations. Clustering of patients in categorical groups and identification of the most effective features for each cluster permits the selection of a suitable classifier for each cluster. In order to identify the best features related to output (i.e., Engel classification), a combination of different feature selections and ranking algorithms are used aside a genetic algorithm search approach. For this purpose, integration of acquired multimodality data is necessary to obtain new effective features that can predict surgical outcome. A method based on supervised data mining and classification of the some clinical, pathological and neuropsychological features of patients is proposed by Armañanzas et.al. (Armañanzas et.al. 2013). The results of this research showed the efficiency of clinical, pathological and neuropsychological features for surgical outcome prediction and necessary investigation of new features on an extended database. A simulation of the epileptogenicity of different brain regions in a mathematical model is proposed by Sinha et.al. (Sinha et.al. 2017) using interictal networks derived from ECoG data which is an invasive test. Feis et.al (Feis et.al, 2013) developed a support vector machine classifier to predict post-surgical seizure outcome using extracted features from brain T1-weighted magnetic resonance images. They investigated men and women patients separately.

Data analysis with advanced computational methods (Siadat, Soltanian-Zadeh, Fotouhi, & Elisevich, 2005) leads to the use of artificial intelligence and machine learning algorithms. Accuracy of machine learning algorithms in an application depends on several factors. One of the challenges is selection of the best subset of available features. To this end, redundant features may be detected and eliminated. This may lead to more accurate, more effective, and faster results. Another challenge is selection of the best clustering approach. Our raw data include 139 instances with 102 attributes. These attributes are composed of video-scalp EEG analysis data based on well-defined standards, outcomes based on Engel classification, base tables (e.g., anti-epileptic drug information, seizure descriptions, medical history), neuropsychology, and Wada tests (Table 3). The large number of attributes may have negative effects on the classification accuracy. Therefore, effective and useful attributes should be found in order to make the classification simpler and more accurate.

In this paper, we introduce six different algorithms for feature selection, clustering and classification using non-invasive and non-imaging data. The main differences among these algorithms reflect different feature selection and ranking approaches and clustering methods. The feature selection and attribute ranking algorithms are explained as are the different clustering approaches combined with a multilayer perceptron classifier to predict the outcome of epilepsy surgery based on Engel classification. Also an algorithm is developed using the features that are extracted from imaging data and the results are compared. The outputs of each feature selection algorithm are reported and the list of selected attributes for each cluster are shown in the supplementary tables.

MATERIAL AND METHODS

Six different algorithms for the classification of localization-related epilepsy patients were developed and the results stored after classification. The general formation of these algorithms is shown in Figure 1. The path of each algorithm expresses the varieties and arrangements of the feature selection and clustering methods used. The paths start from the main raw database and end at the classification results. The formation of algorithms can be briefly expressed as follows:

Algorithm 1: CFS - ReliefF - EM - CFS - MLP
Algorithm 2: CFS - ReliefF - EM - CFS - CSE - MLP
Algorithm 3: CFS - ReliefF - COBWEB stage 1 - CFS - MLP

Figure 1. Six different algorithms proposed for classification of epileptic patients

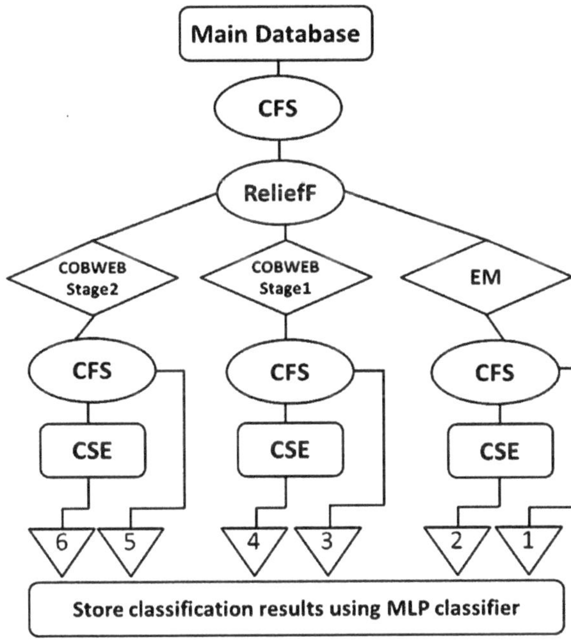

Algorithm 4: CFS - ReliefF - COBWEB stage 1 - CFS - CSE - MLP
Algorithm 5: CFS - ReliefF - COBWEB stage 2 - CFS - MLP
Algorithm 6: CFS - ReliefF - COBWEB stage 2 - CFS - CSE - MLP

First, Correlation-based Feature Selection (CFS) is used in order to select effective attributes and eliminate irrelevant and redundant ones. Then, ReliefF Attribute Evaluation method is used in order to evaluate and rank the attributes and eliminate redundant ones. These feature selection approaches are used in all six algorithms. Afterwards, two kinds of clustering methods that can handle the number of clusters automatically are used.

For algorithms 1 and 2, Expectation Maximization class (EM) was used as the clustering method. For the four remaining algorithms, Incremental Conceptual Clustering (COBWEB) was used. The COBWEB stage 1 is used for algorithms 3 and 4 and the COBWEB stage 2 for algorithms 5 and 6. After clustering, the CFS is used again on each cluster. Next, the classification results for each cluster are stored in algorithms 1, 3 and 5 using Multilayer Perceptron Classifier (MLP). Then, another subset selection approach was used in algorithms 2, 4 and 6, and the classification results stored using MLP. We compare the results of these classifications and select the best features for each cluster through a combination of the results. All of the classification methods are evaluated using the leave-one-out method. The classification output consists of the Engel outcome classification. In this classification, patients fall into one of four classes (1-4), each having a variable number of subclasses (A-D). Therefore, the patients were divided into 13 groups. The description of these classes and subclasses are given in Table 1. Furthermore, because of the importance of determining the class 1 instances, we modified the outputs of instances in the training set so as to appear as numeric values, 1 for class 1 and 2 for other classes and compared the results. Also, a parameter called precision rate is defined that indicates the number of correctly predicted class 1 instances divided by the number of all instances that the classifier predicted to fall in class 1.

The methods used in the above six algorithms are described briefly below.

Correlation-Based Feature Selection (CFS)

The CFS uses a correlation based heuristic to evaluate the features. It takes into account the predictive value of each attribute individually along with the degree of redundancy among them (Witten & Frank, 2005). It determines the merits of the

Table 1. Engel classification of epilepsy patients

Engel Classification of Epileptic Patients		
Class	**Subclasses**	**Description**
1	A	Completely seizure-free since surgery
	B	Non-disabling simple partial seizures only since surgery
	C	Some disabling simple partial seizures after surgery but free of disabling seizures for at least two years
	D	Generalized convulsions with antiepileptic drug withdrawal
2	A	Initially free of disabling seizures but rare seizures now
	B	Rare disabling seizures since surgery
	C	More than rare disabling seizures after surgery but rare for at least two years
	D	Nocturnal seizures only
3	A	Worthwhile seizure reduction
	B	Prolonged seizure-free intervals amounting to greater than half the follow up period, but not less than two years
4	A	Significant seizure reduction
	B	No appreciable change
	C	Seizures worsened

features in terms of their capability to predict the class label and their correlations with the other features. The heuristic is based on the following hypothesis: "Good feature subsets contain features highly correlated with the class, yet uncorrelated with each other." The following equation formalizes the heuristic (Hall, 2000):

$$\text{Merit}_s = \frac{k\overline{r_{cf}}}{\sqrt{k + k(k-1)\overline{r_{ff}}}} \quad (1)$$

This equation quantifies the merit of a feature subset S that includes k features where $\overline{r_{cf}}$ is the average feature-class correlation and $\overline{r_{ff}}$ is the average feature-feature inter-correlation. The nominator quantifies predictability of the feature subset and the denominator quantifies redundancy between features. This process discards redundant attributes which are highly correlated with one or more of the other attributes. The n possible features generate 2^n possible subsets. Testing of these subsets is clearly time-consuming and sometimes even impossible. Thus, we use the CFS method to generate a matrix of feature-class and feature-feature correlations from the training data and search the subset space by different search algorithms. The CFS calculates the correlations globally (i.e., over all training instances) and chooses a subset of features with low redundancy and strong predictability. Afterward, the unselected features are tested one-by-one to determine their efficacy on a local rather than global basis. If the correlation between a feature and a class is more than the highest correlation between it and one of the selected features, the feature is added to the selected subset (Hall, 2000).

ReliefF Attribute Evaluation

The basic Relief attribute evaluation algorithm, as shown below, estimates qualities of attributes based on their potential ability to differentiate between close instances (Kononenko, 1994).

1. Set all weights W[A]:= 0.0;
2. For i:= 1 to m do begin
3. Randomly select an instance R;
4. Find nearest hit H and nearest miss M;
5. For A:= 1 to #all attributes do
6. W[A]:= W[A] – diff(A,R,H)/m + diff(A,R,M)/m;
7. End;

In this method, an instance is selected randomly (R), then Relief selects its two closest neighbors such that one of them is in the same class (*nearest hit* H) and the other is in a different class (*nearest miss* M). Afterward, it computes the quality of attributes W [A] with respect to their values for R, M, and H. The quality that Relief computes for Attribute A expresses an estimate about the following subtraction of probabilities (Kononenko, 1994):

$$W\left[A\right] = P\left(diff.\,value\,of\,A \mid nearest\,inst.\,from\,diff.\,class\right) \\ -P\left(diff.\,value\,of\,A \mid nearest\,inst.\,from\,same\,class\right) \tag{2}$$

Expectation Maximization (EM) Clustering

EM is a statistical approach for clustering that uses the finite Gaussian mixtures model that assumes all features as independent random variables. The algorithm recomputes the parameters to obtain desired convergence. The mixture is composed of **N** probability distributions, each related to a cluster. Each instance allocates a membership probability for each cluster. Denoting the standard deviation as σ and mean value as μ, the Gaussian probability density function may be computed (Wu, Steinbauer, & Kuo, 2005):

$$f\left(x\right) = \frac{1}{\left(\sqrt{2\pi\sigma}\right)} e^{\frac{-\left(x-\mu\right)^2}{2\sigma^2}} \tag{3}$$

The algorithm continues until cluster quality shows no considerable increase. The main parameter that demonstrates cluster quality is the likelihood that is calculated by the multiplication of the sum of the probabilities for each of the instances. For two clusters A and B with instances $x_1, x_2, \ldots, x_n$ where $P_A=P_B=0.5$, the likelihood is:

$$\left[0.5P\left(x_1 \mid A\right) + 0.5P\left(x_1 \mid B\right)\right]\left[0.5P\left(x_2 \mid A\right) + 0.5P\left(x_2 \mid B\right)\right]\ldots\left[0.5P\left(x_n \mid A\right) + 0.5P\left(x_n \mid B\right)\right]$$

The number of clusters can be defined manually or automatically by a simple algorithm that uses cross-validation in the following steps:

1. The number of clusters is set to 1.
2. The training set is randomly split into 10 folds.

3. EM is implemented 10 times using the 10 folds cross-validation.
4. The average log likelihood is calculated over all 10 results.

If the log likelihood has increased, the number of clusters is increased by 1 and the program continues at Step 2 (Wu et al., 2005).

Incremental Conceptual Clustering (COBWEB)

The COBWEB is an incremental approach to perform hierarchical conceptual clustering. The system recruits operators that enable bidirectional travel through the space of hierarchical clustering schemes in order to perform a hill-climbing search in this space. In order to guide this search, a heuristic measure named category utility is used.

A tradeoff between intra-class similarity $P(A_i=V_{ij}|C_k)$ and inter-class dissimilarity $P(C_k|A_i=V_{ij})$ creates the base of category utility where $A_i=V_{ij}$ means attribute-value pair and C_k means a class. A combination of these probabilities can give an overall measure of partition quality. Category Utility (CU) is defined as the rise in the expected number of attribute values that can be guessed correctly ($P(C_k)\sum_i\sum_j P(A_i = V_{ij} \mid C_K)^2$) given a partition $\{C_1, \ldots, C_n\}$ over the expected number of true guesses without such knowledge ($\sum_i\sum_j P(A_i = V_{ij})^2$).

$$CU(\{C_1, C_2, \ldots, C_n\}) = \frac{\sum_{k=1}^{n} P(C_k)\left[\sum_i\sum_j P(A_i = V_{ij} \mid C_k)^2 - \sum_i\sum_j P(A_i = V_{ij})^2\right]}{n} \quad (4)$$

The parameter n in the denominator refers to categories in a partition. In order to make a comparison between various sizes of partitions, the average should be computed over categories. If a special value or all values of an attribute is independent of the class membership, then $P(A_i = V_{ij}|C_k) = P(A_i = V_{ij})$, so, the nominator is zero and that value and the whole attribute is irrelevant for any expression of category makeup (Fisher, 1987).

COBWEB has an ability to adjust the number of classes and structure of hierarchical clustering automatically using the following steps:

1. Clustering with an existing class
2. Generating a new class

3. Splitting a class into several classes
4. Merging two classes into one class

To determine the best host for an instance, COBWEB tests it in each category. Furthermore, the algorithm compares the quality of clustering using an existing class or generates a new singleton class. Also, it includes an operator for splitting and merging of the categories and tests quality of the results to obtain the best structure of clustering (Fisher, 1987).

Multilayer Perceptron Classifier (MLP)

MLP is used for classification of our datasets. Our classifier is composed of an MLP with three hidden layers with 15, 10, and 5 nodes and 1 output node. The architecture of the MLP is designed based on experimental pre-evaluation of the database using 10-fold cross validation. The nodes have sigmoid activation functions except for the output node which is a linear unit. The number of input nodes in each cluster is equal to the number of attributes that are selected for that cluster. The number of selected attributes are mentioned in the results section and the names and explanations of them are mentioned in supplementary tables. A nominal to numeric filter is used for nominal inputs. The output attribute is a numeric value related to the Engel classification of epileptic patients. The numbers between 1 and 13 are used for the patients' Engel classifications after surgery. A filter is used to round the predicted number to the nearest Class & Subclass value by the following algorithm:

- If predicted number <1, rounded number = 1
- If predicted number >13, rounded number = 13
- Else,
- If the decimal term > 0.5, the upper Class & Subclass is selected.
- If the decimal term < 0.5, the lower Class & Subclass is selected.

The method used for the training of this network is simple back propagation (Witten & Frank, 2005). This kind of classifier is used for prediction of the surgery outcome related to the patients of each cluster. In each step, based on the leave-one-out evaluation method, the predicted results are compared with actual surgery results of the patients. The results of such a comparison are mentioned in the Results. Also, the detailed rate of the prediction results related to the each cluster are mentioned in Table 2.

Table 2. Classification results for each of the six proposed algorithms

Path No	Algorithm Description	No of All Clusters	Cluster ID	Classification Results for Each Cluster		Over all Evaluation	
				Correct Predicted Class	Correct Predicted Class and Sub Class	Class	Class and Sub Class
1	CFS-ReliefF-EM-CFS-MLP	3	Cluster1	48.64%	27.02%	47.48%	26.61%
			Cluster2	58.34%	41.67%		
			Cluster3	31.25%	12.5%		
2	CFS-ReliefF-EM-CFS-CSE-MLP	3	Cluster1	38.74%	20.72%	41%	22.3%
			Cluster2	50%	33%		
			Cluster3	50%	31.25%		
3	CFS-ReliefF-COBWEB Stage1-CFS-MLP	3	Cluster1	52.38%	33.33%	56.11%	31.65%
			Cluster2	58.73%	39.68%		
			Cluster3	54.54%	21.81%		
4	CFS-ReliefF-COBWEB Stage1-CFS-CSE-MLP	3	Cluster1	47.61%	28.57%	51.08%	27.34%
			Cluster2	50.8%	26.98%		
			Cluster3	52.73%	27.27%		
5	CFS-ReliefF-COBWEB Stage2-CFS-MLP	7	Cluster4	50%	33.34%	43.89%	23.74%
			Cluster5	22.23%	22.33%		
			Cluster6	40%	10%		
			Cluster7	37.5%	21.9%		
			Cluster8	47.62%	23.8%		
			Cluster9	34.48%	17.24%		
			Cluster10	65.39%	34.62%		
6	CFS-ReliefF-COBWEB Stage2-CFS-CSE-MLP	7	Cluster4	58.34%	33.34%	49.62%	29.63%
			Cluster5	62.5%	50%		
			Cluster6	40%	10%		
			Cluster7	37.5%	31.25%		
			Cluster8	57.14%	38.09%		
			Cluster9	61.54%	26.93%		
			Cluster10	42.30%	23.07%		

Classifier Subset Evaluator (CSE)

This approach evaluates attribute subsets on the training set or a separate hold-out testing set, using a classifier to estimate the merit of a set of attributes. The previously mentioned MLP is used as a classifier for this kind of feature selection and uses a simple Genetic Algorithm as the search method in subset space. A major problem of this classifier is that its training is sometimes very time-consuming. When there are numerous subsets of features, training the classifier for each of them and then testing them one-by-one are costly and sometimes impossible. So, some optimization tools like GA can be used to search the subset space. In spite of this solution, several iterations should be done to obtain good results. This process may take several days using commonly used personal computers. Because of this limitation, this approach is used at the last stage of our proposed algorithm, after decreasing the subset space with the CFS and ReliefF algorithms.

Leave-One-Out Evaluation Method

Leave-one-out is a simple n-fold cross-validation, where *n* is equal to the number of instances of the dataset. At the circle of evaluation, each instance is left out and then the classifier is trained using the remaining instances. Afterwards, the success of classification is judged using the left instance as test data. The correctness of the *n* judgment results represents the success rate of the classification procedure. Two main reasons that make the leave-one-out evaluation method more efficient are described below.

1. In each stage, just one instance of training set is put aside as the test set and the greatest possible dataset is selected for training of the classifier that leads to more accurate classification results.
2. This kind of evaluation is not based on random sampling; all of the instances are judged as a test set. Thus, its deterministic property increases the accuracy of evaluation (Witten & Frank, 2005).

RESULTS

In this section, the feature selection, clustering and classification results are described in two parts. The first part is related to the non-invasive and non-imaging multimodal data of patients. The second part is related to the data and features extracted from MR images of the patients.

Surgical Outcome Prediction Using Non-Invasive and Non-Imaging Multimodal Data

The raw data comprise 139 instances with 101 attributes. The number of attributes was reduced to 63 using CFS. After evaluation and ranking of the attributes, we eliminated 19 of them so that 44 attributes remained. For algorithm 1 and 2, the EM clustering approach is used distributing the instances among three clusters with 111, 12, and 16 members. The CFS was performed again on each cluster and the number of attributes including 23, 30, and 10 were selected for clusters 1, 2, and 3, respectively (Table 4). The classification results of algorithm 1, based on the Leave-One-Out evaluation method, show that 47.48% of the Engel classes and 26.61% of both the Engel classes and subclasses are predicted correctly (Table 2).

For algorithm 2, CSE is used for each cluster and reduced the number of the selected attributes to 15, 7, and 7 for clusters 1, 2, and 3, respectively (Table 5). According to classification results, 41% of Engel classes and 22.3% of both Engel classes and subclasses are predicted correctly (Table 2).

For algorithms 3 to 6, the COBWEB method is used in order to perform a two-stages clustering. The COBWEB distributed the instances into three clusters at stage 1 with 21, 63, and 55 members, and seven clusters at stage 2 with 12, 9, 10, 32, 21, 29, and 26 members.

In algorithm 3, after performing CFS for each cluster of COBWEB stage 1, 22 attributes for cluster 1, 11 attributes for cluster 2, and 10 attributes for cluster 3 were selected (Table 6). By using the CSE on each cluster of COBWEB stage 1, 15 attributes for cluster 1, 9 attributes for cluster 2, and 9 attributes for cluster 3 were selected and used in algorithm 4 (Table 7).

In a same process and with CFS, 10, 7, 9, 10, 13, 8, and 17 attributes were selected for clusters 4 to 7, in the algorithm 5 (Table 8). In addition, by using CFS and CSE, 7, 5, 6, 8, 8, 5, and 8 attributes were selected for clusters 4 to 7, in algorithm 6 (Table 9).

According to the classification results (Table 2), 56.11%, 51.08%, 43.89%, and 49.62% of Engel classes were correctly predicted in algorithms 3, 4, 5, and 6, respectively. Furthermore, 31.65%, 27.34%, 23.74%, and 29.63% of both Engel classes and subclasses were correctly predicted in algorithms 3 to 6, respectively. In order to improve the classification results and selection of the best attributes in each cluster, we investigated the results of classifications (Table 2) and selected the best features that come from the same kind of clustering. Therefore, the algorithms 1 and 2 were combined. The features of clusters 1 and 2 were chosen from the algorithm 1 and the features of cluster 3 were chosen from the algorithm 2. The algorithms 3 and 4 consisted of the COBWEB Stage 1 clustering. However, according to the obtained results (Table 2), the algorithm 3 had better results in each cluster. Therefore, we chose its selected features as the best ones.

With respect to the COBWEB Stage 2 clustering approach and results in Table 2, the features for the clusters 4 to 9 were selected from the algorithm 5 and the features of cluster 10 were selected from the algorithm 6. The overall classification results after combination of the algorithms and choosing the best features are shown in Figure 2 which shows that in combined algorithms 1 and 2, algorithm 3, and combined algorithms 5 and 6, the correct prediction rates of the Engel classes are 49.64%, 56.11%, and 53.68%, respectively whereas, the correct prediction rates of the Engel classes and subclasses are 28.77%, 31.65%, and 31.62%, respectively.

In the case of predicting class 1 instances using the same process of combining the best results of the algorithms that use the same kind of clustering, the following results were obtained. The combination of algorithms 1 and 2 gave a 65.47% correct prediction rate with 72.36% precision. The comparison of algorithm 3 with algorithm 4 showed that algorithm 3 had more accurate results in all three clusters with a 71.42% correct prediction rate and a 70.58% precision rate. With the combination of algorithms 5 and 6, the rate of correct classification of class 1 instances was 70.73%

Figure 2. Overall classification results with combination of the algorithms and choosing the best features

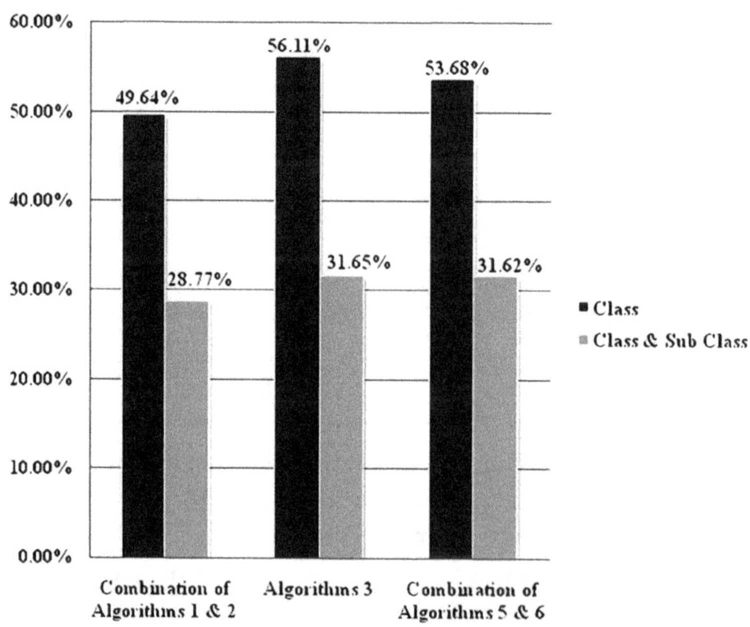

with a 74.35% precision rate. Figure 3 compares the mentioned results for the Engel class 1. Note that algorithm 3 and the combination of algorithms 5 and 6 give more than 70% correct classification for class 1 instances, with more than 70% precision.

Surgical Outcome Prediction Using Imaging Data

In this section, the results of our analysis of the imaging data are presented. To this end, a database including 77 instances with 22 attributes is used. In the present study we used the human brain multi-modality image database system (HBIDS) that was developed by Siadat (Siadat et al. 2005). The HBIDS is composed of several image-processing modules. These modules include anatomical landmark localization and brain structure identification. The imaging modality features included parameters like volume and volume asymmetry, surface area, intensity mean-value and standard deviation, length and width and different texture features, all regarding the left and right hippocampus. The hippocampus is characterized by multiple edges and missing boundaries. The features which are often of interest are volume, surface area, intensity mean-value and standard deviation, length, and width (Jafari-Khouzani et al. 2003). A detailed list of the imaging modality

Figure 3. Overall class 1 classification results and precision of classification with combination of the algorithms and choosing the best features

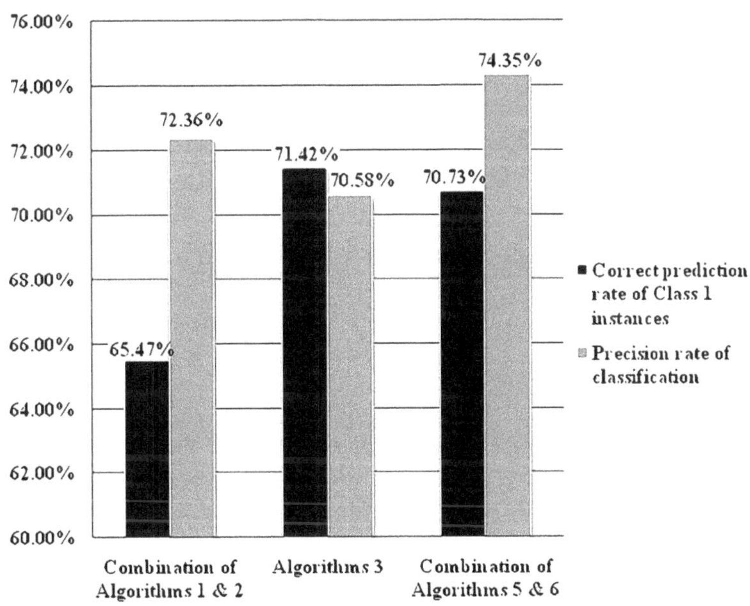

Figure 4. Overall classification results using features that are extracted from image modality data

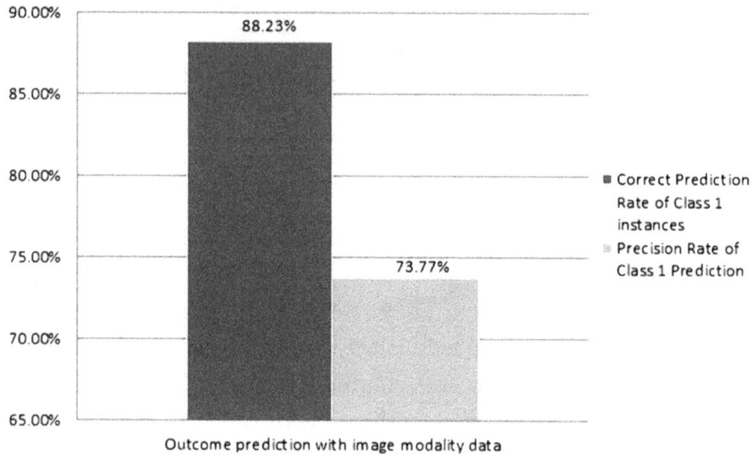

attributes and their brief descriptions and possible values are provided in Table 10. Based on experiences earned from investigation of non-invasive and non-imaging data and with respect to pre-evaluations, an algorithm is designed for prediction of the surgical outcome using features extracted from MRI. In this algorithm, first CFS is done on the database and 22 attributes with highest correlations with the outcome classes selected. Afterwards, CSE is implemented on the database. The 7 attributes selected at the end of the feature selection stage are listed in Table 11. Then, using an MLP classifier and the leave-one-out evaluation method, outcomes are predicted. Using the imaging data and the explained algorithm 64.93% of Engel classes and 46.75% of both Engel class and subclasses are predicted correctly. In the case of predicting class 1 instances using the same process, the following results are obtained. Also, an 88.23% of class 1 instances are predicted correctly (Figure 4). Detailed classification results are given in Table 12.

DISCUSSION

In the present study, we propose several algorithms based on a combination of feature selection, clustering, and classification approaches in order to predict the final condition of localization-related epilepsy patients after surgery with respect to the Engel classification. A unique feature of this study is investigations of non-imaging (i.e., clinical and neuropsychological) data and imaging data (different texture features, all regarding the left and right hippocampus) separately. The results can be used by neurologists to select surgical candidates.

One of the main and fundamental problems in medical data mining is the shortage and limitation of samples. A suitable and up-to-date multimodal epilepsy database is used for this project. Also, by using leave-one-out method, the greatest possible set of samples during the simulation process are used in order to find effective attributes in each cluster and to design more a suitable MLP for them. However, most, individually, do not predict the correct outcome class. A combination of attributes and their values in each cluster generates a better simulation and a more reliable prediction of outcome. An extended population size of samples would lead to increased accuracy in the classification process. The results obtained in this study can be a starting point to detect other, more valuable features for epilepsy surgery candidacy and to define an effective algorithm in order to predict surgical outcome with standard non-imaging tests as means of prognostication without necessarily proceeding to eECoG.

In real multimodal data where the first goal is to find more valuable features and select the best combination of them, just one feature selection method may not lead to optimal results.

In the present study, we used a combination of three types of attribute rankers and feature selectors in order to choose the best attributes. CFS selected the attributes showing the highest correlation with Engel class and the lowest correlation with other attributes. Relief ranked the selected attributes and chose the best ones to decrease the number of attributes. Using the clustering approaches and the CFS again, the best features in the space of the new attributes were selected for each cluster.

Among the proposed algorithms, the main differences are in the clustering methods and using the CSE in the last step. The CSE has a large amount of computations and its training in iterations is very time-consuming. Thus, to search the acceptable space using GA, we put it in the last ring of our algorithm chain. The classification results (Table 2) illustrate that CSE increases classification accuracy in some cases but decreases it in other cases. Therefore, the classification results are stored in two steps in each type of clustering before CSE and after CSE (Figure 1). It aids in picking the best attribute combination for each cluster and designing an MLP for them.

Figure 2 shows that COBWEB Stage 1 in algorithm 3 generates the best results (56.11% for Engel classes and 31.65% for Engel classes and subclasses). In some clusters of COBWEB Stage 2, the correct classification rate is more than that of the algorithm. The superiority of using COBWEB Stage 1 in algorithm 3 is its higher number of samples in the clusters. Thus, it is probable that extension of the database can lead to more accurate results from COBWEB Stage 2.

To predict Engel class 1 cases, algorithm 3 with its 71.42% correct prediction had the best prediction rate and the combination of algorithms 5 and 6 with a 70.73% correct prediction rate had comparable accuracy. However, a combination of algorithms 5 and 6 had better a precision rate (74.35%) in comparison to algorithm 3 (70.58%).

Based on pre-evaluations and experiences from analyzing non-imaging multimodal data, an algorithm was designed and implemented on the image modality data. Among the extracted features from MRI of the patients, 7 most correlated features were selected and an MLP classifier was designed and implemented. The results were promising; 64.93% of Engel classes, 46.75% of both Engel class and subclasses, and 88.23% of the class 1 outcomes were predicted correctly.

In conclusion, this paper shows the ability of clinical, electrographic and neuropsychological data to provide surgical outcome prediction and introduces methods by which this may be achieved. Also, the texture features extracted from MRI data related to the left and right hippocampus have a great potential to predict the surgical outcome. The proposed methodologies can be used to predict surgical outcomes and select patients for surgery using non-invasive multimodal data.

REFERENCES

Antel, S. B., Li, L. M., Cendes, F., Collins, D. L., Kearney, R. E., Shinghal, R., & Arnold, D. L. (2002). Predicting surgical outcome in temporal lobe epilepsy patients using MRI and MRSI. *Neurology*, *58*(10), 1505–1512. doi:10.1212/WNL.58.10.1505 PMID:12034787

Armañanzas, R., Alonso-Nanclares, L., DeFelipe-Oroquieta, J., Kastanauskaite, A., de Sola, R. G., DeFelipe, J., ... Larrañaga, P. (2013). Machine learning approach for the outcome prediction of temporal lobe epilepsy surgery. *PLoS One*, *8*(4), e62819. doi:10.1371/journal.pone.0062819 PMID:23646148

Armon, C., Radtke, R. A., Friedman, A. H., & Dawson, D. V. (1996). Predictors of outcome of epilepsy surgery: Multivariate analysis with validation. *Epilepsia*, *37*(9), 814–821. doi:10.1111/j.1528-1157.1996.tb00033.x PMID:8814093

Berg, A. T., Walczak, T., Hirsch, L. J., & Spencer, S. S. (1998). Multivariable prediction of seizure outcome one year after resective epilepsy surgery: Development of a model with independent validation. *Epilepsy Research*, *29*(3), 185–194. doi:10.1016/S0920-1211(97)00083-1 PMID:9551780

Clusmann, H., Schramm, J., Kral, T., Helmstaedter, C., Ostertun, B., Fimmers, R., ... Elger, C. E. (2002). Prognostic factors and outcome after different types of resection for temporal lobe epilepsy. *Journal of Neurosurgery*, *97*(5), 1131–1141. doi:10.3171/jns.2002.97.5.1131 PMID:12450036

Elisevich, K., Kasunic, K., Hathaway, S. J., Smith, B. J., Stewart, R. W., & Barkley, G. L. (1996). Clinical Care Pathways in a Surgical Epilepsy Program: A Comparison of Costs by Diagnostic Related Groups for Program and Nonprogram Admissions. *Epilepsy Research*, *9*(4), 282–290. doi:10.1016/S0896-6974(96)00021-7

Feis, D. L., Schoene-Bake, J. C., Elger, C., Wagner, J., Tittgemeyer, M., & Weber, B. (2013). Prediction of post-surgical seizure outcome in left mesial temporal lobe epilepsy. *NeuroImage. Clinical*, *2*, 903–911. doi:10.1016/j.nicl.2013.06.010 PMID:24179841

Fisher, D. H. (1987). Knowledge acquisition via incremental conceptual clustering. *Machine Learning*, *2*(2), 139–172. doi:10.1007/BF00114265

Hall, M. A. (2000). Correlation-based feature selection for discrete and numeric class machine learning. *Paper presented at the Proc Seventeenth International Conference on Machine Learning*.

Hennessy, M. J., Elwes, R. D., Honavar, M., Rabe-Hesketh, S., Binnie, C. D., & Polkey, C. E. (2001). Predictors of outcome and pathological considerations in the surgical treatment of intractable epilepsy associated with temporal lobe lesions. *Journal of Neurology, Neurosurgery, and Psychiatry*, *70*(4), 450–458. doi:10.1136/jnnp.70.4.450 PMID:11254766

Jafari-Khouzani, K., Siadat, M. R., Soltanian-Zadeh, H., & Elisevich, K. (2003, May). Texture analysis of hippocampus for epilepsy. In Medical Imaging 2003: Physiology and Function: Methods, Systems, and Applications (Vol. 5031, pp. 279-289). International Society for Optics and Photonics. doi:10.1117/12.480697

Janszky, J., Janszky, I., Schulz, R., Hoppe, M., Behne, F., Pannek, H. W., & .... (2005). Temporal lobe epilepsy with hippocampal sclerosis: Predictors for long-term surgical outcome. *Brain*, *128*(Pt 2), 395–404. doi:10.1093/brain/awh358 PMID:15634733

Janszky, J., Pannek, H. W., Fogarasi, A., Bone, B., Schulz, R., Behne, F., & Ebner, A. (2006). Prognostic factors for surgery of neocortical temporal lobe epilepsy. *Seizure*, *15*(2), 125–132. doi:10.1016/j.seizure.2005.12.002 PMID:16414290

Jeha, L. E., Najm, I. M., Bingaman, W. E., Khandwala, F., Widdess-Walsh, P., Morris, H. H., ... Luders, H. O. (2006). Predictors of outcome after temporal lobectomy for the treatment of intractable epilepsy. *Neurology*, *66*(12), 1938–1940. doi:10.1212/01.wnl.0000219810.71010.9b PMID:16801667

Kononenko, I. (1994). Estimating Attributes: Analysis and Extensions of RELIEF. *Paper presented at the European Conference on Machine Learning*. 10.1007/3-540-57868-4_57

Siadat, M. R., Soltanian-Zadeh, H., Fotouhi, F., & Elisevich, K. (2005). Content-based image database system for epilepsy. *Computer Methods and Programs in Biomedicine*, *79*(3), 209–226. doi:10.1016/j.cmpb.2005.03.012 PMID:15955590

Sinha, N., Dauwels, J., Kaiser, M., Cash, S. S., Brandon Westover, M., Wang, Y., & Taylor, P. N. (2016). Predicting neurosurgical outcomes in focal epilepsy patients using computational modelling. *Brain*, *140*(2), 319–332. doi:10.1093/brain/aww299 PMID:28011454

Spencer, S. S., Berg, A. T., Vickrey, B. G., Sperling, M. R., Bazil, C. W., Shinnar, S., ... Pacia, S. V. (2005). Predicting long-term seizure outcome after resective epilepsy surgery: The multicenter study. *Neurology*, *65*(6), 912–918. doi:10.1212/01.wnl.0000176055.45774.71 PMID:16186534

Tonini, C., Beghi, E., Berg, A. T., Bogliun, G., Giordano, L., Newton, R. W., ... Wiebe, S. (2004). Predictors of epilepsy surgery outcome: A meta-analysis. *Epilepsy Research*, *62*(1), 75–87. doi:10.1016/j.eplepsyres.2004.08.006 PMID:15519134

Uijl, S. G., Leijten, F. S., Arends, J. B., Parra, J., van Huffelen, A. C., & Moons, K. G. (2008). Prognosis after temporal lobe epilepsy surgery: The value of combining predictors. *Epilepsia*, *49*(8), 1317–1323. doi:10.1111/j.1528-1167.2008.01695.x PMID:18557776

Witten, I. H., & Frank, E. (2005). *Data Mining: Practical machine learning tools and techniques* (2nd ed.). San Francisco, CA: Morgan Kaufmann.

Wu, C., Steinbauer, J. R., & Kuo, G. M. (2005). EM Clustering Analysis of Diabetes Patients Basic Diagnosis Index. *Paper presented at the AMIA Annual Symposium Proceedings.*

Yun, C. H., Lee, S. K., Lee, S. Y., Kim, K. K., Jeong, S. W., & Chung, C. K. (2006). Prognostic factors in neocortical epilepsy surgery: Multivariate analysis. *Epilepsia*, *47*(3), 574–579. doi:10.1111/j.1528-1167.2006.00470.x PMID:16529624

APPENDIX

Supplementary Data

Table 3. Non-invasive and non-visual modality attributes' description

Category	Abbreviation	Feature Name	Description	Possible Values
Gender	PERSONAL_INFO. SEX	Sex	Sex	M, F
Seizure Description 1) SPSZ, CPSZ, OR SGTC 2) Habitual SZ 3) Development	SEIZURE_DESCRPT. AGEOFOTSZ	Typical seizure onset Age	Age at which typical seizure begins Typical: the habitual ictal pattern of the patient; habitual refers to the recurrent ictal manifestation	Number
	SEIZURE_DESCRPT. DUROFEPIL	Epilepsy Duration	For how long the patient has epilepsy	Number followed by M (for month) or Y (for Year) Other values are – and null
	SEIZURE_DESCRPT. SPSZ	Simple Partial Seizure	Self-limiting ictal event without loss of cons	Yes, No - Null
	SEIZURE_DESCRPT. SPSZOCCU_Second	Simple Partial Seizure	How often the seizure happens	Number followed by Sec (second), Min (Minute) or Hr (Hour)
	SEIZURE_DESCRPT. CPSZ	Complex Partial Seizure	Ictal event marked by a loss of consciousness and often by stereotypic features.	Yes, No - Null
	SEIZURE_DESCRPT. CPSZOCCU_Second	Complex Partial Seizure		Number followed by Sec (second), Min (Minute) or Hr (Hour)
	SEIZURE_DESCRPT. SGTC	Secondary Generalized Tonic Clonic	Ictal progression to involve both cerebral hemispheres.	Yes, No - Null
	SEIZURE_DESCRPT. SGTCOCCU	Secondary Generalized Tonic Clonic		Number followed by Sec (second), Min (Minute) or Hr (Hour)
	SEIZURE_DESCRPT. SZDEVLOP	Seizure Development	How the seizure evolves over time	CPSZ → SGTC SPSZ → SGTC SPSZ → CPSZ AURA → CPSZ SPSZ → CPSZ → SGTC - Null
	SEIZURE_DESCRPT. SZFRQ_Day	Seizure Frequency	The frequency of habitual seizure	Number followed by (Day, Week, Month, Year)
	SEIZURE_DESCRPT. MONTHSZFREE	# of months seizure free	Longest time interval during which no ictus has manifested	Number
	SEIZURE_DESCRPT. AURAWOSZ	Aura without seizure	The occurrence of a simple partial event without the succeeding habitual ictus	Yes No Null -
	SEIZURE_DESCRPT. AURAWOSZPERC	Aura without seizure percentage	The percentage of the total seizure frequency in which only the aura manifests	Number

continued on following page

Table 3. Continued

Category	Abbreviation	Feature Name	Description	Possible Values
Seizure Description 1) SPSZ, CPSZ, OR SGTC 2) Habitual SZ 3) Development	SEIZURE_DESCRPT. SZDEVPERC	Seizure Development Percentage	The percentage frequency of the said ictus	Number
	SEIZURE_DESCRPT. HABITSZ	Habitual Seizure	Same as typical seizure	SGTC SPSZ CPSZ - Null
	SZDES_AURA. AURAOCCU	Aura Occurrence	The frequency of aura	Number followed by Day, Week, Month, Year
	SEIZURE_DESCRPT. DUROFEPILMY	Epilepsy Duration	For how long the patient has epilepsy	Number followed by M (for month) or Y (for Year) Other values are – and null
Psychiatric History	PSYCHIAT_HIST. PRESDEPRES	Present Depression	The presence of a current state of depression	Yes No - Null
	PSYCHIAT_HIST. PASTDEPRES	Past Depression	The presence of a past state of depression	Yes No - Null
	PSYCHIAT_HIST. PRESANXIETY	Present Anxiety	The presence of a current state of anxiety	Yes No - Null
	PSYCHIAT_HIST. PASTANXIETY	Past Anxiety	The presence of a past state of anxiety	Yes No - Null
	PSYCHIAT_HIST. SUISIDE	Suicide	Willful self-execution	Yes No - Null
	PSYCHIAT_HIST. HALLUCINATION	Hallucination	Occurrence of a visual perception without substance	Yes No - Null
	PSYCHIAT_HIST. SUBS_ABUSE	Substance Abuse	Overconsumption of a particular agent	Yes No - Null
Neuropsychology Tests	NEUROPSYCH. BNT	Boston Naming Test	Formal test of naming ability	Number out of 60
	NEUROPSYCH. IMVMEMW	Wechsler Verbal Memory Immediate	Formal test of immediate verbal recall	Number out of 50
	NEUROPSYCH. DELVMEMW	Wechsler Verbal Memory Delayed		Number out of 50
	NEUROPSYCH. IMVMEM	Wechsler Non-Verbal Memory Immediate	Formal test of immediate perceptual recall	Number out of 41
	NEUROPSYCH. DELVMEM	Wechsler Non-Verbal Memory Delayed	Formal test of delayed perceptual recall	Number out of 41

continued on following page

Table 3. Continued

Category	Abbreviation	Feature Name	Description	Possible Values
Neuropsychology Tests	NEUROPSYCH. IMVMEMRQ	Rey-Osterreith Non-Verbal Memory Immediate	Formal test of immediate recall of complex diagram	Number out of 36
	NEUROPSYCH. DELVMEMRQ	Rey-Osterreith Non-Verbal Memory Delayed	Formal test of delayed recall of complex diagram	Number out of 36
	NEUROPSYCH. CVLT_TOTAL	California Verbal Learning Test Total	Formal test of word acquisition	Number out of 90
	NEUROPSYCH. CVLT_LDFR	California Verbal Learning Test Long Delay Free Recall	Formal test of delayed independent recall of learned word battery	Number
	NEUROPSYCH. CVLT_RETN	California Verbal Learning Test Retention Percentage	Percentage calculation of word retention ability	Number
	NEUROPSYCH. CVLT_RECOG	California Verbal Learning Test Recognition (Discriminatory Percentage)	Percentage calculation of select word recognition	Number
	NEUROPSYCH. CVLT_VERS	California Verbal Learning Test Recognition (Version)	Version of such evaluation	I II
	NEUROPSYCH. FSIQ	Full Scale IQ	Formal full scale assessment of intelligence	Number
	NEUROPSYCH. VIQ	Verbal IQ	Formal assessment of literal intelligence	Number
	NEUROPSYCH. NVIQ	Non-verbal IQ	Formal assessment of perceptual intelligence	Number
Medical History (risk factors)	MEDICAL_HISTORY. MENINGITIS	Meningitis	Infection of meninges (lining of the central nervous system)	Yes No
	MEDICAL_HISTORY. AGEMENINGITIS	Meningitis (Age)	Age of occurrence of meningitis	Number
	MEDICAL_HISTORY. ENCEPHALITIS	Encephalitis	Infection of brain tissue	Yes No
	MEDICAL_HISTORY. AGEENCEPHALITIS	Encephalitis (Age)	Age of occurrence of encephalitis	Number
	MEDICAL_HISTORY. FEBRILESZ	Febrile Seizure	Seizure induced by fever	Yes No
	MEDICAL_HISTORY. AGEFEBRILESZ	Febrile Seizure (Age)	Age at which febrile seizure has occurred	Number
	MEDICAL_HISTORY. HEMORRHAGE	Hemorrhage	Bleeding within cerebral tissue	Yes No

continued on following page

Table 3. Continued

Category	Abbreviation	Feature Name	Description	Possible Values
Medical History (risk factors)	MEDICAL_HISTORY. STROKE	Stroke	Focal loss of circulation within cerebral tissue	Yes No
	AGE_AT_SURGERY. DUR_OF_LATENCY	Latency	During of Latency	Number
	AGE_AT_SURGERY. AGE_AT_SURG	Surgery	Age at Surgery	Number
	AGE_AT_SURGERY. AGE_AT_HEADINJ	Head Injury	Age at Head injury	Number
	MEDICAL_HISTORY. FMLHISEPI	Family History Epilepsy	Familial generational occurrence of epilepsy	Unknown Yes No
	MEDICAL_HISTORY. FMLHISFZ	Family History Febrile Seizure	Familial generational occurrence of seizures with fever	Unknown Yes No
	MEDICAL_HISTORY. FMLHISPTSZ	Family History Partial Temporal Lobe Seizure	Familial generational occurrence of seizures of temporal lobe origin	Unknown Yes No
	MEDICAL_HISTORY. AGMOYRMNGTS	Agmoyrmngts	Month/year designation for age at meningitis	Yes No
	MEDICAL_HISTORY. AGMOYRENCPH	Agmoyrencph	Month/year designation for age at encephalitis	Yes No
	MEDICAL_HISTORY. AGEMOYRFBRIL	Agemoyrfbril	Month/year designation for age at febrile seizure	Yes No
	HANDEDNESS. LRAHANDED	Left or Right Handed	Preferential use of either limb	R L A
	HANDEDNESS. WRITING	Writing	Habitual hand used for writing	R L A
	HANDEDNESS. THROWING	Throwing	Habitual hand used for throwing	R L A
	HANDEDNESS. SWING	Swing	Habitual hand used for swinging (bat or club)	R L A
	HANDEDNESS. SHOOTING	Shooting	Preferential eye used for sighting a target	R L A
	HANDEDNESS. CUTTING	Cutting	Habitual hand preferred for holding scissors	R L A
	HANDEDNESS. BRUSHING	Brushing	Habitual hand used for holding a hairbrush	R L A
	HANDEDNESS. MOTHER	Mother	Handedness of mother	R L A
	HANDEDNESS. FATHER	Father	Handedness of father	R L A
	HANDEDNESS. NOFSIBLINGS	Number of Siblings	Total number of patient's siblings	Number

continued on following page

Table 3. Continued

Category	Abbreviation	Feature Name	Description	Possible Values
Exams	EXAM. MOTORSIDE	Motor Side	Side of loss of power	B, R L, N
	EXAM. ML_PALPEBRAL	Motor Palpebral	Side of asymmetrical eyelid widening	R, L, Y, N
	EXAM. ML_FACE	Motor Face	Side of facial weakness	B, R, L, N
	EXAM. ML_ARM	Motor Arm	Side of upper limb weakness	R, L Y, N, B
	EXAM. ML_LEG	Motor Leg	Side of lower limb weakness	B, N, L, R
	EXAM. SENSIDE	Sensory Side	Side of loss of sensation	R N L
	EXAM. SL_FACE	Sensory Face	Side of facial numbness	R N L
	EXAM. SL_ARM	Sensory Arm	Side of upper limb numbness	R N L
	EXAM. SL_LEG	Sensory Leg	Side of lower limb numbness	R N L
	EXAM. SP_DYSARTHRIA	Speech Dysarthria	Poor articulation of speech	Yes No
	EXAM. VISUALF_LR	Visual Field	Laterality of visual field loss	Yes No L
	EXAM. VISUALHEMI	Visual Hemi	Presence of complete lateral field loss	Yes No L
Electro Encephalography Tests (EEG)	EEG. NUMOFSZ	Total Seizures	Number of seizures of all types	Number
	EEG. SHARP1	Sharp Wave 1	Waveform less than 200ms in duration on EEG identified at site 1	Yes No
	EEG. SH1PERC	Sharp Wave 1 percentage	Percentage estimate of sharp waves at site 1	Number
	EEG. SHARP2	Sharp Wave 2	Same waveform pattern at site 2	Yes No
	EEG. SHARP3	Sharp Wave 3	Same waveform pattern at site 3	Yes No
	EEG. SLOW1	Slow Wave 1	Repetitive extended waveform on EEG at site 1	Yes No
	EEG. SL1LOC	Slow Wave 1 Location	Repetitive extended waveform location on EEG at site 1	T3,Sp1,F7,Sp1-T3,T4,T1,C4,F8,T2,F7-Sp1-T3,Sp2,F4,F2,Sp2-T4,Fp2,F8-Sp2-T4,F4-8,Cz
	EEG. SL1PERC	Slow Wave 1 percentage	Percentage estimate of slow wave at site 1	Number
	EEG. SLOW2	Slow Wave 2	Same waveform pattern at site 2	Yes No

continued on following page

Table 3. Continued

Category	Abbreviation	Feature Name	Description	Possible Values
Electro Encephalography Tests (EEG)	EEG. SL2LOC	Slow Wave 2 Location	Repetitive extended waveform location on EEG at site 2	T3,Sp2-T4,T6,T2,T1,T4,C3,Sp1-T3,F8,F7-Sp1-T3,F3,F8-Sp2-T4,F7,T5,F3-F7,Sp2,Sp1
	EEG. SL2PERC	Slow Wave 2 percentage	Percentage estimate of slow waves at site 2	Number
	EEG. SLOW3	Slow Wave 3	Same waveform pattern at site 3	Yes No
	EEG. POSTOP			Number
Wada Tests	WADA. NOFCORRECTR	Number of Correct Right	Number of correctly recalled items after left carotid injection	Number
	WADA. NOFITEMS	Number of TOTAL items Right	Maximal number of items provided for recall prior to injection	Number
	WADA. NOFCORRECTL	Number of Correct Left	Number of correctly recalled items after right carotid injection	Number
	WADA. NOFITEMSL	Number of TOTAL items Left	Maximal number of items provided for recall prior to injection	Number
	WADA. LANGREPRES	Language Representation	Laterality of language dominance in cerebral hemispheres	L R B
	WADA. TDIFFERENCE	Total Difference		Number
Medication and Surgery	MEDICATION. DOSAGE	Dosage	Amount of individual doses	Number
	MEDICATION. DRUGFRQINT	Drug frequency	Number of times drug is taken during the day	QID, BID, TID, QHS, QD
	SURGERY. LOCATION	Location	Site of surgery within the temporal lobe	10 different values
Outcome	OUTCOME. SZFRQ_CLASS	Engel Class	Postoperative outcome score based on the presence of ictal events and the timing of their appearance	I II III IV
	OUTCOME. SZFRQ_SUBCLASS	Engel Subclass	Subcategories of individual classes to detail the nature of the manifestation	A B C D

Table 4. Selected attributes for Algorithm 1- (CFS-ReliefF-EM-CFS)

No	Cluster 1	Cluster 2	Cluster 3
1	EEG.SHARP3	AGE_AT_SURGERY.AGE_AT_SURG	AGE_AT_SURGERY.AGE_AT_HEADINJ
2	EEG.SL1LOC	AGE_AT_SURGERY.AGE_AT_HEADINJ	NEUROPSYCH.BNT
3	EEG.SL2LOC	EEG.SHARP3	PSYCHIAT_HIST.PRESANXIETY
4	EEG.SL2PERC	EEG.SL1LOC	PSYCHIAT_HIST.PASTANXIETY
5	EXAM.ML_ARM	HANDEDNESS.MOTHER	SEIZURE_DESCRPT.AGEOFOTSZ
6	EXAM.SENSIDE	HANDEDNESS.FATHER	SEIZURE_DESCRPT.SZDEVLOP
7	EXAM.SL_FACE	MEDICAL_HISTORY.AGEMENINGITIS	SEIZURE_DESCRPT.MONTHSZFREE
8	EXAM.SL_ARM	MEDICAL_HISTORY.AGEFEBRILESZ	SEIZURE_DESCRPT.AURAWOSZPERC
9	EXAM.SL_LEG	NEUROPSYCH.IMVMEMRQ	SZDES_AURA.AURAOCCU
10	HANDEDNESS.THROWING	NEUROPSYCH.VIQ	WADA.NOFCORRECTR
11	HANDEDNESS.MOTHER	SEIZURE_DESCRPT.SZDEVLOP	
12	HANDEDNESS.FATHER	SZDES_AURA.AURAOCCU	
13	MEDICAL_HISTORY.MENINGITIS	WADA.LANGREPRES	
14	MEDICATION.DRUGFRQINT		
15	NEUROPSYCH.VIQ		
16	PSYCHIAT_HIST.PRESANXIETY		
17	PSYCHIAT_HIST.PASTDEPRES		
18	SEIZURE_DESCRPT.AGEOFOTSZ		
19	SEIZURE_DESCRPT.CPSZ		
20	SEIZURE_DESCRPT.MONTHSZFREE		
21	SZDES_AURA.AURAOCCU		
22	WADA.NOFCORRECTR		
23	WADA.LANGREPRES		

Table 5. Selected attributes for Algorithm 2- (CFS-ReliefF-EM-CFS-CSE)

No	Cluster 1	Cluster 2	Cluster 3
1	EEG.SHARP3	EEG.SHARP3	PSYCHIAT_HIST. PRESANXIETY
2	EEG.SL1LOC	EEG.SL1LOC	SEIZURE_DESCRPT. AGEOFOTSZ
3	EEG.SL2LOC	HANDEDNESS.MOTHER	SEIZURE_DESCRPT. SZDEVLOP
4	EXAM.SL_FACE	HANDEDNESS.FATHER	SEIZURE_DESCRPT. MONTHSZFREE
5	EXAM.SL_ARM	MEDICAL_HISTORY. AGEMENINGITIS	SEIZURE_DESCRPT. AURAWOSZPERC
6	HANDEDNESS.THROWING	NEUROPSYCH.VIQ	SZDES_AURA.AURAOCCU
7	HANDEDNESS.FATHER	SEIZURE_DESCRPT. SZDEVLOP	WADA.NOFCORRECTR
8	MEDICATION. DRUGFRQINT		
9	NEUROPSYCH.VIQ		
10	PSYCHIAT_HIST. PRESANXIETY		
11	PSYCHIAT_HIST. PASTDEPRES		
12	SEIZURE_DESCRPT. AGEOFOTSZ		
13	SZDES_AURA.AURAOCCU		
14	WADA.NOFCORRECTR		
15	WADA.LANGREPRES		

Table 6. Selected Attributes For Algorithm 3- (CFS-ReliefF-COBWEB Stage1-CFS)

No	Cluster 1	Cluster 2	Cluster 3
1	AGE_AT_SURGERY.AGE_AT_SURG	AGE_AT_SURGERY.AGE_AT_SURG	AGE_AT_SURGERY.AGE_AT_SURG
2	AGE_AT_SURGERY.AGE_AT_HEADINJ	EEG.SL1LOC	EXAM.SENSIDE
3	EEG.SHARP3	EEG.SL2LOC	EXAM.SL_FACE
4	EEG.SL1LOC	EEG.SL2PERC	EXAM.SL_LEG
5	EEG.SL2LOC	EEG.SLOW3	HANDEDNESS.WRITING
6	EXAM.ML_ARM	EXAM.SL_LEG	MEDICAL_HISTORY.MENINGITIS
7	EXAM.SENSIDE	HANDEDNESS.FATHER	MEDICATION.DRUGFRQINT
8	EXAM.SL_FACE	MEDICATION.DRUGFRQINT	PSYCHIAT_HIST.PASTDEPRES
9	EXAM.SL_ARM	SEIZURE_DESCRPT.AGEOFOTSZ	SEIZURE_DESCRPT.DUROFEPILMY
10	EXAM.SL_LEG	SEIZURE_DESCRPT.MONTHSZFREE	WADA.LANGREPRES
11	HANDEDNESS.MOTHER	WADA.LANGREPRES	
12	MEDICAL_HISTORY.MENINGITIS		
13	MEDICATION.DRUGFRQINT		
14	NEUROPSYCH.BNT		
15	NEUROPSYCH.IMVMEMW		
16	NEUROPSYCH.DELVMEMW		
17	NEUROPSYCH.CVLT_RETN		
18	PSYCHIAT_HIST.PASTDEPRES		
19	SEIZURE_DESCRPT.MONTHSZFREE		
20	SZDES_AURA.AURAOCCU		
21	WADA.NOFCORRECTR		
22	WADA.LANGREPRES		

Table 7. Selected Attributes For Algorithm 4- (CFS-ReliefF-COBWEB Stage1-CFS-CSE)

No	Cluster 1	Cluster 2	Cluster 3
1	AGE_AT_SURGERY.AGE_AT_SURG	AGE_AT_SURGERY.AGE_AT_SURG	EXAM.SENSIDE
2	AGE_AT_SURGERY.AGE_AT_HEADINJ	EEG.SL1LOC	EXAM.SL_FACE
3	EEG.SL2LOC	EEG.SL2LOC	EXAM.SL_LEG
4	EXAM.SENSIDE	EEG.SL2PERC	HANDEDNESS.WRITING
5	EXAM.SL_ARM	EEG.SLOW3	MEDICAL_HISTORY.MENINGITIS
6	HANDEDNESS.MOTHER	HANDEDNESS.FATHER	MEDICATION.DRUGFRQINT
7	MEDICAL_HISTORY.MENINGITIS	MEDICATION.DRUGFRQINT	PSYCHIAT_HIST.PASTDEPRES
8	MEDICATION.DRUGFRQINT		
9	NEUROPSYCH.BNT		
10	NEUROPSYCH.IMVMEMW		
11	NEUROPSYCH.CVLT_RETN		
12	SEIZURE_DESCRPT.MONTHSZFREE		
13	SZDES_AURA.AURAOCCU		
14	WADA.NOFCORRECTR		
15	WADA.LANGREPRES		

Table 8. Selected Attributes For Algorithm 5- (CFS-ReliefF-COBWEB Stage2-CFS)

No	Cluster 4	Cluster 5	Cluster 6	Cluster 7	Cluster 8	Cluster 9	Cluster 10
1	AGE_AT SURGERY AGE_AT HEADINJ	AGE_AT_ SURGERY AGE_AT SURG	EXAM.ML_ARM	EXAM.ML_ARM	HANDEDNESS MOTHER	EEG SL1LOC	AGE_AT SURGERY AGE_AT HEADINJ
2	EEG SHARP3	EEG SL2LOC	EXAM .SENSIDE	MEDICAL HISTORY MENINGITIS	HANDEDNESS FATHER	EEG SLOW2	EEG SL1LOC
3	EEG SL1LOC	HANDEDNESS SHOOTING	EXAM SL_FACE	MEDICAL HISTORY AGEFEBRILESZ	MEDICAL HISTORY MENINGITIS	EEG SL2LOC	EEG SL2LOC
4	EEG SLOW2	HANDEDNESS CUTTING	EXAM SL_ARM	MEDICATION DRUGFRQINT	MEDICAL HISTORY AGEFEBRILESZ	MEDICAL HISTORY AGMOYRMNGTS	EEG SL2PERC
5	EEG. SL2LOC	MEDICAL HISTORY MENINGITIS	EXAM SL_LEG	PSYCHIAT HIST PASTANXIETY	MEDICATION DRUGFRQINT	MEDICATION DRUGFRQINT	EXAM ML_ARM
6	EEG. SLOW3	NEUROPSYCH BNT	HANDEDNESS THROWING	PSYCHIAT HIST PASTDEPRES	NEUROPSYCH IMVMEMRQ	SEIZURE DESCRPT SZDEVLOP	EXAM SL_LEG
7	HANDEDNESS WRITING	SEIZURE DESCRPT MONTHSZFREE	MEDICATION DRUGFRQINT	SEIZURE DESCRPT DUROFEPILMY	NEUROPSYCH NVIQ	WADA NOFCORRECTR	MEDICAL HISTORY MENINGITIS
8	MEDICAL HISTORY MENINGITIS		SEIZURE DESCRPT CPSZ	SEIZURE DESCRPT MONTHSZFREE	PSYCHIAT HIST PASTANXIETY	WADA LANGREPRES	MEDICAL HISTORY AGMOYRMNGTS

continued on following page

Table 8. Continued

No	Cluster 4	Cluster 5	Cluster 6	Cluster 7	Cluster 8	Cluster 9	Cluster 10
9	SEIZURE DESCRPT CPSZ		WADA NOFCORRECTR	WADA NOFCORRECTR	PSYCHIAT HIST PASTDEPRES		MEDICAL HISTORY AGEFEBRILESZ
10	WADA LANGREPRES			WADA LANGREPRES	SEIZURE DESCRPT SZDEVLOP		MEDICATION DRUGFRQINT
11					SEIZURE DESCRPT MONTHSZFREE		NEUROPSYCH DELVMEMW
12					WADA NOFCORRECTR		PSYCHIAT HIST PRESANXIETY
13					WADA LANGREPRES		PSYCHIAT HIST PASTANXIETY
14							SEIZURE DESCRPT DUROFEPILMY
15							SZDES AURA AURAOCCU
16							WADA NOFCORRECTR
17							WADA LANGREPRES

Table 9. Selected Attributes For Algorithm 5- (CFS-ReliefF-COBWEB Stage2-CFS-CSE)

No	Cluster 4	Cluster 5	Cluster 6	Cluster 7	Cluster 8	Cluster 9	Cluster 10
1	AGE_AT SURGERY AGE_AT HEADINJ	AGE_AT SURGERY AGE_AT SURG	EXAM.SL FACE	EXAM.ML ARM	HANDEDNESS MOTHER	EEG SL1LOC	AGE_AT SURGERY AGE_AT HEADINJ
2	EEG SHARP3	EEG SL2LOC	EXAM.SL ARM	MEDICAL HISTORY MENINGITIS	MEDICAL HISTORY MENINGITIS	EEG SL2LOC	EEG SL1LOC
3	EEG SL1LOC	HANDEDNESS SHOOTING	HANDEDNESS THROWING	MEDICATION DRUGFRQINT	MEDICATION DRUGFRQINT	MEDICATION DRUGFRQINT	EEG SL2LOC
4	EEG SLOW2	MEDICAL HISTORY MENINGITIS	MEDICATION DRUGFRQINT	PSYCHIAT HIST PASTANXIETY	PSYCHIAT HIST PASTANXIETY	WADA NOFCORRECTR	MEDICAL HISTORY AGMOYRMNGTS
5	EEG SL2LOC	SEIZURE DESCRPT MONTHSZFREE	SEIZURE DESCRPT CPSZ	PSYCHIAT HIST PASTDEPRES	PSYCHIAT HIST PASTDEPRES	WADA LANGREPRES	MEDICATION DRUGFRQINT
6	HANDEDNESS WRITING		WADA NOFCORRECTR	SEIZURE DESCRPT DUROFEPILMY	SEIZURE DESCRPT SZDEVLOP		SEIZURE DESCRPT DUROFEPILMY
7	MEDICAL HISTORY MENINGITIS			SEIZURE DESCRPT MONTHSZFREE	SEIZURE DESCRPT MONTHSZFREE		WADA NOFCORRECTR
8				WADA LANGREPRES	WADA NOFCORRECTR		WADA LANGREPRES

Table 10. Image modality attributes' description

Category	Abbreviation	Feature Name	Description	Possible Values
Normal Tissue Aggregation	NOR_TISS_AGGR. L_F_TEXTUREF1	Left side - Flair Texture feature #1	Texture feature #1 (energy) of the left hippocampus of the brain computed from FLAIR images	Number
	NOR_TISS_AGGR. L_F_TEXTUREF2	Left side - Flair Texture feature #2	Texture feature #2 (energy) of the left hippocampus of the brain computed from FLAIR images	Number
	NOR_TISS_AGGR. L_F_TEXTUREF3	Left side - Flair Texture feature #3	Texture feature #3 (energy) of the left hippocampus of the brain computed from FLAIR images	Number
	NOR_TISS_AGGR. L_F_TEXTUREF4	Left side - Flair Texture feature #4	Texture feature #4 (energy) of the left hippocampus of the brain computed from FLAIR images	Number
	NOR_TISS_AGGR. L_F_TEXTUREF5	Left side - Flair Texture feature #5	Texture feature #5 (energy) of the left hippocampus of the brain computed from FLAIR images	Number
	NOR_TISS_AGGR. L_F_TEXTUREF6	Left side - Flair Texture feature #6	Texture feature #6 (energy) of the left hippocampus of the brain computed from FLAIR images	Number
	NOR_TISS_AGGR. L_F_TEXTUREF7	Left side - Flair Texture feature #7	Texture feature #7 (energy) of the left hippocampus of the brain computed from FLAIR images	Number
	NOR_TISS_AGGR. L_F_AVG_STD	Left side – Flair Average Standard deviation	Standard deviation of intensities of the left hippocampus of the brain computed from FLAIR images	Number
	NOR_TISS_AGGR. L_F_AVG_INTENSITY	Left side – Flair Average Intensity	Average of intensities of the left hippocampus of the brain computed from FLAIR images	Number
	NOR_TISS_AGGR. L_T1_VOLUME	Left side – T1 volume	Volume of hippocampus computed from T1 images	Number
	NOR_TISS_AGGR. R_F_TEXTUREF1	Right side - Flair Texture feature #1	Texture feature #1 (energy) of the right hippocampus of the brain computed from FLAIR images	Number
	NOR_TISS_AGGR. R_F_TEXTUREF2	Right side - Flair Texture feature #2	Texture feature #2 (energy) of the right hippocampus of the brain computed from FLAIR images	Number
	NOR_TISS_AGGR. R_F_TEXTUREF3	Right side - Flair Texture feature #3	Texture feature #3 (energy) of the right hippocampus of the brain computed from FLAIR images	Number
	NOR_TISS_AGGR. R_F_TEXTUREF4	Right side - Flair Texture feature #4	Texture feature #4 (energy) of the right hippocampus of the brain computed from FLAIR images	Number
	NOR_TISS_AGGR. R_F_TEXTUREF5	Right side - Flair Texture feature #5	Texture feature #5 (energy) of the right hippocampus of the brain computed from FLAIR images	Number
	NOR_TISS_AGGR. R_F_TEXTUREF6	Right side - Flair Texture feature #6	Texture feature #6 (energy) of the right hippocampus of the brain computed from FLAIR images	Number
	NOR_TISS_AGGR. R_F_TEXTUREF7	Right side - Flair Texture feature #7	Texture feature #7 (energy) of the right hippocampus of the brain computed from FLAIR images	Number
	NOR_TISS_AGGR. R_F_AVG_STD	Right side – Flair Average Standard deviation	Standard deviation of intensities of the right hippocampus of the brain computed from FLAIR images	Number
	NOR_TISS_AGGR. R_F_AVG_INTENSITY	Right side – Flair Average Intensity	Average of intensities of the right hippocampus of the brain computed from FLAIR images	Number
	NOR_TISS_AGGR. R_T1_VOLUME	Right side – T1 volume	Volume of hippocampus computed from T1 images	Number
	NOR_TISS_AGGR. T1_VOLUME_ASSYM	T1_VOLUME_ASSYM	Difference between volume of the left and right hemisphere hippocampus	Number

Table 11. Selected Attributes For Image Modality Database- (CFS-CSE)

No	Attributes
1	NOR_TISS_AGGR.R_F_AVG_INTENSITY
2	NOR_TISS_AGGR.L_F_TEXTUREF3
3	NOR_TISS_AGGR.L_F_TEXTUREF7
4	NOR_TISS_AGGR.L_F_AVG_INTENSITY
5	NOR_TISS_AGGR.R_F_TEXTUREF4
6	NOR_TISS_AGGR.T1_VOLUME_ASSYM
7	NOR_TISS_AGGR.R_T1_VOLUME

Table 12. Results of leave one out evaluation in outcome prediction using imaging data

	Number of All Instances	Number of Correctly Predicted Class Instances	Number of Correctly Predicted Class and Subclass Instances	Correct Prediction Rate of Class	Correct Prediction Rate of Class and Subclass
Entire Dataset	77	50	36	64.93%	46.75%
Class 1 Instances in Dataset	51	45	33	88.23%	64.7%
Precision of Predicting Class1 Instances	61	45	33	73.77%	54.09%

Chapter 5
Health Information Technology:
Implications for Physician Practice and Professionalism

Erik L. Carlton
West Virginia University, USA

James W. Holsinger Jr.
University of Kentucky, USA

Asos Q. Mahmood
University of Memphis, USA

ABSTRACT

Healthcare reform and health information technology (HIT) are transforming physicians' roles in delivering healthcare. New technologies present physicians with exciting new opportunities and challenges to enhance medical practice, reduce costs, and improve patient experiences, as well as opportunities to develop new competencies and standards of professionalism. The Dreyfus model for skills acquisition may provide a helpful framework. Within the competency context, understanding and leveraging drivers of and the barriers to HIT adoption can promote a learning culture that may more readily assimilate new HIT. Involving physicians in designing and implementing HIT systems could result in increasing physician satisfaction. Supportive staffing and technical assistance may aid physicians in successfully implementing the systems without increasing workload or decreasing professional satisfaction. Understanding the needs of 21st century physicians related to HIT solutions should greatly increase the successful integration of HIT into the 21st century healthcare workplace.

DOI: 10.4018/978-1-5225-8244-1.ch005

INTRODUCTION

The role of physicians in the delivery of healthcare has continued to evolve over the past fifty years. During this period, a growing divergence of professionalism and personal expectations has occurred for physicians often resulting in their inability to meet competing demands. A variety of factors have encroached on autonomy, long the ascendant professional value of physicians. The previous decade has seen a significant shift in practice requirements in the U.S. healthcare system. Health information technology (HIT) has greatly expanded and been at the foundation of the health reforms enacted during this period. While this initially began with the Health Insurance Portability and Accountability Act (HIPAA, 1996), the Health Information Technology for Economic and Clinical Health (HITECH, 2009) provisions of the 2009 American Recovery and Reinvestment Act (ARRA) were a major catalyst to systemic shifts related to HIT and served as a foundation for many of the reforms outlined in the Patient Protection and Affordable Care Act enacted a year later (ACA, 2010). Collectively, these healthcare reform acts sought to restructure health care delivery with improved quality, efficiency, patient-centered care, care integration and coordination, access and affordability of care, and population health as primary motivations for the reforms (Buntin, Jain, & Blumenthal, 2010; Kocher, Emanuel, & DeParle, 2010; Blumenthal, 2009; Blumenthal, 2011a; Blumenthal, 2011b; Geyman, 2015).

As the underlying and practical realities of healthcare systems have evolved, the professional values and practices of physicians have failed to adapt in a corresponding manner. The development of HIT and its application in the practice of medicine both within institutions and also physician office settings may be seen as a major component in the changing medical practice environment. A "professionalism gap" may be present leading to physician dissatisfaction with professional life. In particular, the use of HIT may be especially representative of this gap. Consequently, the profession may be better served by developing a new values framework that conforms to the 21st century healthcare system. To do so will require the forgoing of the 20th century's preferred "independent physician" model in favor of a new professional structure based on teamwork and collaboration. The use (or lack thereof) of HIT both in institutions and in the office setting may be indicative of the quandary in which physicians find themselves as their professional values move from being individual based to being formed through teamwork and collaboration. Convincing established physicians to embrace such a model may be difficult, but opportunities exist for significant progress among a new generation of physicians accustomed to 21st century practice models and HIT.

PROFESSIONAL COMPETENCE

Competence is a core component of every profession, including medicine. Professional competence may be defined as "the habitual and judicious use of communication, knowledge, technical skills, clinical reasoning, emotions, values, and reflection in daily practice for the benefit of the individual and community being served" (Epstein & Hundert, 2002). In the practice of medicine these authors find that acquiring and using knowledge in the practice of medicine, integrating biomedical and psycho-social data, and relating through communicating effectively are important concomitants in the professional practice of medicine. They point out that competence is based on tacit knowledge, which they define as "that which we know but normally do not explain easily, including the informed use of heuristics (rules of thumb), intuition, and pattern recognition" (Epstein & Hundert, 2002). In an editorial, Leach (2002) enumerates the six general competencies of a physician regardless of the specialty practiced: "patient care, medical knowledge, practice-based learning and improvement, interpersonal and communication skills, professionalism, and systems-based practice." The acquisition of skills leading to competence is a developmental process, enhanced over time, and based on understanding experiences resulting in habit formation. As will be discussed later, the utilization of HIT in the practice of medicine is thought to result in a higher quality of health care and is a critical component of competent physician practice in the 21st century. "Physicians need to have the integrity, motivation, and capacity to discern good learning and good health care but should be restless until they get it right" (Leach, 2002).

Professionalism is a key component of professional competence. Several factors can impede physicians in their development of professionalism including, "stress and lack of experience, support, and training [that] can lead to uncertainty about appropriate professional behavior and attitudes" (Brennan & Coles, 2003). The practice of medicine is always changing, and it is clearly important for physicians to stay abreast of current advancements and to develop self-motivation in order to undertake the necessary continuing professional learning (Gibson, Kartsounis, & Kopelman, 2006). The acquisition of skills competence requires being engaged enough in acquiring skills to be accountable. The Dreyfus model of skills acquisition requires moving through a series of five stages in order to become competent. To do so requires "less detachment and greater immersion in particular contexts" (Leach, 2002). The Dreyfus model may be useful in acquiring the skills necessary to become competent in the utilization of HIT.

THE DREYFUS MODEL

The Dreyfus model is a developmental process of skill acquisition, which is based on experiential learning and situated performance. The model was developed based on the study of chess players, air force pilots, and army tank drivers and commanders (Benner, 2004). In *Mind Over Machine*, Dreyfus and Dreyfus (1986) lay out the five stages of skill acquisition. They point out that although some skills may be learned by observing others who are more proficient, most skill acquisition occurs through verbal or written instructions and as such skill acquisition is a learned behavior. "As human beings acquire a skill through instruction and experience, they do not appear to leap suddenly from rule-guided 'knowing that' to experience-based 'know-how'" (Dreyfus & Dreyfus, 1986). They posit that a person learning a new skill passes through a series of five stages in which qualitatively different perceptions of the task being learned or modes of decision-making are identified as skill increases. In applying this model to the acquisition of HIT skills by physicians may require concrete experience in an actual work environment. These stages of skill acquisition have been identified "because (1) each individual, when confronting a particular type of situation in his or her skill domain, will usually approach it first in the manner of the novice, then the advanced beginner, and so on through the five stages, and (2) the most talented individuals employing the kind of thinking that characterizes a certain stage will perform more skillfully than the most talented individuals at an earlier stage in our model" (Dreyfus & Dreyfus, 1986; Dreyfus, 2002; Dreyfus, manuscript; Atherton, 2003). The five stages of the model – novice, advanced beginner, competent, proficient, and expert – are briefly explained in Table 1.

PHYSICIAN PRACTICE SATISFACTION

During the 20th century the key value in the practice of medicine was professional autonomy. "It provided physicians with a sense of pride, accomplishment, and authority, given their position of primacy in the hierarchy of health care professions" (Holsinger & Beaton, 2006). Zuger (2004) noted that by the middle of the 20th century physician autonomy had provided admiring assistants, respectful colleagues, loyal patients, job security, and a large income. However, with the onset of the 21st century significant dissatisfaction with the practice of medicine was being exhibited by physicians, who found themselves plagued by decreased autonomy, a fall in prestige, increased bureaucracy, and personal dissatisfaction with their profession (Zuger, 2004; Dimick et al., 2010). The independent practice of medicine, so significant in the 20th century, "was increasingly characterized by interdependence, rather

Table 1. Five stages of the Dreyfus Model

Stage 1: Novice
The novice recognizes the features and objective facts that are relevant to the particular skill being acquired and acquires an understanding of the rules that determine those actions that are based on the certain facts and features of the particular skill. The key elements of the situation facing the novice are so objectively and clearly defined that the situation in which they are present is immaterial and thus is context-free. The manipulation of context-free elements by specific rules can be defined as information processing.
Stage 2: Advanced Beginner
Once the novice develops a significant amount of experience in handling real situations a marginally acceptable level of skills acquisition should occur. Practical experiences in concrete situations enable the advanced beginner to recognize meaningful elements pertaining to a skill. These new elements are called situational since they may be distinguished from context-free elements. At this stage of skill acquisition the new rules of behavior include both those that are context-free as well as the new situational elements.
Stage 3: Competence
As experience increases, the number of relevant elements the learner recognizes is substantial. Without a sense of what is important in any particular situation, performance provokes anxiety, and the student may question the possibility of skill mastery. At this stage of skill acquisition, it is important to seek new rules and reasoning procedures in order to develop an appropriate new perspective or to decide on a new plan. It is significantly more difficult to arrive at these new rules since there are so many possible situations that can differ from each other so widely. Until this stage the learner is able to rationalize that the rules are inadequate rather than feeling any remorse based on having made a mistake. Here the learner has a sense of being responsible for any disaster that may have occurred. On the other hand, should the learner succeed a sense of elation occurs which is not known to the novice or advanced beginner.
Stage 4: Proficient
At this stage a learner begins to see situations holistically, understands situational priorities, and perceives positive and negative deviations. Consequently, decision-making and skill application becomes less labored. This stage requires that involvement must replace the detached, rule-following of the novice and advanced beginner. Situational discrimination will gradually replace rules and principles and be accompanied by the appropriate associated responses. A remarkable event occurs at this stage for the learner in that the now experienced learner is enabled to see "goals and salient aspects, but not what to do to achieve these goals" (Dreyfus, manuscript).
Stage 5: Expertise
"[A]n expert generally knows what to do based on mature and practiced understanding" (Dreyfus & Dreyfus, 1986). The skills exhibited by an expert simply become a part of the person exhibiting them allowing him or her to be completely unaware of them. An expert under normal conditions does not make decisions or solve problems, but instead an expert simply does what works. Performance using the skills of an expert occurs without reflection and is continuous or ongoing in nature. Intuition is a core process in an expert's use of skills.

than individualism; unfettered authority had been exchanged for ubiquitous checks and balances" (Holsinger & Beaton, 2006). Autonomy, income, and perceived job demands are among the most important predictors of physician job satisfaction (Hoff, Young, Xiang, & Raver, 2015; Scheurer, McKean, Miller, & Wetterneck, 2009). In 1973, more than 85% of practicing physicians surveyed reported that they were not dissatisfied with their choice of a profession. Zuger (2004) found from surveys administered in the late 20th century that, "30% to 40% of practicing physicians would not choose to enter the medical profession if they were deciding on a career again, and an even higher percentage would not encourage their children to pursue a medical career." The National Survey of Physicians (Kaiser Family Foundation, 2002) found that 58% of physicians reported that their enthusiasm for the practice of medicine had declined in the previous five years. The Survey also indicated that 87% of physicians reported a decline in physician morale over the previous five years. Bovier and Perneger (2003) studied physician work satisfaction and found that "physicians were more satisfied with…patient care, professional relations, and personal rewards (intellectual stimulation, opportunities for continuing medical education, enjoyment at work). The lowest satisfaction scores were found in work-related burden (workload, time available for family, friends or leisure, work-related stress, administrative burden) and work-related income, and prestige." More recently, in 2016, a survey was conducted among 17,263 U.S. physicians by Merritt Hawkins team on behalf of The Physicians Foundation. The survey results indicate that about 54% of physicians rate their morale as "somewhat or very negative," 49% are often or always "experience feelings of burn-out," and almost half of them would not recommend medicine as "a career to their children" (The Physician Foundation, 2016). The vast majority of physicians still value "patient relationships" and consider it as "the most satisfying" part of their practice (71%), while 58% reported that "regulatory/ paperwork burdens" are the least satisfying part (The Physician Foundation, 2016). Furthermore, a large portion of physicians (72.1%) feel that their practice has been adversely affected by external factors such as "third party authorizations, treatment protocols, [and] EHR design" (The Physician Foundation, 2016).

In considering the well-being of physicians, the Association of Professors of Medicine (2003) considered burnout to be a syndrome that leads to decreased effectiveness in the practice of medicine. This syndrome consists of a feeling of depersonalization, emotional exhaustion, as well as lowered sense of personal accomplishment. Their paper which included consideration of physician distress found that in a Canadian study including 3500 physicians, 62% of respondents found their workload too heavy and 55% found that they and their families suffered from their choice of medicine as a profession. The consequences of burnout for physicians include "absenteeism, turnover in personnel, feelings of a lack of accomplishment, cynicism, loss of zeal, zest, and enthusiasm, and decreased job satisfaction" (Association of Professors of Medicine, 2003; Alexander, & Ballou, 2018). Significant causes of physician burnout include, among others, the lack of control over the physician's practice environment and work-life balance issues. The former is certainly an issue when efforts are made to institute large integrated clinical information systems and since, at least initially, it is thought that significant amounts of time are required to utilize such systems by physicians, impacting on work-life balance. Also included in dealing with physician burnout are such issues as work schedule and workload, both of which may be heavily impacted by HIT solutions (Shanafelt et al., 2016). Physicians increasingly indicate having a less healthy work-life balance. The percentage of physicians who reported to have a healthy work-life balance in 2014 was only 41%, a significantly lower rate than those who reported so in 2011 (49%). Generally, physicians are not depressed or unhappy at home, they are unhappy at work. (Alexander, & Ballou, 2018).

It is important to note that in multiple reviews (Shanafelt et al., 2016; Hoff et al., 2015; Scheurer et al., 2009), physicians' subjective perceptions of certain aspects of their job and workload are more related to their job satisfaction than more objective measures such as caseload or hours worked. Thus, if physicians perceive certain aspects of their job, such as HIT components, to be burdensome, anxiety-provoking, or dissatisfactory they risk poorer job satisfaction. This resonates with the Dreyfus model of skill acquisition discussed earlier. Physicians have spent years, if not decades, mastering medical practice and becoming medical experts. HIT is new and many physicians may have yet to gain the requisite exposure and experience to achieve comfortable competence, proficiency, or expertise with these new and ever-evolving systems.

The Association of Professors of Medicine (2003) points outs that to promote physician well-being two key approaches, among others, are to "I. Promote Physician Autonomy: Increase physicians' ability to influence their work environment and participate in decisions that affect practice. Provide flexibility and increased physician control over schedule. II. Provide Adequate Support Services: Supply adequate physician coverage to allow time off. Provide adequate and coordinated nursing, secretarial, administrative, social work, and laboratory support in an effort to promote efficient patient care. III. ..." As will be noted later, these are extremely important facets for dealing with physician dissatisfaction with the implementation of major IT solutions.

THE FORMATION OF PHYSICIAN PROFESSIONALISM

During the past quarter century, physician professionalism has been largely based in the needs of physicians. However, changes that have occurred in the practice of medicine and in healthcare itself have resulted in the need for changes in the practice of medicine and in physician values commensurate with societal needs in the 21st century. "Only when the values guiding physician professionalism and societal expectations of the health care system come into greater conformity can we hope to see increased physician satisfaction" (Holsinger & Beaton, 2006). Physician autonomy is no longer an approach that meets the needs of society due largely to the changes that have occurred in the expectations of the healthcare system as viewed through the eyes of society. Many of the difficulties faced in the deployment of large-scale HIT solutions can be found in physician autonomy. In order to develop appropriate physician professionalism for the future, a new values framework for physicians may be required. Such a re-ordering of values should play a major role in the development of successful IT implementation projects.

Leach (2004) has noted the frustration exhibited by physicians who are faced with a large number of constraints. In their review of the literature, they found that six general competencies have been identified that at least frame if not define the practice of medicine: patient care; medical knowledge; practice-based learning and improvement; interpersonal and communication skills; professionalism; and systems-based practice. Virtually all of these competencies can be directly related to the development of IT solutions in both hospitals and physician practice locations. Leach states: "Professionalism is one of the competencies; the community of medicine is currently in active dialogue as it attempts to discern what this word really means" (2004).

In order to develop clarity as to the future of physician professionalism, a new values framework for physicians should markedly assist in the development of physician professionalism. Holsinger and Beaton (2006) adapted Reinhard Priester's values framework originally developed for healthcare in anticipation of the proposed 1992 Clinton healthcare reforms in the United States. His suggestions were not tailored specifically to medical practice, but they serve as a useful substrate in the development of values that are central to the practice of medicine in the 21st century and to the development of a new approach to physician professionalism. "Just as Priester believes that the restructuring of the broader health care system must begin with its underlying values, the reconfiguration of medical professionalism must also start with values" (Holsinger & Beaton, 2006).

Priester identified the most influential values in healthcare in the United States during the last half of the 20th century: (1) professional autonomy and regulatory autonomy; (2) patient autonomy; (3) consumer sovereignty; (4) patient advocacy; (5) access to care; and (6) assurance of quality care (Priester, 1992). In viewing these values, Priester determined that it was no longer possible to view each patient and each physician in isolation from the broader societal context. Since a set of rules had not been agreed upon, a coherent values framework has not been in place. "In practice, professional autonomy has been the most dominant value, while access to care has been subordinate to the others, particularly professional autonomy, patient autonomy, and consumer sovereignty" (Holsinger & Beaton, 2006).

Priester, as a result of his analysis, proposed a new set of values to guide the U.S. healthcare system based on two types – essential and instrumental. He defined essential values as "fundamental for any health care system: without them, a system would be deficient … instrumental values (are) primarily a means to help achieve the essential values" (Priester, 1992). His new values framework (see Table 2) established fair access to care for everyone at the peak of the framework. Priester proposed five essential values – fair access, quality, efficiency, respect for patients, and patient advocacy – along with a set of six instrumental values to support the essential values. These included: (1) personal responsibility; (2) social solidarity; (3) social advocacy; (4) provider autonomy; (5) consumer sovereignty; and (6) personal security.

As noted by Holsinger and Beaton (2006), within Priester's proposed value system can be found the seeds of a new sense of physician professionalism. "To broadly address the inadequacies seen today, the relationship between physicians and society must be directed toward a partnership of mutual respect and quality care and away from absolute physician and patient autonomy" (Holsinger & Beaton, 2006). In the 21st century, it is crucial to link the disparate interest of physician independence to the needs of the community through the concept of collaborative interdependence or teamwork. This point can be made explicitly when dealing with the issues surrounding the development of HIT solutions in hospitals and large physician practices.

Forging a bridge between physicians' values and society's needs will require the adaptation of physician professionalism. The shift from the legacy values of physicians as noted by Priester requires a new generation of essential values (access to care, efficiency, and respect for patients). The result will require physicians to provide leadership, to engage collaboratively, and to develop interdependence in a

Table 2. Priester's proposed value framework for the U.S. Healthcare System

Essential Values	Instrumental Values
Fair Access Quality Efficiency Respect for Patients Patient Advocacy	Personal Responsibility Social Solidarity Social Advocacy Provider Autonomy Consumer Sovereignty Personal Security

Note: Per Priester (1992): "Ordering rules for these values are as follows: (1) Each essential value should be maximized to the degree possible without threatening any other essential value. But fair access should be preeminent. (2) Essential values should be achieved before instrumental values, except insofar as instrumental values are a means to achieve essential values."

manner that would be virtually incomprehensible for their predecessors of a previous generation. "The results should produce a convergence of physician professionalism and societal expectations, as well as increased satisfaction for the physician and greater benefits for patients" (Holsinger & Beaton, 2006). Consequently, physicians will be required to sacrifice authority and control over their medical practice environment in order to develop a team-based and collaborative model of practice. By so doing, physicians will enable the health care system to develop IT solutions in a more positive fashion. The 21st century physician will demonstrate dexterity with HIT as well as distance communication. The implementation of telemedicine and remote monitoring technologies in home health care, primary care, urgent care, and mental/ behavioral health care is just one tangible example of such dexterity (Kvedar, Coye, & Everett, 2014; Gough et al., 2015; Hilty, Chan, Torous, Mahautmr, & Mucic, 2015). Physicians in the 21st century will utilize a variety of flexible practice models, professional interdependence, and HIT to produce the necessary transition away from the independent physician model of the previous century.

PHYSICIAN PERSONALITY FACTORS

An important part of the development of professionalism and competence is based on the individual physician's personality. Among the five major personality factors, conscientiousness includes being organized and self-disciplined, while openness includes being creative and open to change (Firth-Cozens & King, 2006). Both of these personality factors are directly related to professionalism and willingness by physicians to engage in important practice modifications such as utilizing 21st century HIT. However, perfectionism can be a major personality vulnerability requiring a physician to learn coping skills and cognitive strategies to overcome it. Remediation (correction or alleviation) is one approach that may be useful as well in overcoming the aversion to HIT on the part of older, established physicians (Firth-Cozens & King, 2006).

Personal attributes such as conscientiousness, agreeableness, resilience, and a deep learning style may play a significant role in training physicians, especially older ones, in the use of HIT. Lifelong learning is a requirement for the practice of medicine where accelerating advances and a revolution in societal attitudes are occurring, including those directed at medicine as a profession. In defining lifelong learning in medical practice, Stern (2006) argues that it is "a set of self-initiated activities and information-seeking skills that are activated in individuals with a sustained motivation to learn and the ability to recognize their own learning needs." Evidence-based learning is a key to the continuing development of the physician, including a requirement by the physician to understand the need for and use of HIT within the day-to-day practice of medicine (Paice, 2006).

In the 21st century, teamwork is a key dimension of climate/culture linked to high performing physicians in the organized practice of medicine. Teamwork clearly has a significant impact on individual and team performance and viability, as well as innovation, including the use of HIT in the practice setting (West & Spendlove, 2006). Team leadership may be a role accepted by any of the healthcare professions, but it is often perceived that the physician should be the one to fill it. In filling this leadership role, a 21st century physician will need to surrender professional autonomy and develop a new professional structure based on teamwork and collaboration (Firth-Cozens, 2006). In dealing with the implementation of HIT solutions in the healthcare setting, remediation may be required on the part of physicians hampered by a lack of the skills required for successful utilization of such technology. "The development of remedial work needs to focus on improved cooperation between experts in the problem…Stronger professional relationships between a range of disciplines may help to ensure that the doctor is referred to the right source of specialist help" (Cox, King, Hutchinson & McAvoy, 2006). A clear understanding of the use of remediation in expanding the skill sets of physicians having difficulty in utilizing HIT will enhance the probability of a successful implementation of the technology.

PHYSICIANS AND INFORMATION TECHNOLOGY

The past decade has seen an explosion in the number of healthcare organizations that have developed and implemented integrated clinical information systems as the solution to their HIT requirements. However, there have been a significant number of high profile failures as physicians have refused to engage HIT solutions in their workplace. One early study noted, "physicians in the United States are only slowly adopting information technology (IT) tools, despite studies demonstrating their clinical benefits" (Audet et al., 2004). Often, the uptake of healthcare information technologies in physician practices has been a function of regulatory requirements and/or hospital-system alignment. Regardless, adopting IT has been uneven and there is a clear divide between U.S. physicians and their use of IT based on the environment in which they practice and how they are compensated. For U.S. physicians the cost of IT is a critical barrier encountered in its adoption (Vydra, Cuaresma, Kretovics, & Bose-Brill, 2015). It is notable that less than 20% of US physicians in 2004 indicated they utilized an Electronic Medical Records (EMR) system in their office practices, even though more than 90% used the Internet in their personal lives (Audet et al., 2004). Four years later, studies reported that only 17% of practicing physicians and just 12% of hospitals had electronic health records (EHR) systems (DesRoches et al., 2008; Jha et al., 2009). By 2011, one-third of U.S. physicians reported having at least a basic EHR/EMR, including 39% of primary care physicians (Hsiao, Hing, Socey, & Cai, 2011). More recent studies have found that at least 75% of U.S. hospitals have adopted at least a basic EHR system (Adler-Milstein et al., 2015) and 71% of U.S. physicians in ambulatory care practices had adopted some form of EHR system (Heisey-Grove & Patel, 2014). As of 2015, the percentage of office-based physicians using any EHR system reached almost 90%, this means 9 out of 10 physicians in the U.S. are using some form of electronic system. The rates of adoption by primary care physicians were higher (89.6%) than non-primary care physicians (84.4%) (Yang & Hing, 2017). The upward trend in EHR/EMR systems adoption among physicians is mainly related to government regulations and the associated financial incentives or penalties (Heisey-Grove & Patel, 2014).

Adopting and adapting to an EHR system is a significant investment of time and resources. "Adopting various technologies requires an investment of resources for the tools themselves and time to learn how to use and then maintain these systems, which for clinicians translates in time away from direct patient care" (Audet et al., 2004). Notably, physicians working as solo practitioners or in small practices had the highest percentage of uncertainty about or not planning to adopt an EHR system (Heisey-Grove & Patel, 2014; Sowmya et al., 2011; Xierali et al., 2013).

Physicians were requested to rate six barriers to their use of IT: (1) start-up costs including original investment in equipment and training; (2) lack of IT standards at the national, regional, and local levels; (3) insufficient time to develop competency in the use of this new technology; (4) Cost of maintenance of the equipment; (5) questionable evidence of IT usefulness; and (6) insufficient knowledge or training in its use. The most important barriers to IT adoption for U.S. physicians are its start-up costs, the lack of IT standards, and especially the lack of physician time. A key finding reported in this study is that the age and sex of physicians are not significant factors in the utilization of HIT (Audet et al., 2004). While many physicians reported using health IT to improve workflow and healthcare quality (Unertl, Johnson, & Lorenzi, 2012; Asaro & Boxerman, 2008; King, Patel, Jamoom, & Furukawa, 2014; O'Malley, Reschovsky, & Saiontz-Martinez, 2015; Ryan, Bishop, Shih, & Casalino, 2013), many also reported dissatisfactory changes with patient-provider interactions such as interrupted communication, decreased eye contact, and less facetime with patients (Doyle et al., 2012; Makam et al., 2014; Sinsky et al., 2016; Arndt et al., 2017).

Among physicians adopting EHRs post-HITECH (2009), the most important drivers for adoption were (in order): incentive payments or financial penalties, board certification requirements, trusted colleagues using EHRs, electronic exchange capability, technical assistance with EHR implementation, and assistance with selecting an EHR (Heisey-Grove & Patel, 2014; see Figure 1). Among those who did not plan to adopt an EHR, the reasons cited were (again, in order): lack of financial resources, lack of time, privacy and security concerns, and lack of staff (Heisey-Grove & Patel, 2014; see Figure 2).

Other studies have documented the high cost of the installation of IT in American physician offices, a cost that can exceed $100,000. A key point to remember is that in the case of U.S. physicians, 89 percent of the economic benefit derived from the

Figure 1. Percent of physicians citing reasons for adopting an EHR
Source: Heisey-Grove & Patel, 2014

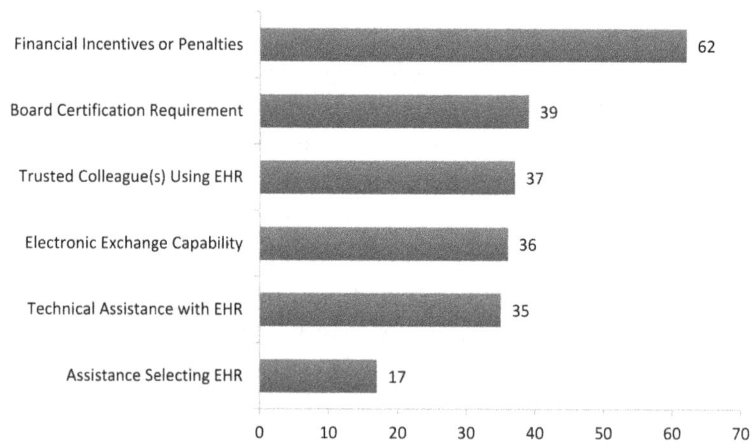

Figure 2. Percent of physicians citing reasons for not planning to adopt an EHR
Source: Heisey-Grove & Patel, 2014

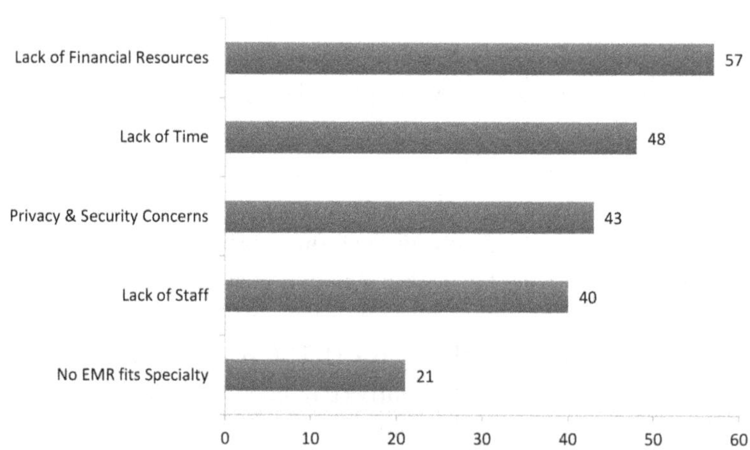

installation of IT in physician offices accrues to others including healthcare insurers (Johnson, 2006). "There is a general lack of capital for system acquisition, and any resultant cost savings would tend to flow to third-party payers, rather than to the clinicians who purchase the systems, resulting in a new financial loss" (Mann, Lloyd-Puryear, & Linzer, 2006). Unlike their American counterparts, physicians in the United Kingdom and Sweden who invest in EHRs are subsidized financially by their governments with the result that by 2004, 58% of physicians in the United Kingdom and 90% of those in Sweden utilized EHR (Audet et al., 2004). "Virtually all Danish physicians use their computers to record their clinical notes and to send and receive clinical electronic messages" (Protti, Edworthy, & Johansen, 2007). Of interest, in the United States nearly 90% of physicians recognize that there are benefits from the use of HIT which include improved patient safety and care as well as improved access to patient clinical information.

Evidence is present that U.S. physicians have been slow to adopt HIT compared to hospitals. Currently, almost all U.S. hospitals (99.1%) use EHR systems and above 95% have computerized physician-order-entry (CPOE) with clinical decision support systems in place (Pedersen, Schneider, & Scheckelhoff, 2017). Still,10% of U.S. physicians in ambulatory care practices have yet to adopt some form of EHR/ EMR system (Yang & Hing, 2017). Even in an era of health care reform, regulatory requirements, and financial incentives and penalties, there is strong evidence of continuing reticence by physicians to adjust to and adopt new healthcare technologies (Heisey-Grove & Patel, 2014). Even among those who adopted earlier EHR systems, there continues to be caution about upgrading to newer systems (Abramson et al., 2012).

Major organizations in the United States (the Leapfrog Group, Institute of Medicine [currently the National Academy of Medicine], and Agency for Healthcare Quality and Research) have advocated for the use of CPOE as a solution to reducing errors and adverse events in the clinical practice of medicine. However, successful implementation may be quite difficult with significant healthcare institutions' efforts failing. Although the ordering of medications is a complex process, the busy environment in which physicians work also results in added risk. "Learning or using a new system is a low priority competing with many other tasks, including direct patient care" (Wu, Abrams, Baker, & Rossos, 2006). A crucial issue facing the implementation of CPOE is the willingness of physicians to adopt the new technology (Abramson et al., 2012). Challenges facing the implementation of CPOE include the requirement to assist physicians in managing the change in their work practices since order entry time is increased as well as the required effort to train all physicians in the use of the system (Wu et al., 2006). Even with expert system support, significant issues arise in the implementation and use of a CPOE system and it is not uncommon for a significant percentage of large healthcare HIT projects to fail (Wears & Berg, 2005).

Since healthcare organizations are simultaneously social as well as technical in nature, it is important to remember that a well designed and implemented HIT project is not simply a technical problem but one that requires working jointly within a sociotechnical system. Commonly ignored within such a system are the dynamics of the organization and its power relationships. In order to develop a successful HIT implementation organizational change must be dealt with successfully. A variety of factors can be shown to be of importance in HIT implementation including technical, personal, organizational, and environmental. Although the financial risk is important, the behavioral and social issues are extremely important since "(o)nce the organization adopts a system, the users need to adopt it" (Ash & Bates, 2005). Of significant concern is the reluctance of physicians to adopt new technology that is perceived to interfere with their workflow and that appears to reduce time from caring for patients.

Regardless of studies that may indicate that CPOE is slower than hand-writing orders, the key issue is the physician's perception that it is slower. In a review of three large HIT implementation projects, two of which failed, Lapointe and Rivard (2006) point out that physician resistance often occurred surrounding the entry of prescriptions which was found to be time-consuming and tedious, requiring physicians to spend more time, up to 1.5 to 2 hours a day, managing their patients' records. The HIT solution was found to be an inefficient method of prescribing medications. Only one healthcare organization was able to correct the difficulties encountered and salvage the investment in the HIT system. These authors determined as the basis of their study that physicians cannot afford to become recalcitrant, but instead must modify their behavior in a manner that is helpful. Recent studies confirm that physicians spend more time on HIT than previously. Arndt and colleagues (2017) conducted a retrospective study among 142 primary care physicians in a single system. They found that the physicians spent almost 6 hours on EHR during workdays which was composed of 4.5 hours during clinic hours and almost 1.5 hours after clinic hours. Clerical and administrative tasks such as "documentation, order entry, billing and coding, and system security" accounted for half of the time spent on EHR (Arndt et al., 2017). Their findings were consistent with another study that was conducted a year earlier (Sinsky et al., 2016). "For every hour physicians provide direct clinical face time to patients, nearly 2 additional hours is spent on EHR and desk work within the clinic day" (Sinsky et al., 2016). At this point, HIT implementation requires physicians to surrender their 20th century concepts of physician autonomy and enter the 21st century putting teamwork and collaboration at the forefront of professionalism. Failure to do is evidenced by the failure of the Cedars-Sinai (Los

Angeles) HIT implementation when physician resistance resulted in the decision to abandon the CPOE effort. "More often, though, resistance is passive, with doctors simply avoiding the technologies" (Haugh, 2004).

In the United States, due to the non-governmental aspects of much of the healthcare system, in contradistinction to countries where health care is provided as a governmental service, governmental agencies providing health care such as the Department of Veterans Affairs (VA) and the Department of Defense medical agencies are the most uniformly committed to HIT solutions. "VA's computerized Patient Record System is now the most widely implemented electronic medical record in a federal health care system…" (Doebbeling, Vaughn, McCoy & Glassman, 2006). In the VA, the usefulness of a cooperative culture between physicians and management has been demonstrated with the needs of both considered resulting in shared decision-making. These authors point out that there are various human factors that need to be taken into consideration during the implementation of an HIT system. One example is the requirement that physicians and other users will require typing skills, a skill that points out to providers that the new system may be seen as a burden. As a result, means to circumvent the full use of the system may occur, including typing less than complete notes. A key point made by these authors is the need to fully understand the culture of medical practice as well as its realities.

A major difference found in the 21st century as compared to the previous one is the current healthcare environment. As new physician graduates arrive on the scene, they come with an entirely different approach to HIT solutions. Having been the first generation born after 1980 they regard the computer as an appliance much as refrigerator or television (Tapscott, 1998). Many physicians in the United States are at least partially trained in the VA, where they are accustomed to using state-of -the-art HIT tools. "Of course, perceived and real slowness or inefficiency in physicians' computer input techniques may always be a barrier to adoption, but the comfort level of the current generation of medical students and young physicians with contemporary human-computer interfaces will likely overcome this barrier" (Berner, Detmer, & Simborg, 2005). Not only are the new 21st century physicians more comfortable with computers than their predecessors, but also due to their education as clinicians they more readily accept that standardization in medical practice will inevitably be the result of the utilization of CPOE and clinical decision support systems.

PHYSICIAN PROFESSIONALISM AND INFORMATION TECHNOLOGY

In order for physicians to fully engage the revolution in health care HIT, significant changes will be required in a variety of areas: (1) the nature of physician professionalism; (2) an understanding of HIT skills acquisition by physicians; (3) the development of physician HIT professional competence; (4) a recognition of the issues of physician dissatisfaction; (5) the interface between physician personality factors and HIT utilization; and (6) physician engagement with HIT. In conclusion, an effort will be made to bring these disparate considerations together in order to provide a basis for the successful implementation of healthcare HIT tools in the 21st century.

All too often in the utilization of HIT, the needs of physicians are ignored. In developing large HIT installations, physicians are treated as a unitary whole with a failure to recognize that physicians will require individual development plans in order to reach a level of readiness that will result in each physician being able to effectively utilize the new system. During the past fifty years, physician autonomy has been a hallmark of clinical practice. This form of professionalism, although it has served the profession well in the past, has become obsolete with such obsolescence being particularly noticeable in the use of such tools. Autonomy has led to the failure of HIT solutions in large health care entities as physicians in powerful positions have rebelled against the use of HIT tools (Lapointe & Rivard, 2006). Re-ordering physician values will lead to a redirection of physician professionalism with the result that autonomy must be subordinated to values such as quality, efficiency, and fair access to the health care system with each playing a major role in the success of large scale HIT solutions (Holsinger & Beaton, 2006).

Fair access to the health care system should be enhanced through the successful use of HIT tools. Through the use of electronic medical records quality care will be improved as each physician will have full access to the patient's record, providing for improved interaction with the physician. Quality, and particularly patient safety, will be markedly enhanced through the use of CPOE tools, which will result in a decrease in medication errors and their related deaths (Kohn, Corrigan & Donaldson, 1999; McAlearney, Chisolm, Schweikhart, Medow, & Kelleher, 2007). HIT tools should improve efficiency in the healthcare system by removing the need for transmission and transcription of physician orders and patient records. In the use of HIT tools by physicians, several of Priester's instrumental values should enhance these essential values, particularly personal responsibility and social solidarity. Physicians should demonstrate their own personal responsibility for the quality and safety of their practice of medicine through the use of HIT, demonstrating social solidarity to their society through working diligently to incorporate the use of HIT tools in their clinical practice. By doing so, they will be engaging in a form of social advocacy, since they will be enhancing the safety and quality of the care they provide (Holsinger & Beaton, 2006).

A major issue that confronts the implementation of HIT tools in healthcare organizations is the need to understand the need for physicians to acquire HIT skills (Anderson, Asher, Whitler & Wilson, 2007). Many already are highly skilled operators who need little or no skills acquisition. Virtually all are proficient at the keyboard and will require little new skills acquisition other than working with and gaining familiarity with the HIT system and its functions (Tapscott, 1998). Older physicians, on the other hand, may require significant training in order to acquire basic computer literacy including the use of the keyboard itself. The Dreyfus Model is a useful approach to understanding the requirements by physicians in the acquisition of HIT skills (Leach, 2004). Prior to implementation of any new system, physicians as a whole need to be at the competent level in order to bring about a successful implementation. Only by continued effort will many physicians reach a level of expert according to the Dreyfus Model. A review of failed system implementations provides significant evidence of lack of skills-based training for physicians as demonstrated by the revolt of powerful physicians (Poon et al., 2004). Use of the Dreyfus Model, first as a diagnostic tool to determine the level of HIT skills of the individual physician, then as a determinant of the point at which physician readiness for implementation has occurred, should assist in bringing system implementation to a successful conclusion.

A key element in the failure of HIT implementation may be determined by recognizing the issues of physician professional dissatisfaction. A major issue of dissatisfaction results from the perceived primacy of the physician in the healthcare system. For many physicians, the use of CPOE represents a fall in professional prestige as the physician is viewed as being engaged in clerical duties (Shanafelt et al., 2016; Zuger, 2004). At this point, the need to assist physicians in understanding that by using HIT tools they are enhancing their practice of medicine by providing legible accessible records of patient care and are making a major difference in the lives of patients by reducing medical errors and the accompanying death toll (Blumenthal, 2017; Kohn, Corrigan & Donaldson, 1999). A major issue for physician satisfaction is not met by CPOE so long as it is perceived to require the use of more physician time than the current paper system (Zitner, 2006). The work-related burden (workload, time available for family, friends or leisure, work-related stress, and administrative burden) must be reduced by the use of HIT tools in order to enhance physician acceptance of such tools as a means for improving the health care system (Loomis,

Ries, Saywell, & Thakker, 2002). Anything that increases workload will increase the likelihood of physician burnout (Association of Professors of Medicine, 2003).

Physician personality factors also play a large role in the acceptance of HIT solutions. As noted earlier, certain personality factors are particularly important including being organized, self-disciplined, creative, and open to change (Firth-Cozens & King, 2006). These personality factors are useful in enabling physicians to conscientiously engage in the necessary personal actions required to creatively utilize HIT tools. They are important attributes of physician professionalism even within the Priester template for 21st century healthcare values. In training physicians with the Dreyfus Model in using HIT, the personal attributes of conscientiousness, agreeableness, resilience and a desire to learn play a significant role in training physicians, particularly older ones. Assisting physicians to understand the evidence behind the use of HIT tools and its importance for society will engage physicians' understanding that evidence-based learning is a key to understanding the need for and use of HIT in the practice of medicine in the 21st century. Teamwork in 21st century health care is a requirement that physicians must understand, particularly due to its importance in the development of HIT solutions in healthcare (Sinsky et al., 2016; Arndt et al., 2017; Panagioti et al., 2017). Engaging in teamwork and collaboration is an important approach in the development of HIT in the clinical setting. However, for some physicians, remediation of skills in order to develop competence in the use of HIT may be required (Firth-Cozens & King, 2006). In sum, physician personality factors play an important role in developing a strategy for physician engagement in the utilization of HIT tools.

CONCLUSION

In order for physicians to fully engage HIT in the 21st century, and for HIT programs to succeed and sustain, physicians must be fully integrated into the design, development, and implementation of such systems (Middleton et al., 2013; Cybulski, 2014). Understanding the nature of the drivers of and barriers to physician engagement with and adoption of health information technologies, including the impact on the professional and personal well-bring, as important implications both for physician practice as well as for the HIT industry (Carlton, et al., 2016). By utilizing Priester's most influential values, physicians can develop a new sense of professionalism which will undergird their engagement with vital healthcare technology in a manner that will result in the successful application of HIT tools in the physician workplace. Utilizing important approaches such as the Dreyfus Model of developing competence in the use of HIT tools will significantly repay the investment of physician time and energy by bringing them to an acceptable level of competence through the use of teamwork and collaboration with not only other healthcare practitioners, but with the HIT staff as well. Bringing physician personality factors into the equation will provide useful support to the HIT implementation effort. The appropriate involvement of physicians in the process of implementation as well as design of HIT systems will result in increasing physician satisfaction by providing the training required to successfully implement the systems without increasing physician workload at the expense of professional satisfaction. Understanding the needs of 21st century physicians in relationship to the development of HIT solutions should greatly increase the successful integration of HIT into the healthcare workplace in the 21st century.

REFERENCES

Abramson, E. L., Patel, V., Malhotra, S., Pfoh, E. R., Osorio, S. N., Cheriff, A., ... Kaushal, R. (2012). Physician experiences transitioning between an older versus newer electronic health record for electronic prescribing. *International Journal of Medical Informatics*, *81*(8), 539–548. doi:10.1016/j.ijmedinf.2012.02.010 PMID:22465355

Adler-Milstein, J., DesRoches, C. M., Kravolec, P., Foster, G., Worzala, C., Charles, D., ... Jha, A. K. (2015). Electronic health record adoption in US hospitals: Progress continues, but challenges persist. *Health Affairs*, *34*(11). doi:10.1377/hlthaff.2015.0992 PMID:26561387

Alexander, A. G., & Ballou, K. A. (2018). Work-Life Balance, Burnout, and the Electronic Health Record. *The American Journal of Medicine*, *131*(8), 857–858. doi:10.1016/j.amjmed.2018.02.033 PMID:29608876

Anderson, D. M., Asher, L. M., Whitler, E. T., & Wilson, E. A. (2007). Physician computer skills: A prerequisite to the future in healthcare services. *The Journal of the Kentucky Medical Association*, *105*, 67–71. PMID:17390734

Arndt, B. G., Beasley, J. W., Watkinson, M. D., Temte, J. L., Tuan, W. J., Sinsky, C. A., & Gilchrist, V. J. (2017). Tethered to the EHR: Primary care physician workload assessment using EHR event log data and time-motion observations. *Annals of Family Medicine*, *15*(5), 419–426. doi:10.1370/afm.2121 PMID:28893811

Asaro, P. V., & Boxerman, S. B. (2008). Effects of computerized provider order entry and nursing documentation on workflow. *Academic Emergency Medicine*, *15*(10), 908–915. doi:10.1111/j.1553-2712.2008.00235.x PMID:18785946

Ash, J. S., & Bates, D. W. (2005). Factors and forces affecting EHR system adoption: Report of a 2004 ACMI discussion. *Journal of the American Informatics Association, 12*(1), 8–12. doi:10.1197/jamia.M1684 PMID:15492027

Atherton, J. S. (2003). *Competence, proficiency and beyond*. Retrieved from http://www.doceo.co.uk/background/expertise.htm

Audet, A., Doty, M. M., Peugh, J., Shamasdin, J., Zapert, K., & Schoenbaum, S. (2004). Information technology: When will they make it into physicians' black bags? *Medscape General Medicine, 6*(4), 2–16. PMID:15775829

Benner, P. (2004). Using the Dreyfus model of skill acquisition to describe and interpret skill acquisition and clinical judgment in nursing practice and education. *Bulletin of Science, Technology & Society, 24*(3), 188–199. doi:10.1177/0270467604265061

Berner, E. S., Detmer, D. E., & Simborg, D. (2005). Will the wave finally break? A brief view of the adoption of electronic medical records in the United States. *Journal of the American Medical Informatics Association, 12*(1), 3–7. doi:10.1197/jamia.M1664 PMID:15492029

Blumenthal, D. (2009). Stimulating the adoption of health information technology. *The New England Journal of Medicine, 360*(15), 1477–1479. doi:10.1056/NEJMp0901592 PMID:19321856

Blumenthal, D. (2011a). Wiring the health system – Origins and provisions of a new federal program (Part One of Two). *The New England Journal of Medicine, 365*(24), 2323–2329. doi:10.1056/NEJMsr1110507 PMID:22168647

Blumenthal, D. (2011b). Implementation of the federal health information technology initiative (Part Two of Two). *The New England Journal of Medicine, 365*(54), 2426–2431. doi:10.1056/NEJMsr1112158 PMID:22187990

Blumenthal, D. (2017). Realizing the value (and profitability) of digital health data. *Annals of Internal Medicine, 166*(11), 842–843. doi:10.7326/M17-0511 PMID:28462419

Bovier, P. A., & Perneger, T. V. (2003). Predictors of work satisfaction among physicians. *European Journal of Public Health, 13*(4), 299–305. doi:10.1093/eurpub/13.4.299 PMID:14703315

Brennan, M. G., & Coles, C. (2003). Developing professional skills. *Lancet, 362*(9394), 1506. doi:10.1016/S0140-6736(03)14716-2 PMID:14602462

Buntin, M. B., Jain, S. H., & Blumenthal, D. (2010). Health information technology: Laying the infrastructure for national health reform. *Health Affairs, 29*(6), 1214–1219. doi:10.1377/hlthaff.2010.0503 PMID:20530358

Carlton, E. L., Holsinger, J. W. Jr, & Anunobi, N. (2016). Physician engagement with health information technology: Implications for practice and professionalism. *International Journal of Computers in Clinical Practice, 1*(2), 51–73. doi:10.4018/IJCCP.2016070103

Cox, J., King, J., Hutchinson, A., & McAvoy, P. (2006). *Understanding doctors' performance*. Oxford: Radcliffe Publishing.

Cybulski, G. R. (2014). Engaging Doctors in the Health Care Revolution. *Harvard Business Review, 92*(10), 20–20. Retrieved from https://hbr.org/2014/06/engaging-doctors-in-the-health-care-revolution PMID:25051859

DesRoches, C. M., Campbell, E. G., Rao, S. R., Donelan, K., Ferris, T. G., Jha, A., ... Blumenthal, D. (2008). Electronic health records in ambulatory care: A national survey of physicians. *The New England Journal of Medicine, 359*(1), 50–60. doi:10.1056/NEJMsa0802005 PMID:18565855

Dimick, M., Hall, M. A., Madison, K., Painter, M., Rodwin, M., Rosenbaum, S., & Tomes, N. J. (2010). *Medical professionalism in the new information age*. Rutgers University Press.

Doebbeling, B. N., Vaughn, T. E., McCoy, K. D., & Glassman, P. (2006). Informatics implementation in the Veterans Health Administration (VHA) Healthcare System to improve quality of care. In *AMIA 2006 Symposium Proceedings* (pp. 204-208). Bethesda: AMIA.

Doyle, R. J., Wang, N., Anthony, D., Borkan, J., Shield, R. R., & Goldman, R. E. (2012). Computers in the examination room and the electronic health record: Physicians' perceived impact on clinical encounters before and after full installation and implementation. *Family Practice, 29*(5), 601–608. doi:10.1093/fampra/cms015 PMID:22379185

Dreyfus, H. L. (2002). Intelligence without representation – Merleau-Ponty's critique of mental representation. *Phenomenology and the Cognitive Sciences, 1*(4), 367–383. doi:10.1023/A:1021351606209

Dreyfus, H. L. (manuscript). *A phenomenology of skill acquisition as the basis for a Merleau-Pontian non-representationalist cognitive science*. Retrieved from http://socrates.berkeley.edu/~hdreyfus/pdf.MerieauPontySkillCogSci.pdf

Dreyfus, H. L., & Dreyfus, S. E. (1986). *Mind over machine: The power of human intuition and expertise in the era of the computer*. New York: Free Press.

Epstein, R. M., & Hundert, E. M. (2002). Defining and assessing professional competence. *Journal of the American Medical Association*, *287*(2), 226–235. doi:10.1001/jama.287.2.226 PMID:11779266

Firth-Cozens, J. (2006). Leadership and the quality of healthcare. In J. Cox, J. King, A. Hutchinson, & P. McAvoy (Eds.), *Understanding doctors' performance* (pp. 123–133). Oxford: Radcliffe Publishing.

Firth-Cozens, J., & King, J. (2006). Are psychological factors linked to performance? In J. Cox, J. King, A. Hutchinson, & P. McAvoy (Eds.), *Understanding doctors' performance* (pp. 61–77). Oxford: Radcliffe Publishing.

Geyman, J. P. (2015). A five-year assessment of the Affordable Care Act: Market forces still trump the common good in US health care. *International Journal of Health Services*, *45*(2), 209–225. doi:10.1177/0020731414568505 PMID:25674797

Gibson, K., Kartsounis, L., & Kopelman, M. (2006). Cognitive impairment and performance. In J. Cox, J. King, A. Hutchinson, & P. McAvoy (Eds.), *Understanding doctors' performance* (pp. 48–60). Oxford: Radcliffe Publishing.

Gough, F., Budhrani, S., Cohn, E., Dappen, A., Leenknecht, C., Lewis, B., ... Bernard, J. (2015). ATA practice guidelines for live, on-demand primary and urgent care. *Telemedicine Journal and e-Health*, *21*(3), 233–241. doi:10.1089/tmj.2015.0008 PMID:25658882

Haugh, R. (2004). Wiring docs. *Hospitals & Health Networks*, *78*(11), 44–46, 55. PMID:15597697

Health Information Technology for Economic and Clinical Health (HITECH) Act, Title XIII of Division A and Title IV of Division B of the American Recovery and Reinvestment Act of 2009 (ARRA), Pub. L. No. 111-5, 123 Stat. 226 (Feb. 17, 2009), *codified at* 42 U.S.C. §§300jj *et seq.*; §§17901 *et seq.* (2009).

Health Insurance Portability and Accountability Act (HIPAA). Pub. L. No. 104-191, § 264, 110 Stat.1936. (1996).

Heisey-Grove, D., & Patel, V. (2014) Physician Motivations for Adoption of Electronic Health Records. ONC Data Brief, no. 21. Office of the National Coordinator for Health Information Technology: Washington DC. Retrieved from https://www.healthit.gov/sites/default/files/oncdatabrief-physician-ehr-adoption-motivators-2014.pdf

Hilty, D., Chan, S., Torous, J., Mahautmr, J., & Mucic, D. (2015). New frontiers in healthcare and technology: Internet- and web-based mental options emerge to complement in-person and telepsychiatric care options. *Journal of Health and Medical Informatics*, *6*(4), 1–14.

Hoff, T., Young, G., Xiang, E., & Raver, E. (2015). Understanding U.S. physician satisfaction: State of the evidence and future directions. *Journal of Healthcare Management*, *60*(6), 409–427. doi:10.1097/00115514-201511000-00007 PMID:26720985

Holsinger, J. W., & Beaton, B. (2006). Physician professionalism for a new century. *Clinical Anatomy (New York, N.Y.)*, *19*(5), 473–479. doi:10.1002/ca.20274 PMID:16506233

Hsiao, C. J., Hing, E., Socey, T. C., & Cai, B. (2011). Electronic health record systems and intent to apply for meaningful use incentives among office-based phsycian practices: United States, 2001-2011. NCHS data brief, No. 79. Hyattsville, MD: National Center for Health Statistics. Retrieved from http://www.cdc.gov/nchs/data/databriefs/db79.htm

Jha, A., DesRoches, C. M., Campbell, E. G., Donelan, K., Rao, S. R., Ferris, T. G., ... Blumenthal, D. (2009). Use of electronic health records in U.S. hospitals. *The New England Journal of Medicine*, *360*(16), 1628–1638. doi:10.1056/NEJMsa0900592 PMID:19321858

Johnson, B. (2006). Hospitals, physicians, and information technology. *Trustee*, *59*(5), 23, 27.

Kaiser Family Foundation. (2002). *National survey of physicians part III: doctors' opinions about their profession, March, 2002*. Retrieved from https://kaiserfamilyfoundation.files.wordpress.com/2013/01/highlights-and-chart-pack-2.pdf

King, J., Patel, V., Jamoom, E. W., & Furukawa, M. F. (2014). Clinical benefits of electronic health record use: National findings. *Health Services Research*, *49*(1pt2), 392–404. doi:10.1111/1475-6773.12135 PMID:24359580

Kocher, R., Emanuel, E. J., & DeParle, N. M. (2010). The Affordable Care Act and the future of clinical medicine: The opportunities and challenges. *Annals of Internal Medicine*, *153*(8), 536–539. doi:10.7326/0003-4819-153-8-201010190-00274 PMID:20733178

Kohn, L. T., Corrigan, J. M., & Donaldson, M. S. (Eds.). (1999). *To err is human: Building a safer health system*. Washington: National Academy Press.

Kvedar, J., Coye, M. J., & Everett, W. (2014). Connected health: A review of technologies and strategies to improve patient care with telemedicine and telehealth. *Health Affairs*, *33*(2), 194–199. doi:10.1377/hlthaff.2013.0992 PMID:24493760

Lapointe, L., & Rivard, S. (2006). Getting physicians to accept new information technology: Insights from case studies. *Canadian Medical Association Journal*, *174*(11), 1572–1578. doi:10.1503/cmaj.050281 PMID:16717265

Leach, D. C. (2002). Competence is a habit. *Journal of the American Medical Association*, *287*(2), 243–244. doi:10.1001/jama.287.2.243 PMID:11779269

Leach, D. C. (2004). Professionalism: The formation of physicians. *The American Journal of Bioethics*, *4*(2), 11–12. doi:10.1162/152651604323097619 PMID:15186669

Loomis, G. A., Ries, J. S., Saywell, R. M., & Thakker, N. R. (2002). If electronic medical records are so great, why aren't family physicians using them? *Journal of Family Medicine*, *51*, 636–641. PMID:12160503

Makam, A. N., Lanham, H. J., Batchelor, K., Moran, B., Howell-Stampley, T., Kirk, L., ... Halm, E. A. (2014). The good, the bad and the early adopters: Providers' attitudes about a common, commercial EHR. *Journal of Evaluation in Clinical Practice*, *20*(1), 36–42. doi:10.1111/jep.12076 PMID:23962319

Mann, M. Y., Lloyd-Puryear, M. A., & Linzer, D. (2006). Enhancing communication in the 21st century. *Pediatrics*, *117*(Supplement 3), S315–S319. doi:10.1542/peds.2005-2633K PMID:16735258

McAlearney, A. S., Chisolm, D. J., Schweikhart, S., Medow, M. A., & Kelleher, K. (2007). The story behind the story: Physician skepticism about relying on clinical information technologies to reduce medical errors. *International Journal of Medical Informatics*, *76*(11-12), 836–842. doi:10.1016/j.ijmedinf.2006.09.021 PMID:17112779

Middleton, B., Bloomrosen, M., Dente, M. A., Hashmat, B., Koppel, R., Overhage, J. M., ... Zhang, J. (2013). Enhancing patient safety and quality of care by improving the usability of electronic health record systems: Recommendations from AMIA. *Journal of the American Medical Informatics Association*, *20*(e1), e2–e8. doi:10.1136/amiajnl-2012-001458 PMID:23355463

O'Malley, A. S., Reschovsky, J. D., & Saiontz-Martinez, C. (2015). Interspecialty communication supported by health information technology associated with lower hospitalization rates for ambulatory care–sensitive conditions. *Journal of the American Board of Family Medicine*, *28*(3), 404–417. doi:10.3122/jabfm.2015.03.130325 PMID:25957373

Paice, E. (2006). The role of education and training. In J. Cox, J. King, A. Hutchinson, & P. McAvoy (Eds.), *Understanding doctors' performance* (pp. 78–90). Oxford: Radcliffe Publishing.

Panagioti, M., Panagopoulou, E., Bower, P., Lewith, G., Kontopantelis, E., Chew-Graham, C., ... Esmail, A. (2017). Controlled interventions to reduce burnout in physicians: A systematic review and meta-analysis. *JAMA Internal Medicine*, *177*(2), 195–205. doi:10.1001/jamainternmed.2016.7674 PMID:27918798

Patient Protection and Affordable Care Act (PPACA), 42 U.S.C. § 18001. (2010).

Pedersen, C. A., Schneider, P. J., & Scheckelhoff, D. J. (2017). ASHP national survey of pharmacy practice in hospital settings: Prescribing and transcribing—2016. *American Journal of Health-System Pharmacy*, *74*(17), 1336–1352. doi:10.2146/ajhp170228 PMID:28743758

Poon, E. G., Blumenthal, D., Jaggi, T., Hououour, M. M., Bates, D. W., & Kaushal, R. (2004). Overcoming barriers to adopting and implementing computerized physician order entry systems in U.S. hospitals. *Health Affairs*, *23*(4), 184–190. doi:10.1377/hlthaff.23.4.184 PMID:15318579

Priester, R. (1992). A values framework for health system reform. *Health Affairs*, *11*(1), 84–107. doi:10.1377/hlthaff.11.1.84 PMID:1577390

Protti, D., Edworthy, S., & Johansen, I. (2007). Adoption of information technology in primary care physician offices in Alberta and Denmark, Part 1: Historical, technical and cultural forces. *Healthcare Quarterly*, *10*(3), 95–102. PMID:17626551

Ryan, A. M., Bishop, T. F., Shih, S., & Casalino, L. P. (2013). Small physician practices in New York needed sustained help to realize gains in quality from use of electronic health records. *Health Affairs*, *32*(1), 53–62. doi:10.1377/hlthaff.2012.0742 PMID:23297271

Scheurer, D., McKean, S., Miller, J., & Wetterneck, T. (2009). U.S. physician satisfaction: A systematic review. *Journal of Hospital Medicine*, *177*(8), 883–888. PMID:20013859

Shanafelt, T. D., Dyrbye, L. N., Sinsky, C., Hasan, O., Satele, D., Sloan, J., & West, C. P. (2016, July). Relationship between clerical burden and characteristics of the electronic environment with physician burnout and professional satisfaction. *Mayo Clinic Proceedings*, *91*(7), 836–848. doi:10.1016/j.mayocp.2016.05.007 PMID:27313121

Shanafelt, T. D., Sloan, J. A., & Habermann, T. M.Association of Professors of Medicine. (2003). The well-being of physicians. *The American Journal of Medicine*, *114*(6), 513–519. doi:10.1016/S0002-9343(03)00117-7 PMID:12727590

Sinsky, C., Colligan, L., Li, L., Prgomet, M., Reynolds, S., Goeders, L., ... Blike, G. (2016). Allocation of physician time in ambulatory practice: A time and motion study in 4 specialties. *Annals of Internal Medicine*, *165*(11), 753–760. doi:10.7326/M16-0961 PMID:27595430

Sowmya, R. R., DesRoches, C. M., Donelan, K., Campbell, E. G., Miralles, P. D., & Jha, A. K. (2011). Electronic health records in small physician practices: Availability, use, and perceived benefits. *Journal of the American Medical Informatics Association*, *18*(3), 271–275. doi:10.1136/amiajnl-2010-000010 PMID:21486885

Stern, D. T. (2006). *Measuring medical professionalism*. Oxford University Press.

Tapscott, D. (1998). *Growing up digital: The rise of the next generation*. New York: McGraw-Hill.

The Physician Foundation. (2016). 2016 Survey of America's Physicians; Practice Patterns & Perspectives. Retrieved from https://www.merritthawkins.com/uploadedFiles/Physicians%20Foundation%202016%20Survey%20of%20Americas%20Physicians.pdf

Unertl, K. M., Johnson, K. B., & Lorenzi, N. M. (2012). Health information exchange technology on the front lines of healthcare: Workflow factors and patterns of use. *Journal of the American Medical Informatics Association, 19*(3), 392–400. doi:10.1136/amiajnl-2011-000432 PMID:22003156

Vydra, T.P., Cuaresma, E., Kretovics, M., & Bose-Brill, S. (2015). Diffusion and use of tethered personal health records in primary care. *Perspective in Health Information Management,* (Spring), 1-16.

Wears, R. L., & Berg, M. (2005). Computer technology and clinical work: Still waiting for Godot. *Journal of the American Medical Association*, *293*(10), 1261–1263. doi:10.1001/jama.293.10.1261 PMID:15755949

West, M., & Spendlove, M. (2006). The impact of culture and climate in healthcare organizations. In J. Cox, J. King, A. Hutchinson, & P. McAvoy (Eds.), *Understanding doctors' performance* (pp. 91–105). Oxford: Radcliffe Publishing.

Wu, R. C., Abrams, H., Baker, M., & Rossos, P. G. (2006). Implementation of a computerized physician order entry system of medications at the University Health Network – Physicians' perspectives on the critical issues. *Healthcare Quarterly*, *9*, 106–109. PMID:16548441

Xierali, I. M., Phillips, R. L., Green, L. A., Bazemore, A. W., & Puffer, J. C. (2013). Factors influencing family physician adoption of electronic health records (EHRs). *Journal of the American Board of Family Medicine*, *26*(4), 399–393. doi:10.3122/jabfm.2013.04.120351 PMID:23833153

Yang, N., & Hing, E. (2017). Table of Electronic Health Record Adoption and Use among Office-based Physicians in the U.S., by Specialty: 2015 National Electronic Health Records Survey. *CDC*. Retrieved from https://www.cdc.gov/nchs/data/ahcd/nehrs/2015_nehrs_ehr_by_specialty.pdf

Zitner, D. (2006). Physicians will happily adopt information technology. *Canadian Medical Association Journal*, *174*(11), 1583–1584. doi:10.1503/cmaj.060470 PMID:16717267

Zuger, A. (2004). Dissatisfaction with medical practice. *The New England Journal of Medicine*, *350*(1), 69–75. doi:10.1056/NEJMsr031703 PMID:14702431

Chapter 6
Predicting Patient Turnover:
Lessons From Predicting Customer Churn Using Free-Form Call Center Notes

Gregory W. Ramsey
Morgan State University, USA

Sanjay Bapna
Morgan State University, USA

ABSTRACT

Predicting patient turnover within health services is beneficial for resource planning. In this chapter, patient turnover is viewed as a form of customer churn. As such, the authors examine whether free-form notes are useful for solving the classification problem typically associated with customer churn. The authors show that classifiers which incorporate free-form notes, using natural language processing techniques, are up to 11% more accurate than classifiers that are solely developed using structured data. In addition, the authors show that free-form notes aggregated for each account perform better than treating each note separately. It is suggested that hospitals and chronic disease management clinics can use structured data and free-form notes from electronic health records to predict which patients are likely to cease receiving care from their facilities. Classification tools for predicting patient churn are of interest to hospital administrators; such information can aid in resource planning and facilitates smoother handoffs between care providers.

DOI: 10.4018/978-1-5225-8244-1.ch006

INTRODUCTION

Customers who cease using a firm's service or product, also referred to as customer churn, end their paying relationship with the firm for voluntary or involuntary reasons (Lin, Tzeng, & Chin, 2011). This issue is of great concern to commercial entities because acquiring and retaining customers is costly for most businesses Hospitals and other healthcare facilities can benefit by predicting which patients will churn, or turnover, and when it will occur. Instead of concerns for costs of acquiring patients these facilities need to anticipate churn to help in resource planning, to help with patient handoffs between providers of care, and to coordinate patient follow-ups (Park et al., 2016).

Modeling and predicting churn have been studied using a number of modeling techniques, such as logistic regression, neural networks, decision trees, and others (e.g., Burez & Van den Poel, 2009; Coussement & Van den Poel, 2008; Jiayin, Yangming, Yingying, & Shuang, 2006; Lu et al., 2014; Neslin, Gupta, Kamakura, Lu, & Mason, 2006; Milošević, Živić, & Andjelković, 2017; Pendharkar, 2009; Vafeiadis et al., 2016; Verbeke, Martens, Mues, & Baesens, 2011). The majority of these models are constructed using structured data, data which is typically maintained within corporate and/or administrative databases. Approximately 85% of data within firms is either unstructured or semi-structured (Negash, 2004). A distinction is made between unstructured data (e.g., a free-form note that is captured without any associated context) and semi-structured data (e.g., a free-form note that is captured and associated with a particular patient's account, thus establishing a context) (Negash, 2004). Semi-structured data is voluminous within the healthcare environment (Berg, 2001; Kontio et al., 2014; Miettinen & Korhonen, 2008; Srinivas, Rani, & Govrdhan, 2010). Some churn models based on structured data are briefly discussed in this paper, however, the focus of this paper is on investigating the usefulness of including semi-structured data (free-flowing text) in models for identifying and determining the likelihood of recipients of services to churn.

The paper is organized in the following manner. First, a literature review is presented in three parts, which are: (a) discussion of types and issues associated with patient churn, (b) identification of some of the more popular methods for modeling churn, and (c) a presentation of text mining techniques that will be applied to develop a churn model based on semi-structured data. Second, the methodology for developing and testing different churn models is reported. Third, results of a series of prediction experiments are presented. Finally, in the discussion and conclusion section, the findings from the experiments applied to possible real-world opportunities for predicting patient churn are presented

LITERATURE REVIEW

In this section, the authors review the literature on churn, applications of churn in the healthcare domain, models utilized to determine churn of customers, and text mining as applied to churn models.

Churn

Customer satisfaction, and the ensuing loyalty that comes about from that satisfaction, leads to profitable outcomes for companies (Reichheld, Teal & Smith, 1996). Loyal customers are unlikely to discontinue the product or service, or switch to competing products and services as long as switching barrier costs remain the same (Johnes, Mothersbaugh, & Betty, 2002). Churn can be managed to maximize profit by examining the lifetime value of a customer (Lemmens & Gupta, 2017). Retention campaigns and promotions to customers likely to churn may increase the profitability of the company, however, the customers likely to churn may not be as profitable as all other customers (Jahromi, Stakhovych, & Ewing, 2014). However, under some circumstances customer churn is a positive occurrence (Dechant et al., 2018), that while sought still needs to be planned for. Connection to other members in a social network can also determine who is likely to churn in domains where a group of members are strongly connected to each other in the same group (Richter, Yom-Tov, & Slonim, 2010).

Patient Churn

In the healthcare domain, patient churn as discussed in literature can be categorized under three themes (Duffield, Diers, Aisbett, & Roche, 2009; Duffield et al., 2011; Duffield, Roche, Diers, Catling-Paull, & Blay, 2010; Gill & Krentz, 2009; Needleman, Buerhaus, Mattke, Stewart, & Zelevinsky, 2002; Needleman et al., 2011; Needleman, Buerhaus, Stewart, Zelevinsky, & Mattke, 2006; Schaffer et al., 2018): (1) effects of patient churn on resource allocations, (2) relationship between patient churn and adverse events within units of care, and (3) implications for individual and public health management of chronic diseases.

Patient churn, which is often referred to as patient turnover, has numerous definitions with no clear metric for measuring it (Duffield, et al., 2011). Within hospitals, patients have clear statuses of being admitted, discharged, or transferred; similarly in the context of a health clinic, patients either receive services from the clinic or not. While the statuses are explicit, consensus is lacking on how to transform the statuses into a clearly defined metric for measuring churn. Unruh and

Fottler (2006) defined patient churn as the inverse of the length of stay, which is a definition that appears to be gaining traction in the literature.

Most literature (see citations listed above) on patient churn centers on measuring churn for some organizational unit rather than predicting churn at the level of an individual patient. Churn is of concern because the requirements for nursing staff resources increase with churn (Duffield, et al., 2009; Duffield, et al., 2011; Duffield, et al., 2015; Park et al., 2010; Unruh & Fottler, 2006; VanFosson, Yoder & Jones, 2017). When churn and concomitant resources are not properly coupled the occurrence of adverse events increases (Needleman, et al., 2011). Additionally, when nurse staffing levels are not managed to match patient churn there are increased reports of nursing burnout, low morale, increased rates of failure to rescue (FTR) patients, and reduced staff retention (Duffield, et al., 2011; Needleman, et al., 2002; Needleman, et al., 2011). These applications of patient churn are relevant from an aggregate perspective of patient churn. However, there are many domains where predicting which specific patient is likely to churn are also important. Patient churn within a public health or disease management clinic is of concern because patients who cease using facilities services potentially expose themselves and the public to health risks (Gill & Krentz, 2009) and also creates the "free rider" problem where there is no incentive for an insurer to invest in a cure because the patient may go elsewhere (Schaffer et al., 2018). This paper focuses on applications that will enable identification of specific patients that are likely to churn.

Churn Models

Businesses apply a number of tools and techniques for identifying service recipients that are likely to churn. For instance, customer relationship management (CRM) systems provide technologies for cultivating and managing customer relationships. These types of technologies afford companies means to gather data for maintaining and growing paying relationships with customers (Tuzhilin, 2012), but these data have to be modeled to predict the likelihood of churn and to identify where interventions are required to retain customers (Ngai, Xiu, & Chau, 2009). Predictive actionable models within these systems allow firms to treat customers differently based on their perceived value and individual needs (Tuzhilin, 2012). Electronic health records (EHR) and the systematic capture of patient data in electronic format provide new opportunities to manage patient care in ways that are similar to how CRM systems are used to manage customers. This section identifies some of the more popular approaches that have been used to build predictive churn models for commercial purposes and then directs attention to key developments in text processing that will be used to create an alternative churn model which can be applied to healthcare applications.

The majority of existing churn models have been created using the following approaches (Neslin, et al., 2006; Milošević, Živić, & Andjelković, 2017): (1) logistic or linear regression (e.g., Gustafsson, Johnson, & Roos, 2005; Mutanen, Ahola, & Nousiainen, 2006), (2) decision trees (e.g., Lemmens & Croux, 2006), (3) expert informed variable selection (e.g., Lima, Mues, & Baesens, 2009), (4) discriminant analysis (e.g., Xie & Li, 2008), (5) self-reported use of theory (e.g., Madden, Savage, & Coble-Neal, 1999; Miguéis et al., 2012), and (6) models derived from machine learning (Vafeiadis et al., 2015). Common to these approaches is a reliance on structured data for primary model features. The importance of data preparation algorithms prior to running the churn models also significantly impacts the results of the models (Coussement, Lessman, & Verstraeten, 2017).

The use of structured data in churn models has several advantages, such as predefined fields for obtaining attributes and predetermined ranges of values. In the healthcare domain, structured data has been utilized for various purposes for analytical models (Murphy et al., 2013; Sun, Rumshisky, & Uzuner, 2013), including churn models (Morid, Sheng, & Abdelrahman, 2017). But these models also have drawbacks and/or limitations. For instance, Gustafsson, Johnson et al. (2005) gathered telecommunications customer data using periodic surveys. While this data source was useful for constructing a churn model, it required collecting data via post-service call surveys, a time consuming process with added cost. Another example of limitations with a churn model based solely upon structured data was brought to light by Mutanen, Ahola et al. (2006). Their model predicted churn of retail banking customers using a logistic regression model with 70% predictive accuracy, but the model required constant updates in the choice of independent variables to maintain predictive accuracies. With the rise of unstructured and semi-structured data within firms, there is now a push to exploit this potential source of business intelligence so that it can be converted into actionable knowledge (Grover & Davenport, 2001; Negash, 2004), which includes building more robust churn models.

A last example of churn models based on structured data comes from Hadden et al. (2006b; 2006a; 2007). They used complaint data that was captured within structured data fields to construct their models. Tuzhilin (2012) suggests that use of semi-structured sources provides firms with a means to assess both objective and subjective sentiments as is often found within CRM systems. These subjective, semi-structured sources of customer information are examined within this study to extract service recipients' information using text mining techniques. The next portion of the literature review identifies literature within text mining that is relevant for developing churn models based on subjective, semi-structured data.

Text Mining

Natural language processing (NLP) is a computational process for interpreting and manipulating natural language speech and text (Chowdhury, 2003). A subfield within NLP is text mining, which is using computers to discover, extract, and process previously unknown information contained within written resources (Gupta & Lehal, 2009; Nassirtoussi et al., 2014). Text mining is a difficult process because interpretation of text is highly contextual, redundant and subject to misspelling and idiomatic substitutions (Cohen et al., 2014; Gupta & Lehal, 2009; Li et al., 2015; Pletscher-Frankkild et al., 2015). A fundamental technique within text mining is classification which is used to predict which class a specific entity belongs to, based on the textual information captured about that entity.

Several studies have examined and developed methods for text classification (Ikonomakis, Kotsiantis, & Tampakas, 2005; Joachim, 1999; Nigam, McCallum, Thrun, & Mitchell, 2000). Text at the highest level falls under two headings, facts and opinions (Liu, 2010). For this body of work the authors are interested in opinions and other types of subjective text; specifically, studies which identify and assess the existence of subjective material (Liu, 2010; Pang & Lee, 2008).

Subjective material is context-sensitive and often expresses opinions that can be used to predict a service recipient's intention to enable actions likely to be directed towards the recipient (Park, Lee, & Han, 2007). Liu (2010) reported that the opinion scoring of text is often formulated as a text classification problem. A common approach for classifying opinions is scoring along a continuum with ordinal measures, for example applying a Likert-like scale along a dimension of an opinion (Kontio et al., 2014; Liu, 2010). The unstructured nature of free-form text creates problems of high dimensionality, particularly when the size of the corpus is large (B. Tang, Shepherd, Milios, & Heywood, 2008).

Since a corpus of text documents can contain several thousands of words, dimensionality reduction plays an important role in text mining. Several approaches to dimensionality reduction in text mining have been reported (Underhill, 2007). A common approach to dimensionality reduction uses eigenvalues and eigenvectors as done in Principle Component Analysis (PCA), Singular Value Decomposition (SVD), Multi-dimensional scaling (MDS). In these approaches, a document can be represented as a linear combination of all the dimensionally reduced semantic features. A criticism of such approaches is that these methods are unable to represent interprctablc semantics features and that all semantic features are assumed to be part of a document (Lee & Seung, 1999). Another approach to dimensionality reduction, vector quantization (VQ), can represent semantic features; however, only one semantic feature can be represented in any one document. In this paper, the authors use non-matrix factorization (NMF) as a dimension reduction technique. NMF dimensionality reduction allows for several, but not necessarily all, interpretable semantic features to be attributed to documents. In facial image processing, NMF has been shown to represent interpretable parts of faces (lips, eyes, mouth), which neither PCA nor VQ have been able to represent (Lee & Seung, 1999).

NMF is a collection of algorithms that start with a matrix representation of all documents (represented as columns) and all words in the corpus (represented by rows), the starting matrix is decomposed into the product of a matrix representing a set of latent features and a matrix of feature weights. NMF is a non-negative, additive parts-based representation of the starting matrix; however the feature and the weights matrices are of a lower dimension than the starting matrix, consequently it is easier to represent and process the alternate form of subjective material (Lee & Seung, 1999; Saha & Sindhwani, 2012). This transformation has an added benefit in that the latent features are robust to context-sensitive usage of terms (Lee & Seung, 1999).

NMF is an appropriate transformation to apply to free-form notes for the following reasons: (1) the transformation learns the semantic features of the text, including recurring abbreviations used by healthcare providers or call center representatives, (2) the transformation disambiguates polysemous words (e.g., lead paint versus lead position), and (3) the transformation does not learn syntactic relationships between parts resulting in greater generalizability of the transforms (Lee & Seung, 1999).

The NMF algorithm has been implemented on several platforms and described in numerous published articles. Interested individuals are referred to literature for details on specific implementations (e.g., Fogel, Young, Hawkins, & Ledirac, 2007; Peers & Dutre, 2006; Shahnaz, Berry, Pauca, & Plemmons, 2006; Z. Tang, Wang, Zhang, Wei, & Zhao, 2011).

In a large corpus, as can be found in a repository of call center notes or EHRs, the dimensionality of the classification problem is high (B. Tang, et al., 2008). Consequently, using a transformation technique such as NMF is required to create tractable models. This study extends the literature on predictive modeling for churn management by applying a NMF transformation to free-form text notes captured within EHRs and call center CRM systems. This study advances the literature by categorizing service recipients' accounts for the likelihood of churning based on text-derived predictive models.

METHODOLOGY

Dataset

The dataset used in this study was obtained from the Wharton Customer Analytics Initiative (WCAI). WCAI partnered with a publically-traded subscription broadcast firm to provide data on a sampling of customers' transactions covering a timespan from August 2001 to February 2012. Approximately 79% of customer accounts had called into a service center from which free-form text notes were recorded. Many of these customers had multiple notes recorded at different times.

The free-form notes constitute a noisy data source because portions of some notes were redacted to protect customer privacy, many notes contain misspelled words, and extraneous characters were inserted by customer service representatives to format or emphasize certain portions of the notes. The average number of tokens (this includes words, abbreviations, codes, etc.) was 28 with a standard deviation of 15, the median number of tokens was 27. The number of unique tokens in the corpus was 396,190.

Below is a sample note from the dataset used in this study. The note is presented in the form in which it appeared in the dataset, our explanations (in lower case) and our interpretation (in upper case) of what has been written are shown within square brackets.

Taber ZZZZZ [<last name>] ci [CALLED IN] to cancel XXXXXXXXXXXX bec [BECAUSE] of the cost [.] [I, as the customer service agent] offered half off [the subscription cost] for X [<some number>] yr [YEARS]. [The] cust [CUSTOMER] accepted [the] offer and agreed w [WITH] t [THE] c [CONDITIONS.] [The] cust [CUSTOMER] will call back w [WITH] the cc [CREDIT CARD] info [INFORMATION.] so pls [PLEASE] refund the XX XX [<some dollar amount>] when he calls back

In the paragraph below is a sample note obtained from an EHR. This is typical of notes found in patient records, some individual notes may be longer and many are shorter. Note that while more is explicitly stated within the patient's note and, in the current note, nothing needs to be interpreted as to what given statements mean; however, this is not always the case.

pt [PATIENT] is a 57yo [YEAR OLD] f [FEMALE] who is followed at gh [GENERAL HOSPITAL – sometimes the abbreviation is used for growth hormone] by dr [DOCTOR] XXXXXX. she arrived a&ox3 [ALERT & ORIENTED TO PERSON, PLACE, TIME] via amb [AMBULANCE] from XXXXXX ew [EMERGENCY

WARD] for further eval [EVALUATION]/monitoring. today pt [PATIENT] was at home and states that her legs felt weak and she fell to the ground striking her head on the kitchen floor. pt [PATIENT] states that she did not have loc. [LOSS OF CONSCIOUSNESS] 911 was called and pt [PATIENT] taken to XXXXXX hosp. [HOSPITAL] she sustained a lac [LACERATION] to the back of her head that was sutured. she did rec [RECEIVE] tet [TETANUS] tox [TOXOID BOOSTER] per rn. [REGISTERED NURSE] per report she has been a&ox3 [ALERT & ORIENTED TO PERSON, PLACE, TIME]. she had labs [LABORATORY BLOOD TEST] drawn which showed inr [INTERNATIONAL NORMALIZED RATIO - clotting factor] to be 24, hct [HEMATOCRIT] 25.4, na [SODIUM] 132, k [POTASSIUM] 5.1, dig [DIGOXIN] 2.4 w/elevated bun/creat. [BLOOD UREA NITROGEN/CREATININE] she had head ct [COMPUTERIZED TOMOGRAPHY] done which was reported to be neg. [NEGATIVE] she was also noted to have bp [BLOOD PRESSURE] that dropped to 70's--pt [PATIENT] cont'd [CONTINUED TO BE] a&ox3 [ALERT & ORIENTED TO PERSON, PLACE, TIME], she was started on dopa [DOPAMINE] up to 8mcg, she was given 1 unit ffp. [FRESH FROZEN PLASMA] she was transfered to ccu [CRITICAL CARE UNIT]for further monitoring. (Source: physionet.org/works/DeidentifiedMedicalText)

The notes in the WCAI-sourced database are similar in structure to notes captured in free-form fields within EHRs. First, because of HIPAA requirements and the need to safeguard protected health information, much of the free-form data that would be available to commercial developers of churn models would contain redacted text, as represented by repeating letters in the above text samples. Second, many of the words which are typed into patient records are entered using standard and non-standard abbreviations. Both of these attributes make EHR free-form notes like customer service notes found in the current dataset.

Customer accounts, in the dataset provided to us, had one of five statuses, the statuses of interest were active and cancelled, while the other statuses were used by the company as interim steps between active and cancelled statuses. A total of 1,520,507 customer account records were sampled with 1,102,000 unique accounts. Some customer accounts had multiple records to track multiple broadcast devices. For accounts with more than one device it was possible to have a mixture of active and cancelled statuses. Such accounts with multiple devices were eliminated to prevent introducing confounders in models thus reducing the number of unique accounts to 824,212. From the unique accounts with single devices, 381,299 accounts had one or more free-form notes entered by a customer service representative. The breakdown on the number of accounts with notes was: 210,326 (55.2%) had an active status, 166,196 (43.6%) had a cancelled status, and 4,777 (1.2%) had other statuses. The accounts for single devices with notes having either an active or cancelled status were used for model building and testing. The number of notes on active and cancelled accounts is shown in Figure 1.

An additionally selection criterion was used for sampling records, all accounts with reactivation dates present were excluded because it presented a potential source of confounding predictions. This reduced the number of accounts to examine to 194,865.

Procedure

The predictive models were constructed and tested using a 4-step process using Oracle's Data Miner with custom pre-processing programs written in PL/SQL. Each step is described below.

- **Cleanse Data:** Notes associated with customer accounts were randomly sampled to determine the quality of notes. This information was used to

Figure 1. Graph showing the distribution of the number of notes on customer accounts. The solid line represents accounts with an active status, whereas the dashed line represents accounts with a cancelled status.

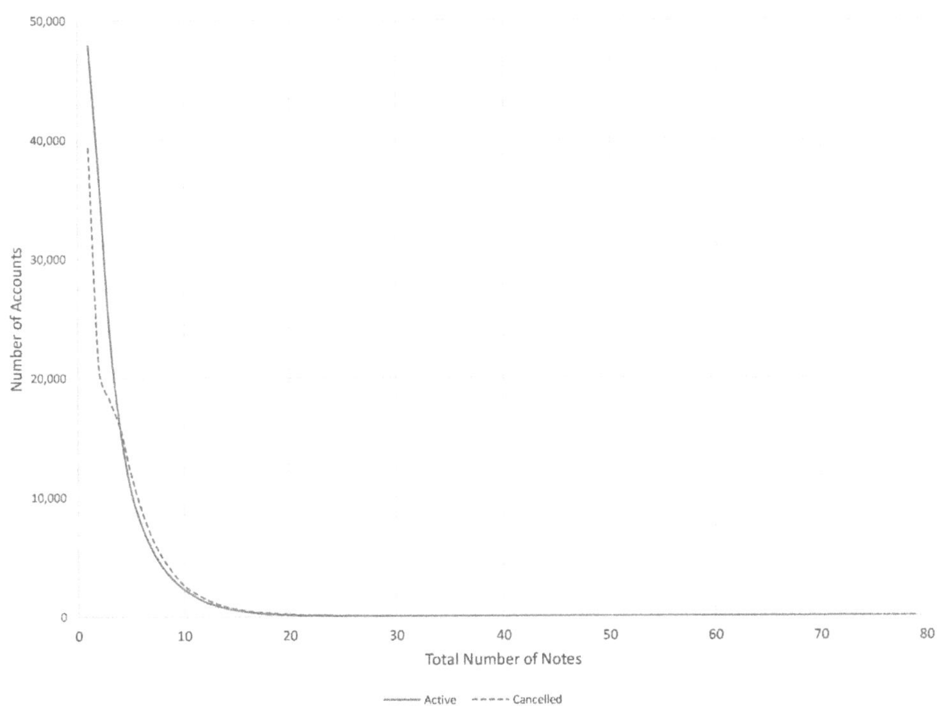

identify the types of data cleansing steps that were needed to pre-process the data. Particular attention was placed on: identifying the structure of notes; determining the frequency of redacted portions of text; determining the extent and use of symbols, abbreviations, misspellings, and other non-language textual representations. Results of these data analyses were used to create data cleansing routines which were run on all note fields.

The notes data are noisy because of non-standard customer representative abbreviations and numerous misspellings. No attempts were made to correct spelling or to decode abbreviations. The cleansing process consisted of removing non-language textual representations and structuring notes so that they had a similar format. Structuring of the notes included removing symbols and repeated characters that were included in the notes as a means of highlighting or separating topics, and removing all redacted text (often represented using repeating upper case characters).

- **Prepare Notes:** Cleansed notes were transformed using NMF. Notes were prepared in one of two ways. Method 1, each note was treated as a separate document. Method 2, all notes for a given account were combined to form a single note, essentially create a bag-of-words for each account. Transforms for both themes and tokens were examined. A theme is the identification of higher-level conceptual categories to which words are mapped, whereas tokens are simpler representations of strings of characters (typically words). A limit was placed on each document to identify 50 or fewer tokens/themes for describing each document, with a constraint of 10,000 or fewer tokens/themes for the entire corpus. Models were constructed and tested with and without the use of stoplists[1]. The NMF transformation was applied to reduce the dimensionality and noise associated with the data.
- **Sample Data:** Cleansed data were sampled to create training and testing datasets that contained 5,000 and 20,000 accounts respectively. The data were randomly sampled from the available 301K records with notes selecting those accounts without reactivations presents (a reactivation is a case where a customer cancels and later restarts service). After sampling, the datasets were examined to verify that the active to cancelled status ratios mirrored those in the data pool. All notes recorded on or after the reported cancellation dates were eliminated because in many cases the word "cancel" or similar words were used in the notes; this step was taken to prevent from creating biased models. The final number of records available for sampling was 195K. For the models using the separate notes there were 30,748 notes in the modeling set and 124,326 notes in the testing set.

- **Train and Test Models:** Two sets of models were trained and tested. Each set of models was comprised on three classifiers, the algorithms used were: were decision trees, support vector machine, and naïve bays. The first set of models used data from individual note entries on each given account. These model runs were referred to as using *separate* data. The second set of models used the data in a recast format where all notes on each customer's account were aggregated into a single note, in addition the total number of notes and the average number of days between notes was added to the resulting note. These model runs were referred to as using *aggregated* data. Other attributes were tested to determine if additional attributes should be included in the model to improve the predictive accuracy. Since the zip code information was available, median zip code income information from the Census 2010 data was merged to obtain the better predictive accuracy for the models.

Using the training dataset, models were developed to predict individual customer's probability of churning. The test dataset was used to evaluate the generalizability of the developed models. See Figure 2.

Model evaluation consisted of comparing each model with the other developed models.

The six churn models were developed and compared to each other. See Table 1 below for a listing of attributes used in the models. The first set of experiments (structured model) examined the predictive power of structured data for predicting account status. The second set of experiments (notes derived models) examined the predictive capability of models constructed using transformed free-form notes. Additional information was included in these models: for the separate notes a note sequence identifier was included, for the aggregated notes the average number of days between notes and the number of notes were included. The third set of experiments examined the benefits of combining both structured and semi-structured data in models when predicting account status.

Settings were tested to find which parameters were best for the notes data. Term frequency was used where each term was counted and inversely weighted according to the frequency with which it appeared across documents in the corpus.

The Status Label is the target variable for predicting (active or cancelled); Transformed Notes are free-form customer service notes after using the NMF transformation. Transformed Composite Notes were formed by aggregating all notes on an account into a single note and then applying the NMF transformation.

Figure 2. Graphical depiction of the model development and testing process

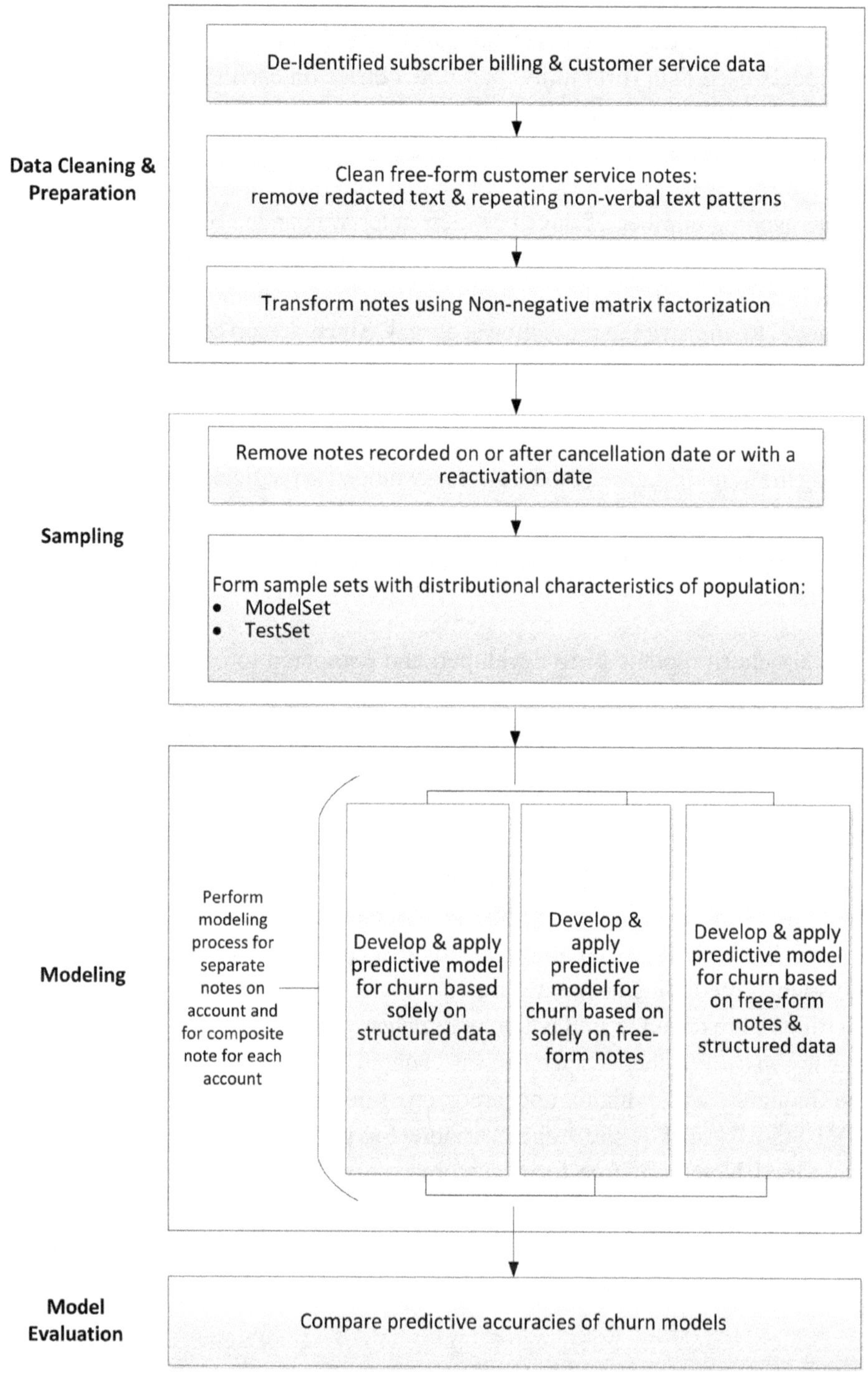

Table 1. Listing of attributes used in the modeling experiments

<table>
<tr><th>Data Used in Classifier</th><th>Structuring of Notes</th><th>Data Fields Included</th></tr>
<tr><td rowspan="2">structured</td><td>separate</td><td>average balance
average income
note sequence no.
note type
status label</td></tr>
<tr><td>aggregated</td><td>average balance
average income
note type
average days between notes
number of notes on account
status label</td></tr>
<tr><td rowspan="2">notes</td><td>separate</td><td>transformed notes
notes sequence no.
status label</td></tr>
<tr><td>aggregated</td><td>transformed composite note
average days between notes
number of notes on account
status label</td></tr>
<tr><td rowspan="2">structured + notes</td><td>separate</td><td>average balance
average income
transformed notes
notes sequence no.
note type
status label</td></tr>
<tr><td>aggregated</td><td>average balance
average income
transformed composite note
note type
average days between notes
number of notes on account
status label</td></tr>
</table>

RESULTS

For the experiments three data mining classifiers were applied to develop the models: support vector machine (SVM), decision tree, and Naïve Bayes. Table 2 presents the predictive confidence[2], precision, recall, F1, accuracy measures, and area under the receiver operating characteristic (ROC) curve for each experiment performed using each of the classifiers.[3]

F1, which is the harmonic average of precision and recall, indicates that the Naïve Bayes classifier using free-form notes yielded the highest predictive accuracy of all the experiments. In an ideal predictive model the area under the ROC curve would be 1.0. The area under the ROC curve obtained with the Support Vector

Table 2. Data mining metrics for the various decision tree classifiers

Algorithm	Data	Notes Structure	Predictive Confidence %	Area Under Curve	Max Overall Accuracy %	Max Average Accuracy %	Model Accuracy %	Precision	Recall	F1
Support Vector Machine	structured	separate	19.9	0.64	61	60	60	0.620	0.540	0.577
		aggregated	19.1	0.65	64	61	57	0.721	0.475	0.573
	notes	separate	23.4	0.66	62	62	62	0.619	0.644	0.631
		aggregated	36.7	0.75	71	69	69	0.766	0.694	0.729
	structured + notes	separate	33.9	0.73	67	67	67	0.687	0.642	0.664
		aggregated	41.0	0.78	73	71	71	0.786	0.707	0.744
Decision Tree	structured	separate	32.8	0.71	67	67	66	0.683	0.632	0.656
		aggregated	26.3	0.71	68	64	68	0.818	0.399	0.537
	notes	separate	18.2	0.61	59	59	59	0.591	0.643	0.616
		aggregated	16.1	0.60	62	58	58	0.684	0.557	0.614
	structured + notes	separate	32.8	0.71	67	67	66	0.683	0.632	0.656
		aggregated	26.3	0.71	68	64	68	0.818	0.399	0.537
Naïve Bayes	structured	separate	32.8	0.73	67	67	66	0.675	0.673	0.674
		aggregated	30.1	0.71	67	65	65	0.748	0.629	0.683
	notes	separate	25.2	0.67	63	63	63	0.688	0.617	0.651
		aggregated	36.9	0.75	71	69	69	0.768	0.689	0.727
	structured + notes	separate	34.4	0.73	67	67	67	0.636	0.619	0.627
		aggregated	38.1	0.76	71	69	69	0.774	0.694	0.732

Machine classifier for the aggregate notes model reached 0.78, the highest for all of the tested classifiers.

Figures 3 through 5 show the ROC curves for the experiments conducted with the models using the various classifiers. The ROC curve shows the tradeoff between correct classifications (true positives) obtained as the threshold for incorrect classifications (false positives) is varied. In the figures below, the ROC curves show performance of the classification models for the three classifiers when active and cancelled statuses are considered for both separate and aggregate notes.

Figure 2 shows that the decision tree predictive models does not perform well with notes. Figures 3 and 4 show that notes and structured data when incorporated in churn models developed based on Naïve Bayes or SVM classifiers yielded results that were better than those obtained using solely structured data. In conclusion, these experiments reveal that incorporating notes information improves the overall accuracy of classifiers. Moreover, aggregating the notes improves the performance further. Thus, notes can be mined in EHR applications to improve churn prediction.

Figure 3. ROC curve for a decision tree model predicting accounts canceling service

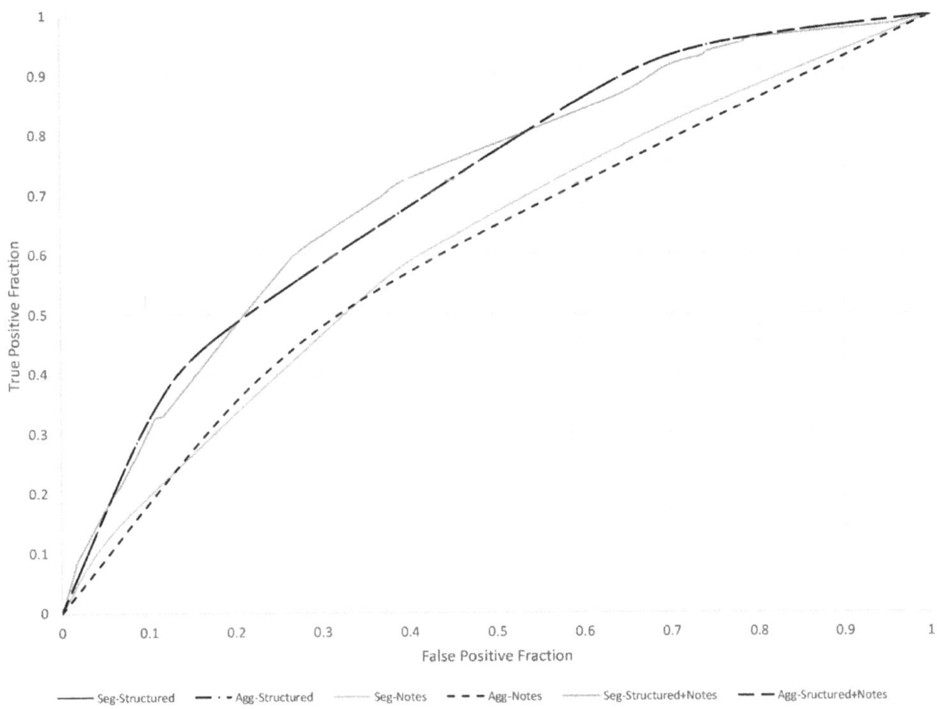

DISCUSSION AND CONCLUSION

The experiments conducted using the decision tree, support vector machine, and Naïve Bayes classifiers to test the usefulness of free-form notes in predicting service recipient (patients or customers) churn demonstrated that notes data does add value to churn models. With the exception of the decision tree algorithm, all models performed well for predicting churn. The best performing classifier was SVM, where free-form notes increased classifier accuracy (i.e., churn prediction) up to 11% over models without free-form text.

In a prior paper (Ramsey & Bapna, 2014) experiments were conducted using accounts sampled with reactivations present. In contrast, in this paper, only records without reactivations were analyzed thereby leading to a reduction in the dataset size which led to the prediction problem becoming harder, leading to the decreased performance for the repeated experiments.

In a healthcare context, predicting cancelled status is beneficial, because predicted cancelled accounts indicate that a patient will be either leaving a nursing unit or a health clinic. When patients are leaving nursing units the workload of nursing staff

Figure 4. ROC curve for a Naïve Bayes model predicting accounts canceling service

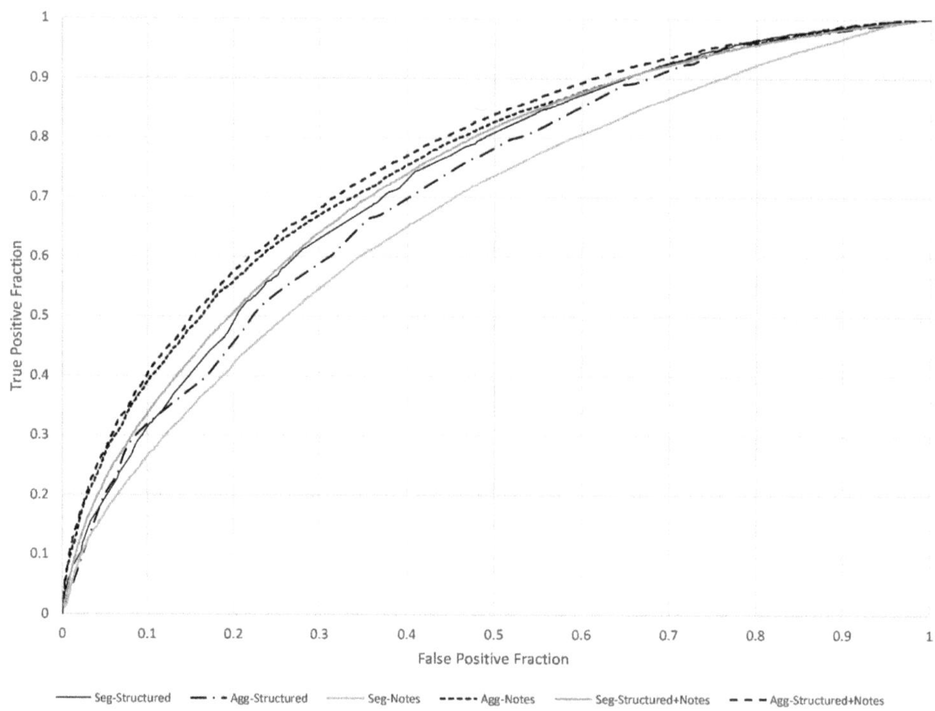

increases as they must attend to discharge orders, arrange to have rooms prepared for new patients, and orient new patients. The ability to automatically cull EHR notes to predict patient turnover can help administrators make better workforce plans. Better workforce planning and patient discharge planning lead to increased staff satisfaction, fewer adverse events, and opportunities for better planned patient handoffs.

If health clinics are able to more accurately identify customers that are likely to churn then they can take preemptive action to prevent losing the patient or to facilitate a transfer of the patient to a new clinic. Incorporating free-form text in models for churn can help health clinics better target patients that are worth engaging to prevent churn. By taking action with patients predicted to transition to a cancelled status, health clinic personnel can reduce patients who could otherwise enter a "lost to follow up" status. Additionally, for patients with communicable diseases, such as HIV/AIDS, the ability to predict who is about to enter a cancelled status allows health workers to take action to prevent them from reaching that status, thus helping with public health disease management.

Figure 5. ROC curve for a support vector machine model predicting accounts canceling service

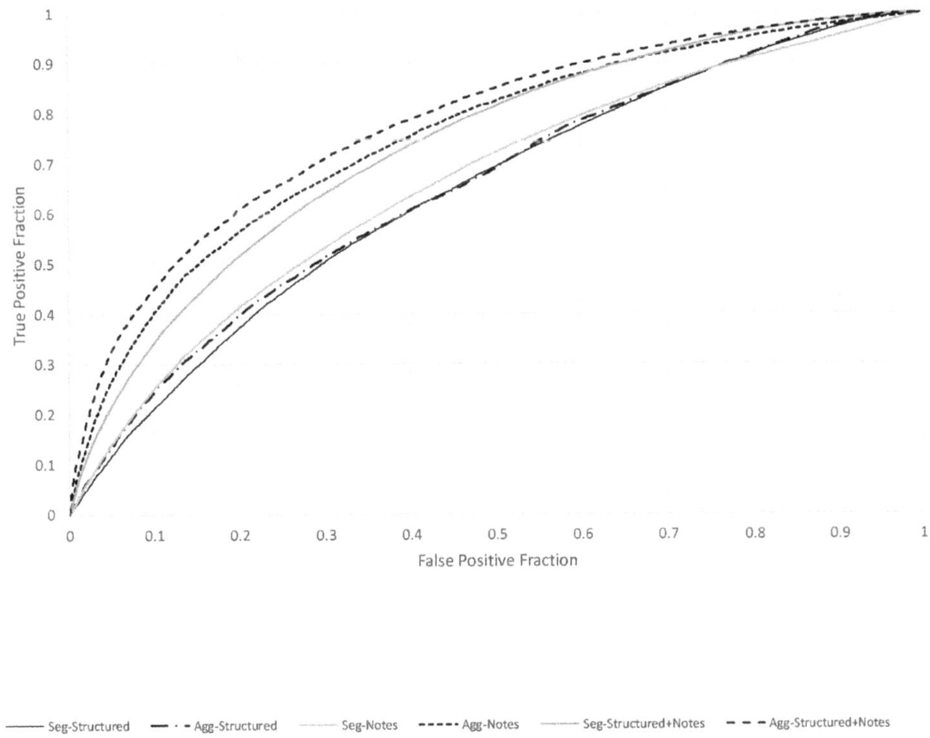

LIMITATIONS

A limitation with this study is customer service notes were used as opposed to actual patient notes from an EHR. In a future study when de-identified patient data are available, the experiments performed in this paper will be repeated to determine if the findings and conclusions reached in this paper continue to hold.

ACKNOWLEDGMENT

The authors thank the Wharton Customer Analytics Initiative (WCAI) for providing access to the data and subject matter experts needed to complete this study.

REFERENCES

Applebaum, A. (2001). The constant customer. *Gallup Management Journal*, *17*, 1–5.

Berg, M. (2001). Implementing information systems in health care organizations: Myths and challenges. *International Journal of Medical Informatics*, *64*(2), 143–156. doi:10.1016/S1386-5056(01)00200-3 PMID:11734382

Burez, J., & Van den Poel, D. (2009). Handling class imbalance in customer churn prediction. *Expert Systems with Applications*, *36*(3), 4626–4636. doi:10.1016/j.eswa.2008.05.027

Chowdhury, G. G. (2003). Natural language processing. *Annual Review of Information Science & Technology*, *37*(1), 51–89. doi:10.1002/aris.1440370103

Cohen, R., Aviram, I., Elhadad, M., & Elhadad, N. (2014). Redundancy-aware topic modeling for patient record notes. *PLoS One*, *9*(2), e87555. doi:10.1371/journal.pone.0087555 PMID:24551060

Coussement, K., Lessmann, S., & Verstraeten, G. (2017). A comparative analysis of data preparation algorithms for customer churn prediction: A case study in the telecommunication industry. *Decision Support Systems*, *95*, 27–36. doi:10.1016/j.dss.2016.11.007

Coussement, K., & Van den Poel, D. (2008). Churn prediction in subscription services: An application of support vector machines while comparing two parameter-selection techniques. *Expert Systems with Applications*, *34*(1), 313–327. doi:10.1016/j.eswa.2006.09.038

Dechant, A., Spann, M., & Becker, J. U. (2018). Positive Customer Churn: An Application to Online Dating. *Journal of Service Research.*

Duffield, C., Diers, D., Aisbett, C., & Roche, M. (2009). Churn: Patient turnover and case mix. *Nursing Economics*, *27*(3), 185. PMID:19558079

Duffield, C., Diers, D., O'Brien-Pallas, L., Aisbett, C., Roche, M., King, M., & Aisbett, K. (2011). Nursing staffing, nursing workload, the work environment and patient outcomes. *Applied Nursing Research*, *24*(4), 244–255. doi:10.1016/j.apnr.2009.12.004 PMID:20974086

Duffield, C., Roche, M., Diers, D., Catling-Paull, C., & Blay, N. (2010). Staffing, skill mix and the model of care. *Journal of Clinical Nursing*, *19*(15-16), 2242–2251. doi:10.1111/j.1365-2702.2010.03225.x PMID:20659202

Duffield, C. M., Roche, M. A., Dimitrelis, S., Homer, C., & Buchan, J. (2015). Instability in patient and nurse characteristics, unit complexity and patient and system outcomes. *Journal of Advanced Nursing*, *71*(6), 1288–1298. doi:10.1111/jan.12597 PMID:25511970

Fogel, P., Young, S. S., Hawkins, D. M., & Ledirac, N. (2007). Inferential, robust non-negative matrix factorization analysis of microarray data. *Bioinformatics (Oxford, England)*, *23*(1), 44–49. doi:10.1093/bioinformatics/btl550 PMID:17092989

Gill, M., & Krentz, H. (2009). Unappreciated epidemiology: The churn effect in a regional HIV care programme. *International Journal of STD & AIDS*, *20*(8), 540–544. doi:10.1258/ijsa.2008.008422 PMID:19625584

Grover, V., & Davenport, T. H. (2001). General perspectives on knowledge management: Fostering a research agenda. *Journal of Management Information Systems*, *18*(1), 5–22. doi:10.1080/07421222.2001.11045672

Gupta, V., & Lehal, G. S. (2009). A survey of text mining techniques and applications. *Journal of Emerging Technologies in Web Intelligence*, *1*(1), 60–76. doi:10.4304/jetwi.1.1.60-76

Gustafsson, A., Johnson, M. D., & Roos, I. (2005). The effects of customer satisfaction, relationship commitment dimensions, and triggers on customer retention. *Journal of Marketing*, *69*(4), 210–218. doi:10.1509/jmkg.2005.69.4.210

Hadden, J., Tiwari, A., Roy, R., & Ruta, D. (2006). Churn prediction using complaints data. *Paper presented at the Proceedings Of World Academy Of Science, Engineering and Technology.*

Hadden, J., Tiwari, A., Roy, R., & Ruta, D. (2006). Churn prediction: Does technology matter. *International Journal of Intelligent Technology*, *1*(1), 104–110.

Hadden, J., Tiwari, A., Roy, R., & Ruta, D. (2007). Computer assisted customer churn management: State-of-the-art and future trends. *Computers & Operations Research*, *34*(10), 2902–2917. doi:10.1016/j.cor.2005.11.007

Ikonomakis, M., Kotsiantis, S., & Tampakas, V. (2005). Text classification using machine learning techniques. *WSEAS Transactions on Computers*, *4*(8), 966–974.

Jahromi, A. T., Stakhovych, S., & Ewing, M. (2014). Managing B2B customer churn, retention and profitability. *Industrial Marketing Management*, *43*(7), 1258–1268. doi:10.1016/j.indmarman.2014.06.016

Jiayin, Q., Yangming, Z., Yingying, Z., & Shuang, S. (2006, December 12-15). TreeLogit Model for Customer Churn Prediction. *Paper presented at the IEEE Asia-Pacific Conference on Services Computing APSCC '06.*

Joachims, T. (1999). Transductive inference for text classification using support vector machines. *Paper presented at the machine learning-international workshop then conference.*

Johnes, M., Mothersbaugh, D. L., & Betty, S. E. (2000). Switching barriers and repurchase intentions in service. *Journal of Retailing*, *76*(2), 259–274. doi:10.1016/S0022-4359(00)00024-5

Kontio, E., Airola, A., Pahikkala, T., Lundgren-Laine, H., Junttila, K., Korvenranta, H., ... Salanterä, S. (2014). Predicting patient acuity from electronic patient records. *Journal of Biomedical Informatics*, *51*, 35–40. doi:10.1016/j.jbi.2014.04.001 PMID:24726853

Lee, D. D., & Seung, H. (1999). Learning the parts of objects by non-negative matrix factorization. *Nature*, *401*(6755), 788–791. doi:10.1038/44565 PMID:10548103

Lemmens, A., & Croux, C. (2006). Bagging and boosting classification trees to predict churn. *JMR, Journal of Marketing Research*, *43*(2), 276–286. doi:10.1509/jmkr.43.2.276

Lemmens, A., & Gupta, S. (2017). *Managing churn to maximize profits*. Cambridge, MA: Harvard Business School. doi:10.2139srn.2964906

Li, Y., Algarni, A., Albathan, M., Shen, Y., & Bijaksana, M. A. (2015). Relevance feature discovery for text mining. *IEEE Transactions on Knowledge and Data Engineering*, *27*(6), 1656–1669. doi:10.1109/TKDE.2014.2373357

Lima, E., Mues, C., & Baesens, B. (2009). Domain knowledge integration in data mining using decision tables: Case studies in churn prediction. *The Journal of the Operational Research Society*, *60*(8), 1096–1106. doi:10.1057/jors.2008.161

Lin, C.-S., Tzeng, G.-H., & Chin, Y.-C. (2011). Combined rough set theory and flow network graph to predict customer churn in credit card accounts. *Expert Systems with Applications*, *38*(1), 8–15. doi:10.1016/j.eswa.2010.05.039

Liu, B. (2010). Sentiment analysis and subjectivity. In Handbook of Natural Language Processing (pp. 627-666).

Lu, N., Lin, H., Lu, J., & Zhang, G. (2014). A customer churn prediction model in telecom industry using boosting. *IEEE Transactions on Industrial Informatics*, *10*(2), 1659–1665. doi:10.1109/TII.2012.2224355

Madden, G., Savage, S. J., & Coble-Neal, G. (1999). Subscriber churn in the Australian ISP market. *Information Economics and Policy*, *11*(2), 195–207. doi:10.1016/S0167-6245(99)00015-3

Miettinen, M., & Korhonen, M. (2008, June 17-19). Information Quality in Healthcare: Coherence of Data Compared between Organization's Electronic Patient Records. *Paper presented at the 21st IEEE International Symposium on Computer-Based Medical Systems CBMS '08.*

Miguéis, V. L., Van den Poel, D., Camanho, A. S., & Cunha, J. F. (2012). Modeling partial customer churn: On the value of first product-category purchase sequences. *Expert Systems with Applications*, *39*(12), 11250–11256. doi:10.1016/j.eswa.2012.03.073

Milošević, M., Živić, N., & Andjelković, I. (2017). Early churn prediction with personalized targeting in mobile social games. *Expert Systems with Applications*, *83*, 326–332. doi:10.1016/j.eswa.2017.04.056

Morid, M. A., Sheng, O. R., & Abdelrahman, S. (2017). Leveraging Time Series Data in Similarity Based Healthcare Predictive Models: The Case of Early ICU Mortality Prediction. Retrieved from https://arxiv.org/ftp/arxiv/papers/1704/1704.07499.pdf

Murphy, D. R., Laxmisan, A., Reis, B. A., Thomas, E. J., Esquivel, A., Forjuoh, S. N., ... & Singh, H. (2013). Electronic health record-based triggers to detect potential delays in cancer diagnosis. *BMJ Qual Saf.*

Mutanen, T., Ahola, J., & Nousiainen, S. (2006). Customer churn prediction-a case study in retail banking. *Practical Data Mining: Applications, Experiences and Challenges, 13.*

Nassirtoussi, A. K., Aghabozorgi, S., Wah, T. Y., & Ngo, D. C. L. (2014). Text mining for market prediction: A systematic review. *Expert Systems with Applications*, *41*(16), 7653–7670. doi:10.1016/j.eswa.2014.06.009

Needleman, J., Buerhaus, P., Mattke, S., Stewart, M., & Zelevinsky, K. (2002). Nurse-staffing levels and the quality of care in hospitals. *The New England Journal of Medicine*, *346*(22), 1715–1722. doi:10.1056/NEJMsa012247 PMID:12037152

Needleman, J., Buerhaus, P., Pankratz, V. S., Leibson, C. L., Stevens, S. R., & Harris, M. (2011). Nurse staffing and inpatient hospital mortality. *The New England Journal of Medicine*, *364*(11), 1037–1045. doi:10.1056/NEJMsa1001025 PMID:21410372

Needleman, J., Buerhaus, P. I., Stewart, M., Zelevinsky, K., & Mattke, S. (2006). Nurse staffing in hospitals: Is there a business case for quality? *Health Affairs*, *25*(1), 204–211. doi:10.1377/hlthaff.25.1.204 PMID:16403755

Negash, S. (2004). Business Intelligence. *Communications of the Association for Information Systems*, *13*, 177–195. doi:10.17705/1CAIS.01315

Neslin, S., Gupta, S., Kamakura, W., Lu, J., & Mason, C. (2006). Defection detection: Measuring and understanding the predictive accuracy of customer churn models. *JMR, Journal of Marketing Research*, *XLIII*(May), 204–211. doi:10.1509/jmkr.43.2.204

Ngai, E. W., Xiu, L., & Chau, D. (2009). Application of data mining techniques in customer relationship management: A literature review and classification. *Expert Systems with Applications*, *36*(2), 2592–2602. doi:10.1016/j.eswa.2008.02.021

Nigam, K., McCallum, A. K., Thrun, S., & Mitchell, T. (2000). Text classification from labeled and unlabeled documents using EM. *Machine Learning*, *39*(2), 103–134. doi:10.1023/A:1007692713085

Pang, B., & Lee, L. (2008). Opinion Mining and Sentiment Analysis. *Foundations and Trends in Information Retrieval*, *2*(1-2), 1–135.

Park, D.-H., Lee, J., & Han, I. (2007). The effect of on-line consumer reviews on consumer purchasing intention: The moderating role of involvement. *International Journal of Electronic Commerce*, *11*(4), 125–148. doi:10.2753/JEC1086-4415110405

Park, S. H., Blegen, M. A., Spetz, J., Chapman, S. A., & De Groot, H. (2012). Patient turnover and the relationship between nurse staffing and patient outcomes. *Research in Nursing & Health*, *35*(3), 277–288. doi:10.1002/nur.21474 PMID:22457013

Peers, P., & Dutre, P. (2006). *Update Rules for a Weighted Non-negative FH*G Factorization*. Heverlee, Belgium: Katholieke Universiteit Leuven.

Pendharkar, P. C. (2009). Genetic algorithm based neural network approaches for predicting churn in cellular wireless network services. *Expert Systems with Applications*, *36*(3, Part 2), 6714–6720. doi:10.1016/j.eswa.2008.08.050

Pletscher-Frankild, S., Palleja, A., Tsafou, K., Binder, J. X., & Jensen, L. J. (2015). Diseases: Text mining and data integration of disease–gene associations. *Methods (San Diego, Calif.)*, *74*, 83–89. doi:10.1016/j.ymeth.2014.11.020 PMID:25484339

Ramsey, G. W., & Bapna, S. (2014). A Technique to Exploit Free-Form Notes to Predict Customer Churn. *International Journal of Computational Models and Algorithms in Medicine*, *4*(1), 1–16. doi:10.4018/ijcmam.2014010101

Reichheld, F. F., Teal, T., & Smith, D. K. (1996). The loyalty effect: Vol. 1. *No. 3* (pp. 78–84). Boston, MA: Harvard Business School Press.

Richter, Y., Yom-Tov, E., & Slonim, N. (2010, April). Predicting customer churn in mobile networks through analysis of social groups. In *Proceedings of the 2010 SIAM international conference on data mining* (pp. 732-741). Society for Industrial and Applied Mathematics. 10.1137/1.9781611972801.64

Roumani, Y. F., May, J. H., Strum, D. P., & Vargas, L. G. (2013). Classifying highly imbalanced ICU data. *Health Care Management Science*, *16*(2), 119–128. doi:10.100710729-012-9216-9 PMID:23132123

Saha, A., & Sindhwani, V. (2012). Learning evolving and emerging topics in social media: A dynamic NMF approach with temporal regularization. *Paper presented at the Proceedings of the 5th International Conference on Web Search and Data Mining (WSDM)*. 10.1145/2124295.2124376

Schaffer, S. K., Messner, D., Mestre-Ferrandiz, J., Tambor, E., & Towse, A. (2018). Paying for Cures: Perspectives on Solutions to the "Affordability Issue." *Value in Health*, *21*(3), 276–279. doi:10.1016/j.jval.2017.12.013 PMID:29566833

Shahnaz, F., Berry, M. W., Pauca, V. P., & Plemmons, R. J. (2006). Document clustering using nonnegative matrix factorization. *Information Processing & Management*, *42*(2), 373–386. doi:10.1016/j.ipm.2004.11.005

Srinivas, K., Rani, B. K., & Govrdhan, A. (2010). Applications of Data Mining Techniques in Healthcare and Prediction of Heart Attacks. *International Journal on Computer Science and Engineering*, *2*(02), 250–255.

Sun, W., Rumshisky, A., & Uzuner, O. (2013). Evaluating temporal relations in clinical text: 2012 i2b2 challenge. *Journal of the American Medical Informatics Association*, *20*(5), 806–813. doi:10.1136/amiajnl-2013-001628 PMID:23564629

Tang, B., Shepherd, M., Milios, E., & Heywood, M. I. (2008). Comparing and combining dimension reduction techniques for efficient text clustering.

Tang, Z., Wang, S., Zhang, X., Wei, W., & Zhao, Y. (2011). Lexicographical framework for image hashing with implementation based on DCT and NMF. *Multimedia Tools and Applications*, *52*(2-3), 325–345. doi:10.100711042-009-0437-y

Tuzhilin, A. (2012). Customer relationship management and Web mining: The next frontier. *Data Mining and Knowledge Discovery*, 1–29.

Underhill, D. G. (2007). Exploring Dimensionality Reduction for Text Mining: DTIC Document.

Unruh, L. Y., & Fottler, M. D. (2006). Patient turnover and nursing staff adequacy. *Health Services Research*, *41*(2), 599–612. doi:10.1111/j.1475-6773.2005.00496.x PMID:16584467

Vafeiadis, T., Diamantaras, K. I., Sarigiannidis, G., & Chatzisavvas, K. C. (2015). A comparison of machine learning techniques for customer churn prediction. *Simulation Modelling Practice and Theory*, *55*, 1–9. doi:10.1016/j.simpat.2015.03.003

VanFosson, C. A., Yoder, L. H., & Jones, T. L. (2017). Patient turnover: A concept analysis. *Advances in Nursing Science*, *40*(3), 300–312. doi:10.1097/ANS.0000000000000171 PMID:28266962

Verbeke, W., Martens, D., Mues, C., & Baesens, B. (2011). Building comprehensible customer churn prediction models with advanced rule induction techniques. *Expert Systems with Applications*, *38*(3), 2354–2364. doi:10.1016/j.eswa.2010.08.023

Xie, Y., & Li, X. (2008). Churn prediction with Linear Discriminant Boosting algorithm. *Paper presented at the 2008 International Conference on Machine Learning and Cybernetics*.

ENDNOTES

1 A stoplist is a set of words that are excluded from text processing either because they do not add useful information or because they confuse the meaning of other words.

2 Predictive confidence is a measure of improvement in predictions compared to the performance of a naïve model that predicts the dominant target value

3 Precision is Tp/(Tp + Fp); Recall is Tp/(Tp + Fn); F1 is (2*Precision*Recall)/(Precision + Recall), and; Accuracy = (Tp + Tn) / (Tn + Tp + Fp + Fn). Key: Tp – true positives (i.e., a correct cancellation prediction), Tn – true negative (i.e., a correct non-cancellation prediction), Fp – false positive (i.e., incorrect cancellation prediction), Fn – false negative.

Chapter 7
Exploring Diseases Relationships:
An Ontology-Based Spreading Activation Approach

Said Fathalla
Alexandria University, Egypt & Bonn University, Germany

Heba Mohamed
Alexandria University, Egypt & Bonn University, Germany

Yaman Kannot
Arab Academy for Science, Technology, and Maritime Transport, Egypt

ABSTRACT

Developing an efficient algorithm for traversing large ontologies is a key challenge for many semantic-based applications. This chapter introduces an approach, spreading activation over ontology (SAOO), to explore the relationship between two human diseases using an ontology-based spreading activation approach. SAOO comprises two phases: semantic matching and diseases relatedness detection. In the semantic matching phase, user-submitted diseases are semantically identified in the ontology graph using the proposed matching algorithm. Semantic matching conducts more analysis in the matching process, which comprises term normalization; phrase analysis, and word sense disambiguation. In the diseases relatedness detection phase, the URIs of these diseases are passed to the relatedness detector to detect the relationship connecting them. SAOO improves healthcare systems by considering semantic domain knowledge and a set of SWRL rules to infer diseases relatedness. We present a use case that outlines how SAOO can be used to explore relationships between vaccines in the vaccine ontology.

DOI: 10.4018/978-1-5225-8244-1.ch007

INTRODUCTION

In the era of extraordinary large-scale data analysis empowered by the vast amount of biological information produced every day, biomedical research plays a key role. Therefore, there is a great demand to explore effective methods for biomedical data integration and knowledge management (Goble & Stevens, 2008). The semantic web gives the meaning of knowledge making software systems perform intelligent tasks instead of users (Berners-Lee, Hendler, & Lassila, 2001) using a semantic knowledgebase called Ontology. The ontology is a repository in which information is organized and used in semantic-based applications in order to support reasoning process such as detecting inconsistencies, identifying subsumption relationships, and instance classification (Said Fathalla and Christoph Lange, 2018a; Shadbolt, Hall, & Berners-Lee, 2006). Developing an efficient algorithm for traversing large ontologies is a key challenge for many semantic-based systems. This chapter introduces an ontology-based spreading activation approach, called SAOO (Spreading Activation over Ontology), in order to explore the relationship between two human diseases, i.e., the relatedness. If a relationship exists, the set of diseases connecting them is provided. For instance, is there a relation between "*Pedophilia*" and "*Voyeurism*"? If so, what is the relatedness? An interesting feature of finding relations between diseases is the treatment of the real cause of a disease, which might be because of the existence of another disease (Fathalla & Kannot, 2017a). For instance, Gallstones disease, bile forms solid particles (stones) in the gallbladder, might be caused by "*Hemolytic Anemia*" disease so crushing gallstones is not a solution or treatment because the stones will develop again (Trotman, Bernstein, Bove, & Wirth, 1980). Therefore, the objectives of detecting the relatedness between diseases are:

- **Causality:** Possibly, the existence of disease might result in another disease to occur. For example, *Hereditary Spherocytosis* diseases are an autosomal preponderant anomaly of erythrocytes that causes gallstones. *Pigmented* gallstones occur in approximately half of the untreated patients,
- **Complications of Diseases:** A disease can increase the complications of another disease, e.g., Diabetes and HCV hepatitis,
- **Treatments Prescription:** A treatment prescription for a disease can change when there is a relationship between this disease and another one, e.g., HCV hepatitis and hypertension.

The methodology of the proposed approach is divided into two phases: semantic matching and diseases relatedness detection. In the semantic matching phase, user-submitted diseases are semantically identified in the ontology graph using the proposed matching algorithm. In the diseases relatedness detection phase, the URIs of these diseases are passed to the relatedness detector which in turn detects the relationship using the bidirectional spreading activation algorithm on the disease ontology and returns the set of diseases connecting them. The idea behind the use of bidirectional search is to find a path starting from the source node, i.e., the first disease, and the goal node, i.e., the second disease until an intersection occurs. In other words, it runs two simultaneous searches: forward from one node and backward from the other. When the two search frontiers meet, the algorithm will reconstruct a path, represent the set of diseases connect them. The knowledge base here is the disease ontology and Semantic Web Rule Language (SWRL) rules. In order to support the inference process, a set of SWRL rules is defined. From these rules, new relationships could be discovered from instance data, which did not explicitly exist in the ontology. Usage of SWRL rules extends the expressivity of OWL semantics (Tsarkov, Riazanov, Bechhofer, & Horrocks, 2004).

The rest of this chapter is organized as follows. Section 2 introduces broad definitions and discussions of the topic of this study. Section 3 presents a review of the literature. Section 4 provides a brief description of the disease ontology. Section 5 presents the architecture of the proposed approach. Section 6 illustrates the methodology of the SAOO by showing a case study. Section 7 outlines a use case for the usage of SAOO. Section 8 introduces future work directions. Finally, Section 9 presents the conclusions.

BACKGROUND

In this section, broad definitions and discussions of the topic of this study are provided, which are needed to understand this chapter. Starting by giving definitions of some terms related to ontology, then providing a description of how spreading activation works.

Usually, computers were used to perform tasks with none sort of intelligence or semantics thus there is a necessity to make computers as intelligent as human (Antoniou & Harmelen, 2004). The defect of non-Semantic applications is painted by the statement "lack of semantics" particularly when the talk is concerning information retrieval. Semantic Web technologies, the extension of the World Wide Web through standards by the World Wide Web Consortium (W3C), provide a set of standards to facilitate the representation, publication, linking, and querying of heterogeneous data available in the web (Shadbolt et al., 2006). In particular, the Resource Description Framework (RDF) (Hayes, 2004) enables triple-based assertions of named properties, RDF Schema (RDFS) (W3C, 2014), the extension of RDF, provides a data-modeling vocabulary for RDF data, and the Web Ontology Language (OWL) (Hitzler, Parsia, Patel-schneider, & Rudolph, 2009) represent rich and complex knowledge about things, including restrictions to classes and properties. The goal of the semantic web is to extend the automation in processing web-based data and to enhance the interoperability of web-based information systems (Payne & Lassila, 2004).

Biomedical Ontologies

Beyond the name, ontology is concerning with providing the definition of entities and the relations among them in a specific domain, i.e. effective knowledge modeling. The main purpose of developing ontology is to use it as a semantic knowledge base representation for identifying concepts in a specific domain and discover concepts semantics and the relationships between them (Fathalla & Kannot, 2017b). Ontologies can be used beneficially in semantic-based systems in various communities within computer science, such as information retrieval (Fathalla, Hassan, & El-Sayed, 2012; Oberle, 2014), scholarly communication (Fathalla, Vahdati, Auer, & Lange, 2017; Said Fathalla and Christoph Lange, 2018b), healthcare (Feigenbaum, Herman, Hongsermeier, Neumann, & Stephens, 2007) and bioinformatics (Fathalla, 2018). Ontologies do not provide shareable and reusable knowledge only, but also add new knowledge to the domain. Below a group of definitions that are used as a basis for the mathematical formulation of the term ontology and its components (Fonseca, Davis, & Câmara, 2003):

Definition 1: (Triple) A term is a triple $\tau = [\eta, \delta, A]$, $\tau \in T$, where η is a string of characters containing the name of the term, δ is a string of characters containing its definition and A is a set of attribute domains $A_1, A_2, \ldots, A_n$, each associated to a value set V_i.

Definition 2: (Relation) A relation φ: $T \rightarrow T$, $\varphi \in \Phi$: is a function from T to T such that for every term $\tau_1 \in T$, there is a term $\tau_1 = \varphi(\tau_1)$, $\tau_2 \in T$.

Definition 3: (Semantic relation) A semantic relation σ between two concepts is one of the relations among the set of semantic relations Σ = {Hypernym, Hyponymy (is-a), Meronomy (i.e., part of), Synonymy}. In linguistics, a hyponym is a word whose semantics is enclosed inside another word which called its hyperonym or its hypernym. In other words, a hyponym has the same *type of* relationship with its hypernym. For instance, dog, cat, and cow are all hyponyms of Mammals (their hypernym); that, in turn, could be a hyponym of animal (Fromkin, V., Rodman, R., & Hyams, 2013).

Definition 4: (Co-hyponyms) Given a concept C, has two hyponyms A and B, then A and B are identified as co-hyponyms.

In the field of health informatics, ontology is used for the representing and organizing medical vocabularies. In the past ten years, there has been a rapid rise in the use of ontologies in the field of bioinformatics (Oberle, 2014). Biomedical ontologies are becoming increasingly popular in the bioinformatics community as the focus of the recent research on analyzing the vast amount of information resulting every day in a semantic form which gives better results rather non-semantic formats, such as tables, text, and XML. These ontologies are used as a controlled vocabulary to annotate entities (i.e., diseases, genes, etc.) in order to discover the interlinking relations. For instance, the Gene Ontology (GO), which has become a *de facto* standard in this domain. In fact, biomedical ontologies play a key role in biomedical research, whereas their success lies in defining vocabularies in a semantic representation enabling getting the intended meaning of them (Hoehndorf, Schofield, & Gkoutos, 2015). In addition, the provision of machine-understandable format that enables reasoning makes it easy to infer new knowledge. As robust, well-formed and standard ontological resources are developed as complex reasoning about the biomedical knowledge we can have. Below are some of the famous medical-related ontologies:

Disease Ontology (DO)[1] is a biomedical resource of standardized common and rare disease concepts with stable identifiers organized by disease etiology. The purpose, enhancement, and statistics of the Disease Ontology (DO) are described in detail in the next section. *Vaccine Ontology* (VO)[2] is a biomedical ontology in the domain of vaccine and vaccination. VO has been developed through collaboration with vaccine researchers and many national and international centers and programs. It aims to represent vaccines data such as vaccines data type, vaccine components ...etc. VO is represented in the Web Ontology Language (OWL) and edited using the Protégé-OWL. In the recent release of 01-04-2018, VO contains 5,926 terms and relationships. VO can be utilized for various applications, e.g., analysis and prediction of protective immune network based on literature mining, and in analyzing clinical vaccines data (He et al., 2009). *The Infectious Disease Ontology* (IDO)[3] is a general scientific classification, terminology, and reasonable representation of entities pertinent to all contagious diseases. IDO ontologies are designed as a set of interoperable ontologies that will together provide coverage of the infectious disease domain. At the core of the set is a general Infectious Disease Ontology (IDO-Core) of entities relevant to both biomedical and clinical aspects of most infectious diseases. IDO-Core is the superior-level ontology that hosts terms of general relevance across the domain, while extension ontologies host terms to a certain part of the domain.

IDO is now applied through disease-specific IDO extensions for the investigation of seven diseases, which are infective endocarditis, dengue fever, influenza, malaria, and other vector-borne diseases, Staphylococcus aureus bacteremia, tuberculosis, and brucellosis. In the latest release of 03-11-2017, IDO contains 518 terms and relationships. *The Ontology for Biomedical Investigations* (OBI)[4] is an integrated ontology for the description of life-science and clinical investigations. OBI is an ontology that supports terms with properly defined characteristics to portray all parts of how investigations in the biological and medical domains are managed. OBI is developed in OWL and to date, OBI has created 2366 classes and 40 relations along with textual and formal definitions (Bandrowski et al., 2016). *The Ontology for General Medical Science* (OGMS)[5] is based on the papers toward an ontological treatment of disease and diagnosis and on carcinomas and other pathological entities. OGMS was previously called the Clinical Phenotype Ontology. OGMS supports definitions for the top-level terms such as disease, entity, sign, symptom, and healthcare process. The number of terms provided in OGMS latest release in 20-09-2011 is 194 term. There are various projects that utilize OGMS ontology, such as Adverse Event Reporting Ontology (AERO)[6], Blood Ontology (BLO)[7], Beta Cell Genomics database[8], etc.

Spreading Activation

In 1975, Collins and Loftus proposed a technique, inspired from psycholinguistics and semantic priming, called Spreading Activation which runs on semantic networks for information retrieval purposes (Collins & Loftus, 1975). The basic idea behind spreading activation is that it runs on a semantic network, which comprises of a set of nodes connected by edges, by activating graph nodes with a certain "activation value" and the activation is spread to the adjacent nodes like an electric current moving through a set of connected wires. The concepts are nodes which have an activation value and the relations between them are represented by edges between these nodes. The initial nodes are activated with a certain value defined by the user and the weight for each edge is set depending on the context model. An activation value is assigned to each node in the graph and then the algorithm spreads to the nodes with the higher activation value. The algorithm runs in a set of iterations, or cycles, and terminates when a stopping condition is reached.

LITERATURE REVIEW

There is a considerable amount of literature on biomedical knowledge management and medical decision making. Biomedical knowledge available on the web is increasing considerably as most of the biomedical research papers are published online. Semantic matching is a technique used to identify information which is semantically matched in structured data. Many diverse solutions of the match have been proposed so far, several examples of individual approaches addressing the matching problem can be found in (Dhamankar, Lee, Doan, Halevy, & Domingos, 2004) and (Do & Rahm, 2002). In their cutting-edge paper of 2004, Kanavos, Theodoridis, & Tsakalidis (2014) proposed a metasearch engine over PubMed[9]. It provides accurate clustering of results according to their specific topic using a biomedical ontology, named MeSH[10] in addition to RxNorm[11] that is a US-specific terminology in medicine that semantically links clinical drugs vocabularies and supports the interoperation between them. Ngo, Cao, & Le (2010) proposed an ontology-based model for semantic annotation and searching using a vector space model. It takes advantage of ontological features of both named entities and WordNet vocabularies and develops a spreading activation algorithm for query expansion. As anticipated, their experiments demonstrate that the proposed model is better than the solely keyword-based model and better than the models using only WordNet or named entities. In addition, it merges various ontologies to improve the semantic search process. De Maio et al. (2011) proposed a project named ODINO which uses a fuzzy knowledge approach for disease diagnosis that supports medical decision making. Medical knowledge is defined according to the physician's expertise and represents relations between medical disease and its symptomatology. ODINO has three main features which are a faceted search of diseases through taxonomy constraints, disease catalog browsing, and preliminary medical diagnosis. Many efforts have been made to represent medical information as a semantic knowledgebase for further processing by semantic applications. Despite the existence of many medical ontologies, one of its important reuse and integration of ontologies is to establish suitable mappings between their concepts. In recent years there has been growing interest in ontology matching and integration (Euzenat, Meilicke, Stuckenschmidt, Shvaiko, & Trojahn, 2011; Shvaiko & Euzenat, 2013, Shvaiko & Euzenat, 2013). Giunchiglia, Yatskevich, & Shvaiko. (2007) surveyed the state of the art of ontology matching and addressed some important challenges for ontology matching. In addition, they analyzed the results of recent ontology matching evaluations.

The rest of this section presents the preliminary research investigating foundational issues in the biomedical ontologies research as well as the development of ontological resources. Hoffman, Arnoldi, & Chuang. (2005) present a curated resource, the Clinical Bioinformatics Ontology (CBO), an ontology for describing genomics concepts, which is reuses existing clinical vocabularies to include molecular diagnostics and cytogenetics concepts. In 2005, the CBO contains 4,069 concepts, associated with 8,463 relationships (Hoffman et al., 2005) and reaches 12,000 concepts in 2015 (Turgeon, 2015). Spasić & Ananiadou. (2005) present a measure of similarity among biomedical terms using the biomedical information retrieved from an ontology. They approximate the edit distance defined as the minimal cost incurred by the changes between two concepts. Many studies have focused on the role played by ontologies in integrating various biomedical resources. Marshall, Su, McDonald, Eggers, & Chen. (2006) proposed a feature decomposition tagger in order to identify key features in extracted relation name strings. Ohno-Machado et al. (2017) presented DataMed, a web service for medical datasets linking, which supports the findability and accessibility of biomedical datasets. Zhao, Zhang, Li, & Chen. (2018) propose a method, called FCA-Map, to identify and validate mappings across biomedical ontologies in terms of object properties. Dumontier et al. (2014) presented an ontology, The Semanticscience Integrated Ontology (SIO), to facilitate biomedical knowledge discovery through ontology-based data integration. SIO describes two key entities; objects and processes, and their attributes in the biomedical domain.

THE DISEASE ONTOLOGY

The semantic web uses RDF data model to describe data models, including concepts and relationships between them. Köhler et al. (2014) and Guo, Fan, Ai, & Croft. (2016) discuss in their research that the human disease data is a cornerstone of biomedical research, therefore, there is an enormous need for a consistent representation of human disease for robust data. Creating a biomedical knowledge base in the form of ontologies creates a rigid knowledgebase for semantic annotation of biomedical data through defining concepts and relations connecting them (Hoehndorf, Dumontier, & Gkoutos, 2013). The disease ontology (DO) used in this work has been developed as a standardized ontology for representing human diseases. The objective of DO is to provide the biomedical community with a convenient, reusable and robust knowledgebase of human disease concepts, phenotype characteristics, and related medical vocabulary disease concepts. It is a collaborative effort of researchers at Northwestern University, Center for Genetic Medicine, the University of Maryland School of Medicine, and Institute for Genome Sciences. DO does not include progression (early, late, metastasis, stages) or manifestations (transient, acute, chronic) of disease as part of the definition of disease (Kibbe et al., 2015). The human disease ontology concentrates on representing predominant and rare disease concepts captured across biomedical resources with the mission of providing a disease interface between data resources through ongoing support of disease terminology needs. Major enhancements to the DO database since 2012 have been made including: the content of DO has had 192 revisions, including the addition of 760 terms and 32% of all terms now include definitions, improved data structure, new areas of community-based efforts, new community partners and a switch to web ontology language (OWL). The current version of the DO website provides a comprehensive resource to perform full-text searching on the DO as well as exploring and visualizing relationships between terms. The Disease Ontology content is available via the Creative Commons Public Domain Dedication CC 1.0 Universal license[12]. The DO project has had a considerable influence on the development of biomedical resources, as evidenced by 466 Google Scholar citations to DO's paper in 2012 (Schriml et al., 2012). The Disease Ontology database has been updated to the latest ontology as of 03-07-2018, available in the GitHub repository[13] of DO, by adding about 600 definitions, created logical definitions linking disease and anatomy terms for DO's nervous system, respiratory system and the thoracic disease branches (Bello et al., 2018). Currently, DO comprises of 17363 classes, 90 object properties, 36 annotation properties, and 160724 axioms. Disease names are represented by English labels provided using the "*rdfs:label*" annotation property while human readable, English language definitions are provided using the Open Biomedical Ontologies (OBO) property IAO_0000115. Figure 1 illustrates a partial view of the class and properties taxonomies of the DO.

METHODOLOGY

The methodology of the proposed work is divided into two phases: *Semantic Matching* and *Diseases Relatedness Detection* as shown in Figure 2. In the Semantic Matching phase, semantically search for the user submitted diseases to identify whether these diseases exist in the ontology using concepts that are semantically related to query concepts. The output of this phase is whether the diseases are found in the ontology or not. In case of finding, the URIs of both diseases are retrieved. In the Diseases Relatedness Detection phase, the URI for each disease is passed to the relatedness detector to find out whether they are related. If they are related, the

Figure 1. Partial view of a class (left side) and properties taxonomies (right side) in DO

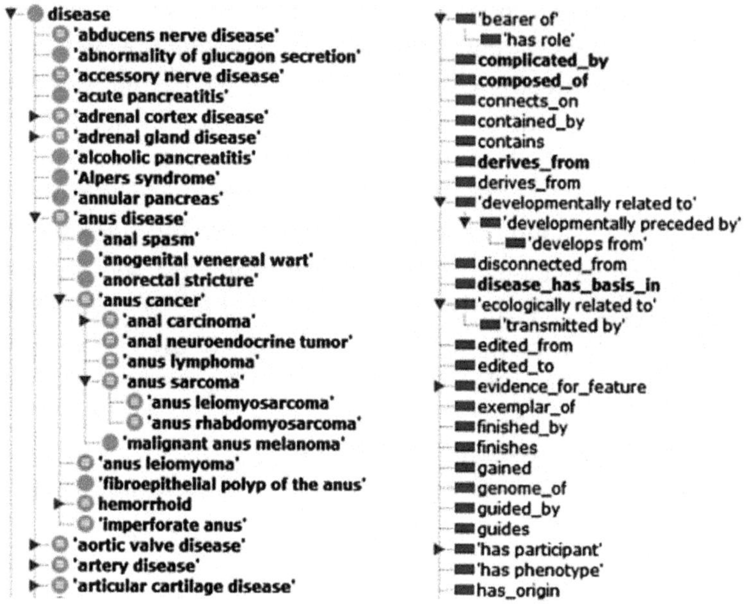

algorithm returns the set of diseases connecting them forming a path from the first disease to the second. Inference on the Semantic Web is used to improve the quality of data integration in the ontology by combining rules and ontologies to discover new relationships, detect possible inconsistencies and infer logical consequences from a set of asserted facts or axioms. A standard way to infer new information on the Semantic Web is to define inference rules (Hayes, 2004).

Inference Rules

In the beginning, a set of SWRL (Semantic Web Rule Language) rules (Horrocks et al., 2004) has been defined (Equations 1-4) in order to support the inference process by discovering new relationships and inferring new knowledge from instance data and class descriptions, which did not explicitly exist in a knowledge graph.

$$Hyponym(?a,?b) \wedge Hpomnym(?b,?c) \rightarrow Hyponym(?a,?c) \quad (1)$$

$$Synonym(?a,?b) \rightarrow Synonym(?b,?a) \quad (2)$$

$$Synonym(?a,?b) \rightarrow swrl:equal(?b,?a) \tag{3}$$

$$Hypernyms(?a,?b) \wedge Hypernyms(?c,?b) \rightarrow Hyponym(?a,?c) \tag{4}$$

Inference engines can infer logical consequences from a set of asserted facts or axioms together with any optional ontology information, axioms, and rules associated with the reasoner. The main use of this technique is to support the use of languages which allow additional facts to be inferred from instance data and class descriptions such as RDFS and OWL. There are three types of reasoners:

- *Transitive reasoner* provides support for storing and traversing property chains or transitivity axioms. This implements just the transitive and reflexive properties.
- *RDFS rule reasoner* implements a configurable subset of the RDFS entailments.
- *Generic rule reasoner* supports user-defined rules. Also, forward chaining, backward chaining, and hybrid execution strategies are supported.

Semantic Matching

The main objective of this phase is to semantically identify user-submitted diseases in the ontology. It is assumed that, when searching for a concept, it is also important to match synonyms of that concept. For example, the synonyms of the disease "*Hyperuricemia*" are "*Hyperuricaemia*" and "*Uricacidemia*" therefore, diseases describing these concepts are also considered as well. The matching process is based on calculating the similarity between concepts. The similarity between two nodes is defined as the maximum information content among all common ancestors from the taxonomical knowledge modeled in biomedical ontologies (Sánchez & Batet, 2011). The matching process is performed by the proposed matching algorithm (see Algorithm 1).

The matching algorithm iterates through ontology resources and matches input diseases. When a match is found, the URI of the disease is stored (URI[0]). This process is repeated for the second disease as well. Otherwise, the disease is not found in the ontology and the algorithm returns null. Semantic matching conducts more analysis in the matching process. This analysis comprises term normalization; phrase analysis, word sense disambiguation, and the matching may be performed on phrase level and word sense level (Li & Xu, 2014).

Algorithm 1. Matching algorithm

```
Input:
1.        Ontology O
2.        String disease1
3.        String disease2
Output: URI of both diseases when matched, null if not.
Steps:
begin
α ← false
β ← false
For each (Resource R in O) do
α = Semantic_Matching (R, disease1)
If (α ≠ false) then
URI [0] = Resource.getURI(R);
   Else
                Print ("Disease 1 not found")
                Return null
   End if
   β = semantic_matching (R, disease2)
   If (β ≠ false) then
            URI [1] = Resource.getURI(R);
   Else
                Print ("Disease 2 not found")
                Return null
   End if
End for
End
```

Diseases Relatedness Detection

In diseases relatedness detection phase, the relatedness between two diseases is detected using bidirectional spreading activation on ontology graph. The idea of a bidirectional search is to cut back the search time by looking out forward from the beginning and backward from the goal at the same time. When the two search frontiers meet, the algorithm will reconstruct one path that extends from the beginning state through the frontier intersection to the goal. The merit of bidirectional search

Figure 2. Architecture of the proposed approach

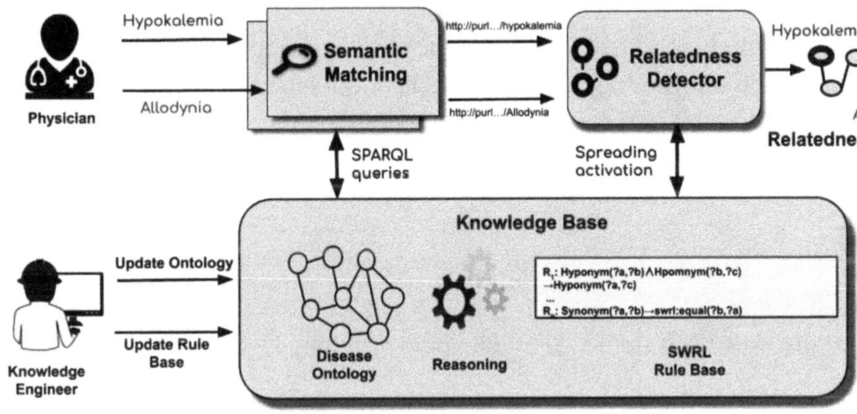

is its speed and it requires less memory (Poole & Mackworth, 2010). After the identification of the input diseases in the ontology graph, the spreading activation begins with these two initial nodes as starting nodes. Then, the spreading process begins to activate node(s) according to the proposed relatedness detector algorithm (see Algorithm 2).

Algorithm 2. Diseases Relatedness Detection

begin
$a_i \leftarrow 1.0$ //activation value for the initial node
$T \leftarrow 1.0$ //threshold
$cycle \leftarrow 1.0$ //iteration cycles
while (Termination condition not true)
    For each (Link ij connected to the target node j) **do**
        $a_j \leftarrow a_j + a_j * w_{ij}$ // w_{ij} relatedness weight
            If ($a_j > 1.0$) **then** $a_j = 1.0$
            If ($a_j < 0.0$) **then** $a_j = 0.0$
        If ($a_j > T$) **then** $a_j.visited = true$
    End For
  $cycle \leftarrow cycle + 1$
 End while
End

Assumptions:

1. Diseases are represented as nodes in the ontology graph,
2. All nodes in the ontology have activation values of zero,
3. Starting nodes take an activation value of 1.0,
4. Relations between diseases are represented by edges between nodes.

Input:

1. Disease ontology,
2. Two diseases URIs, returned by semantic matching algorithm.

Output:

1. A path connecting the two input diseases, i.e., the relatedness.

Steps:

CASE STUDY

The proposed approach can be used to identify relations between diseases in the disease ontology. As an example, consider a query containing the two diseases, "*Alcoholic liver cirrhosis*" and "*Portal hypertension*". The result of relatedness detection is a set of diseases connecting them. As shown in Figure 3, the relatedness between "*Alcoholic liver cirrhosis*" and "*Portal hypertension*" diseases are detected by the intersection node "*Gastrointestinal system disease*". The query is processed in the following steps:

1. **User Input:** The user submits the two diseases as a string.
2. **Query Preprocessing:** Including:
    a. **Intelligent Tokenization and Stop List Elimination:** First, the query string is tokenized by breaking it down into understandable segments. Usually, a token is defined as an alpha-numeric string that separated by white space or punctuation. Second, eliminating all stop words. Those terms have little value in describing the user's intention. A stop word list typically consists of those word classes that do not contain important significance to be used in the query, such as articles (an, a), conjunctions

Figure 3. The relatedness path between "Alcoholic liver cirrhosis" and "Portal hypertension" diseases detected by the proposed approach

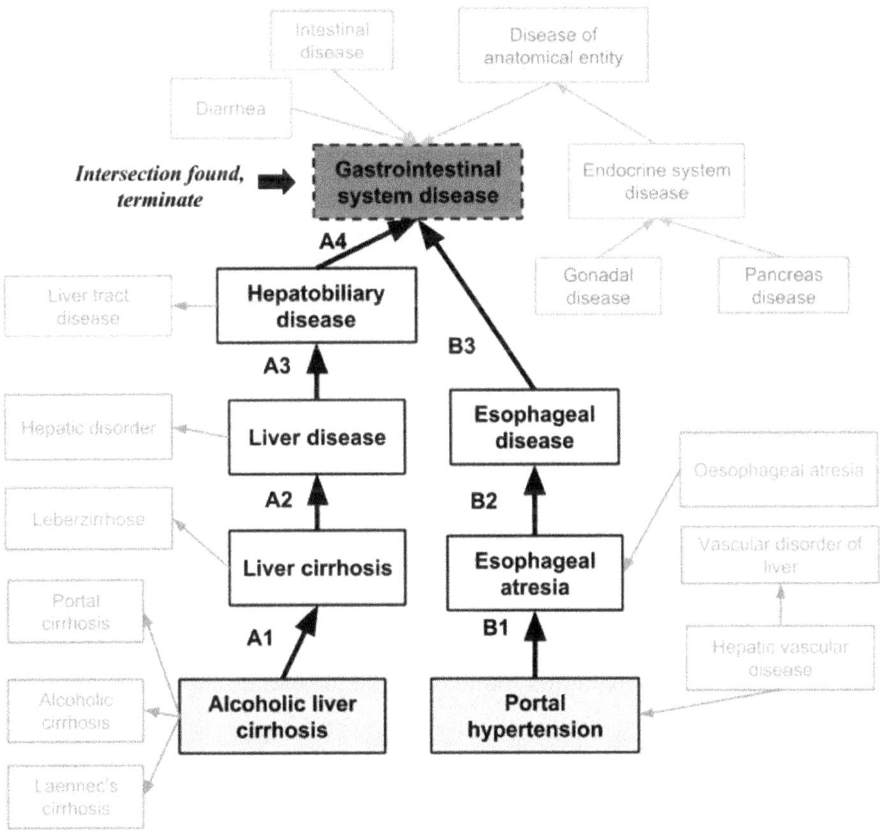

(and, thus), interjections (oh, but), prepositions (at, on), pronouns (he, she), and forms of the "to be" verb (is, are).

b. **Stemming:** Stemming removes word suffixes: both inflectional suffixes (*-s, -es, -ed*) and derivational suffixes (*-able, -aciousness, -ability*) are stemmed.

3. **Formulate Semantic Query:** Formulate a semantic query using SPARQL and executes it against the ontology which performs the semantic matching process based on the inference rules presented in section 5.1 (Fathalla et al., 2012). By incorporating these rules, semantically matched diseases could be found using Jena reasoners (Jena, 2015). These rules have been divided into three types: Transitive Rules, Symmetric Rules, and Co-Reflexive Rules. As an example

of the symmetric rule, if the disease "*Hyperuricemia*" is related to the disease "*Hyperuricaemia*" via hasSynonym property, then, it could be inferred that "Hyperuricaemia" must also be related to "*Hyperuricemia*" via hasSynonym property. In other words, if "*Hyperuricemia*" is a synonym of "*Hyperuricaemia*", then "*Hyperuricaemia*" must be a synonym of "Hyperuricemia". hasSynonym property is also a Co-Reflexive property, because the synonym of a disease is also the same disease. As an example of the transitive rule, if a disease "*Heart failure*" has a synonym "*Weak heart*" and "*Weak heart*" itself has a synonym "*CHF*" then it could be inferred that "Heart failure" has synonym "CHF".

4. **Disease Relatedness Detection:** The diseases relatedness is detected by using the relatedness detector if the diseases have been found in the matching process. Figure 3 illustrates the relatedness path between "Alcoholic liver cirrhosis" and "*Portal hypertension*" diseases detected by the proposed approach. The whole spreading process is summarized in Table 1. The algorithm runs in the following steps:
    a. Begin with two initial nodes "*Alcoholic liver cirrhosis*" and "*Portal hypertension*", (marked in light gray),
    b. The first cycle of the activation process will active one node from each of the starting nodes which are "*Liver Cirrhosis*" (from node 1) and "*Esophageal atresia*" (from node 2),
    c. There is no intersection found between the two diseases then proceed to the next cycle.
    d. The second cycle of activation process will activate "*Liver disease*" and "*Esophageal disease*" diseases from the first and second path respectively,
    e. No intersection found, then continue to the next cycle,

Table 1. Summarization of the spreading process

Action	Node
1st Initial Node	Alcoholic liver cirrhosis
2nd Initial Node	Portal hypertension
The path from node 1	Alcoholic liver cirrhosis - Liver cirrhosis - Liver disease - Hepatobiliary disease - Gastrointestinal system disease
The path from node 2	Portal hypertension - Esophageal atresia - Esophageal disease - Gastrointestinal system disease
Intersection	Gastrointestinal system disease

f. The third cycle of the activation process will activate "*Hepatobiliary disease*" and "*Gastrointestinal system disease*" from the first and the second path respectively,
g. No intersection found, then continue to the next cycle,
h. The fourth cycle node "*Gastrointestinal system disease*" is activated from the first path and no node activated from the second path,
i. The algorithm detects an intersection node "*Gastrointestinal system disease*" and stops.

USE CASE

This section presents a use case that depicts how the proposed approach can be used to explore the relations between vaccines using the vaccine ontology.

Vaccine: Vaccine Relationship

In this use case, we describe how the proposed approach could be used to detect the relation, e.g., conflicts, between vaccines. Vaccine Ontology is designed for vaccine data standardization, integration, and analysis. VO has been developed following the OBO Foundry principles (Smith et al., 2007). It focuses on vaccines components, vaccine allergen, and categorization. VO does not contain only the description of vaccines, but it also includes a description of different genes, such as viral gene, cattle gene, and gene of bacteria, vaccinee, i.e., an organism that is vaccinated with a vaccine. The relationships between vaccines and diseases relay on several properties, which relate vaccines to each other. Table 2 lists some of these

Table 2. Some of the VO properties

Label	Definition
has vaccine allergen	Specifies a relation between a vaccine and a vaccine allergen.
has vaccine component	Defines a relation between a vaccine and its component.
has vaccine contraindication	Specifies contraindication of a vaccine.
has vaccine virmugen	Specifies a relation between a vaccine and a vaccine virmugen.
infection_of	A relation between a disorder and an infectious pathogen.
interacts with	Holds between two entities in which the processes executed by the two entities are causally connected.

Table 3. Summarization of the spreading process

Action	Node
1st Initial Node	Hexavax
2nd Initial Node	Poliovax
The path from node 1	Hexavax - Inactivated Poliomyelitis vaccine - Poliovirus vaccine
The path from node 2	Poliovax - Poliovirus vaccine
Intersection	Poliovirus vaccine

properties along with its URI, label, and definition. We will give two examples of exploring the relationship between two vaccines (Example 1) and the case of the existence of two different relationships between two vaccines (Example 2).

Example 1: (*Exploring the relationship between two vaccines*)

In this example, the vaccines relatedness is detected by SAOO on VO ontology graph if the vaccines have been found in the matching process. Figure 4 illustrates the relatedness path between "*Hexavax*" and "*Poliovax*" vaccines detected by the proposed approach. The whole spreading process is summarized in Table 3. The algorithm starts with two initial nodes "*Hexavax*" and "*Poliovax*". The algorithm runs in the following steps:

1. Begin with two initial nodes "*Hexavax*" and "*Poliovax*", (marked in light gray),
2. The first cycle of the activation process will active one node from each of the starting nodes which are "*Inactivated Poliomyelitis vaccine*" (from node 1) and "*Poliovirus vaccine*" (from node 2),
3. There is no intersection found between the two diseases then proceed to the next cycle.
4. The second cycle of activation process will activate "*Poliovirus vaccine*" from the first path and the nodes "*Viral vaccine*" or "*Inactivated viral vaccine*" might be activated, based on a predefined threshold,
5. The algorithm detects an intersection node "*Poliovirus vaccine*" and stops.

Example 2: (*More than one relationship between two vaccines*)

In this example, the algorithm starts with two initial nodes "*Poliovax*" and "*Imovax Polio*" vaccines (see Figure 5). In the first cycle of the activation process

Figure 4. The relatedness path between "Hexavax" and "Poliovax" vaccines detected by the proposed approach

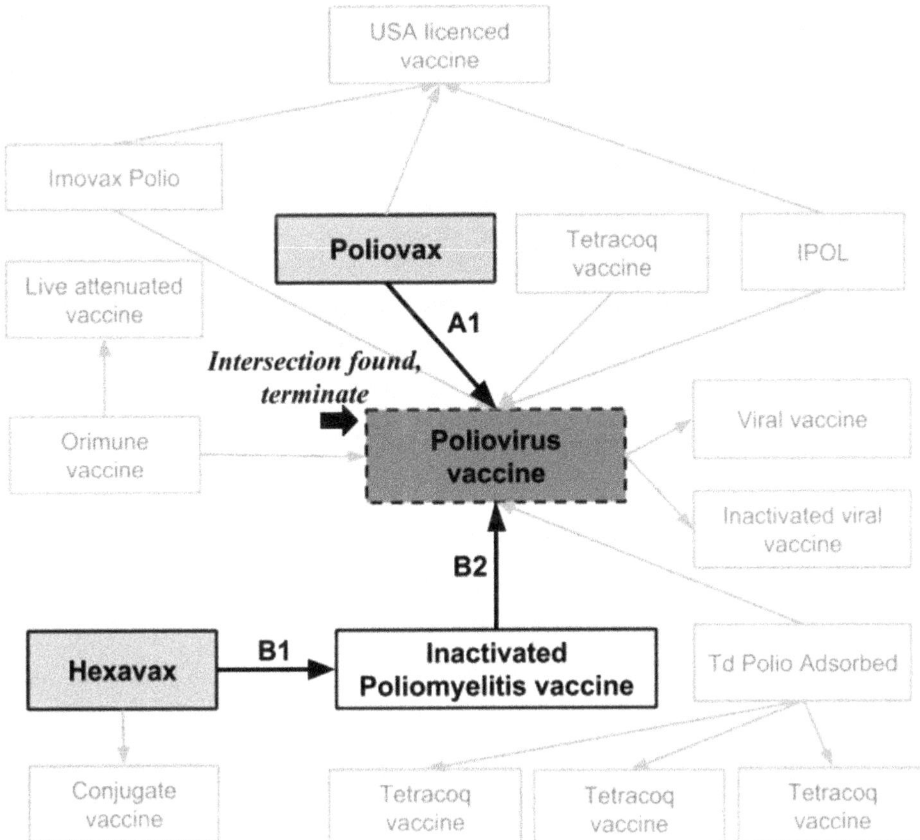

will active one node from each of the starting nodes which are "*Poliovirus vaccine*" (from node 1) and "*USA licensed vaccine*" (from node 2). The algorithm detects two intersections then stops.

FUTURE TRENDS

For future work, authors are planning to develop an algorithm to detect the relatedness between more than two diseases using multiple-goal search algorithms and provide the relatedness graph between them not only a simple path. In addition, a set of relationships is returned to the user which is a subset of the power set of the input

Figure 5. The relatedness path between "Poliovax" and "Imovax Polio" vaccines detected by the proposed approach

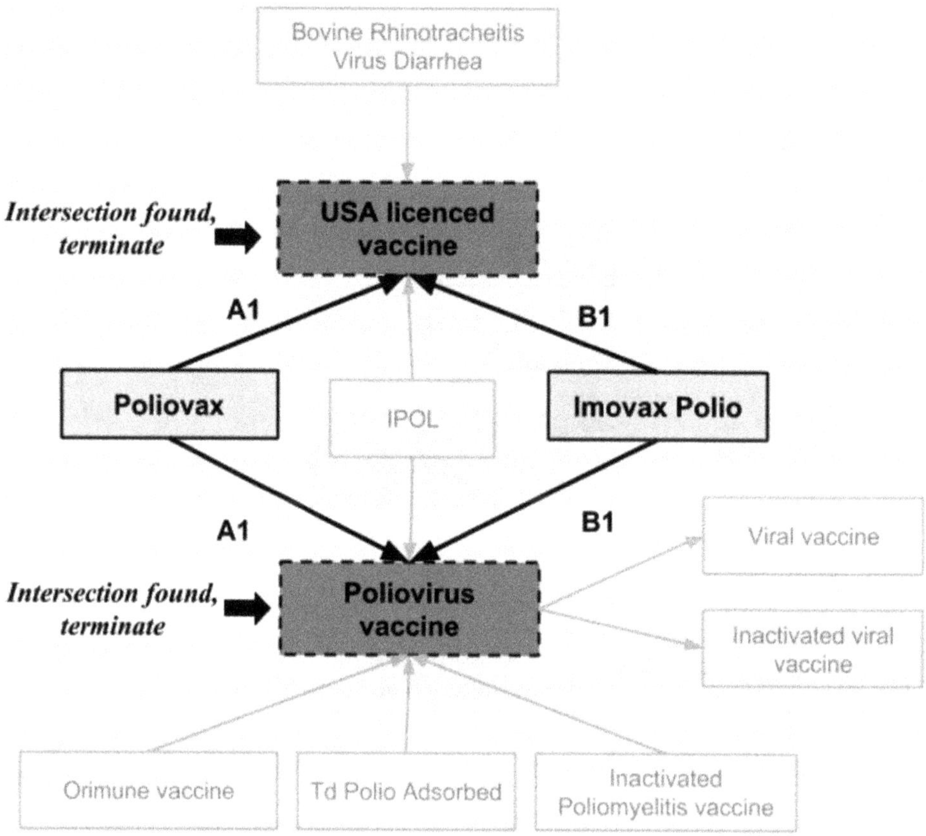

diseases. In other words, which of the submitted diseases is related to the others? Another direction to extend this work is to search for more relationships not only the first-detected relationship. This direction could lead to finding more strong relationships between human diseases. Finally, it is planned to integrate different ontologies in the medical domain using ontology matching and integration techniques.

CONCLUSION

This chapter proposes a novel approach, SAOO (Spreading Activation over Ontology), in order to detect the relationship, i.e., relatedness, between two human diseases by applying spreading activation algorithm based on bidirectional search technique over a well-formed disease ontology. The idea behind the use of bidirectional search is to find a path starting from the source node, i.e., the first diseases, and from the goal node, i.e., the second disease until an intersection occurs. The methodology of the proposed work is divided into two phases: semantic matching and diseases relatedness detection. A set of SWRL rules has been defined in order to support the inference process which helps in discovering new relationships which did not explicitly exist in the ontology. The leading causes of detecting the relatedness between diseases are: 1) Causality: possible, a disease can cause another disease, 2) Complications of diseases: a disease can increase the complications of another disease, 3) Treatments prescription: treatment recipes for a disease can change when there is a relationship between it and another disease. The proposed approach improves healthcare systems by considering semantic domain knowledge and a set of inference rules to infer diseases relatedness. Applying SAOO approach on medical ontologies can have several advantages: 1) it eases the process of discovering the cause of a disease which might be related to another disease that causes this disease, 2) it can be used to find the relationship between any two entities in the biomedical ontologies such as diseases and vaccines. For example, SAOO can be used to explore relationships between vaccines in the vaccine ontology.

ACKNOWLEDGMENT

Said Fathalla would like to acknowledge the Ministry of Higher Education (MoHE) of Egypt for providing a scholarship to conduct this study as well as the University of Bonn, Germany for offering all facilities and tools required to do this work.

REFERENCES

W3C. (2014). RDF Schema 1.1. World Wide Web Consortium.

Antoniou, G., & van Harmelen, F. (2004). *Semantic Web Primer*. The MIT Press.

Bandrowski, A., Brinkman, R., Brochhausen, M., Brush, M. H., Bug, B., & Chibucos, M. C. ... Zheng, J. (2016). The Ontology for Biomedical Investigations. *PLoS One*. doi:10.1371/journal.pone.0154556

Bello, S. M., Shimoyama, M., Mitraka, E., Laulederkind, S. J. F., Smith, C. L., Eppig, J. T., & Schriml, L. M. (2018). Disease Ontology: Improving and unifying disease annotations across species. *Disease Models & Mechanisms, 11*(3), dmm032839. doi:10.1242/dmm.032839 PMID:29590633

Berners-Lee, T., Hendler, J., & Lassila, O. (2001). The Semantic Web. *Scientific American, 284*(5), 34–43. doi:10.1038cientificamerican0501-34 PMID:11323639

Collins, A. M., & Loftus, E. F. (1975). A spreading-activation theory of semantic processing. *Psychological Review, 82*(6), 407–428. doi:10.1037/0033-295X.82.6.407

De Maio, C., Loia, V., Fenza, G., Gallo, M., Linciano, R., & Morrone, A. (2011). Fuzzy knowledge approach to automatic disease diagnosis. In *IEEE International Conference on Fuzzy Systems*. 10.1109/FUZZY.2011.6007498

Dhamankar, R., Lee, Y., Doan, A., Halevy, A., & Domingos, P. (2004). iMAP: discovering complex semantic matches between database schemas. In *Proceedings of the 2004 ACM SIGMOD International Conference on Management of Data - SIGMOD '04* (pp. 383–394). 10.1145/1007568.1007612

Do, H.-H., & Rahm, E. (2002). COMA: a system for flexible combination of schema matching approaches. In *Proceedings of the 28th international conference on Very Large Data Bases* (pp. 610–621). 10.1016/B978-155860869-6/50060-3

Dumontier, M., Baker, C. J. O., Baran, J., Callahan, A., Chepelev, L., & Cruz-Toledo, J. … Hoehndorf, R. (2014). The semanticscience integrated ontology (SIO) for biomedical research and knowledge discovery. *Journal of Biomedical Semantics*. doi:10.1186/2041-1480-5-14

Euzenat, J., Meilicke, C., Stuckenschmidt, H., Shvaiko, P., & Trojahn, C. (2011). Ontology Alignment Evaluation Initiative: Six Years of Experience. *Journal on Data Semantics, XV*, 158–192. doi:10.1007/978-3-642-22630-4_6

Fathalla, S. (2018). Detecting Human Diseases Relatedness: A Spreading Activation Approach Over Ontologies. *International Journal on Semantic Web and Information Systems, 14*(3), 120–133. doi:10.4018/IJSWIS.2018070106

Fathalla, S., Hassan, Y., & El-Sayed, M. (2012). A hybrid method for user query reformation and classification. In *22nd International Conference on Computer Theory and Applications, ICCTA 2012* (pp. 132–138). 10.1109/ICCTA.2012.6523559

Fathalla, S., & Kannot, Y. (2017a). A Bidirectional-Based Spreading Activation Method for Human Diseases Relatedness Detection Using Disease Ontology. In *Conference on Computational Collective Intelligence Technologies and Applications* (pp. 14–23). Springer. 10.1007/978-3-319-67074-4_2

Fathalla, S., & Kannot, Y. (2017b). A Bidirectional-Based Spreading Activation Method for Human Diseases Relatedness Detection Using Disease Ontology. *International Journal of Computers in Clinical Practice*, *2*(1), 14–23. doi:10.4018/IJCCP.2017010104

Fathalla, S., & Lange, C. (2018a). EVENTSKG: A Knowledge Graph Representation for Top-Prestigious Computer Science Events Metadata. In *International Conference on Computational Collective Intelligence*. Springer. 10.1007/978-3-319-98443-8_6

Fathalla, S., Vahdati, S., Auer, S., & Lange, C. (2017). Towards a knowledge graph representing research findings by semantifying survey articles. In *International Conference on Theory and Practice of Digital Libraries,* LNCS (Vol. 10450, pp. 315–327). Springer. 10.1007/978-3-319-67008-9_25

Feigenbaum, L., Herman, I., Hongsermeier, T., Neumann, E., & Stephens, S. (2007). The semantic web in action. *Scientific American, 297*(6), 90–97. doi:10.1038cient ificamerican1207-90 PMID:18237102

Fonseca, F., Davis, C., & Câmara, G. (2003). Bridging ontologies and conceptual schemas in geographic information integration. *GeoInformatica*, *7*(4), 355–378. doi:10.1023/A:1025573406389

Fromkin, V., Rodman, R., & Hyams, N. (2013). *An introduction to language*. Cengage Learning.

Giunchiglia, F., Yatskevich, M., & Shvaiko, P. (2007). Semantic Matching : Algorithms and Implementation. *Journal on Data Semantics*. doi:10.1007/978-3-540-74987-5_1

Goble, C., & Stevens, R. (2008). State of the nation in data integration for bioinformatics. *Journal of Biomedical Informatics*, *41*(5), 687–693. doi:10.1016/j.jbi.2008.01.008 PMID:18358788

Guo, J., Fan, Y., Ai, Q., & Croft, W. B. (2016). Semantic Matching by Non-Linear Word Transportation for Information Retrieval. In *Proceedings of the 25th ACM International on Conference on Information and Knowledge Management - CIKM '16* (pp. 701–710). ACM. 10.1145/2983323.2983768

Hayes, P. (2004). RDF Semantics. *W3C Recommendation.*

He, Y., Cowell, L., Diehl, A. D., Mobley, H. L., Peters, B., & Ruttenberg, A. … others. (2009). VO: vaccine ontology. In *The 1st International Conference on Biomedical Ontology (ICBO 2009) Nature Proceedings* (Vol. 2009).

Hitzler, P., Parsia, B., Patel-schneider, P. F., & Rudolph, S. (2009). OWL 2 Web Ontology Language Primer. *W3C Recommendation.* Retrieved from http://www.w3.org/TR/owl2-primer/

Hoehndorf, R., Dumontier, M., & Gkoutos, G. V. (2013). Evaluation of research in biomedical ontologies. *Briefings in Bioinformatics, 14*(6), 696–712. doi:10.1093/bib/bbs053 PMID:22962340

Hoehndorf, R., Schofield, P. N., & Gkoutos, G. V. (2015). The role of ontologies in biological and biomedical research: A functional perspective. *Briefings in Bioinformatics, 16*(6), 1069–1080. doi:10.1093/bib/bbv011 PMID:25863278

Hoffman, M., Arnoldi, C., & Chuang, I. (2005). The clinical bioinformatics ontology: A curated semantic network utilizing RefSeq information. *Pacific Symposium on Biocomputing*. PMID:15759621

Horrocks, I., Patel-schneider, P. F., Boley, H., Tabet, S., Grosof, B., & Dean, M. (2004). SWRL : A Semantic Web Rule Language Combining OWL and RuleML. *W3C.*

Kanavos, A., Theodoridis, E., & Tsakalidis, A. (2014). A PubMed Meta search engine based on biomedical entity mining. In *Proceedings - International Workshop on Database and Expert Systems Applications, DEXA*. 10.1109/DEXA.2014.32

Kibbe, W. A., Arze, C., Felix, V., Mitraka, E., Bolton, E., Fu, G., ... Schriml, L. M. (2015). Disease Ontology 2015 update: An expanded and updated database of Human diseases for linking biomedical knowledge through disease data. *Nucleic Acids Research, 43*(D1), D1071–D1078. doi:10.1093/nar/gku1011 PMID:25348409

Köhler, S., Doelken, S. C., Mungall, C. J., Bauer, S., Firth, H. V., Bailleul-Forestier, I., ... Robinson, P. N. (2014). The Human Phenotype Ontology project: Linking molecular biology and disease through phenotype data. *Nucleic Acids Research, 42*(D1), D966–D974. doi:10.1093/nar/gkt1026 PMID:24217912

Li, H., & Xu, J. (2014). Semantic Matching in Search. *Foundations and Trends® in Information Retrieval, 7*(5), 343–469. doi:10.1561/1500000035

Marshall, B., Su, H., McDonald, D., Eggers, S., & Chen, H. (2006). Aggregating automatically extracted regulatory pathway relations. *IEEE Transactions on Information Technology in Biomedicine*, *10*(1), 100–108. doi:10.1109/TITB.2005.856857 PMID:16445255

Ngo, V. M., Cao, T. H., & Le, T. M. V. (2010). Combining named entities with WordNet and using query-oriented spreading activation for semantic text search. In *2010 IEEE-RIVF International Conference on Computing and Communication Technologies: Research, Innovation and Vision for the Future, RIVF 2010*. 10.1109/RIVF.2010.5633401

Oberle, D. (2014). How ontologies benefit enterprise applications. *Semantic Web*, *5*(6), 473–491. doi:10.3233/SW-130114

Ohno-Machado, L., Sansone, S. A., Alter, G., Fore, I., Grethe, J., & Xu, H. … Kim, H. E. (2017). Finding useful data across multiple biomedical data repositories using DataMed. *Nature Genetics*. doi:10.1038/ng.3864

Payne, T. R., & Lassila, O. (2004). Semantic Web Services. *IEEE Intelligent Systems*, *19*(4), 14–15. doi:10.1109/MIS.2004.29

Poole, D. L., & Mackworth, A. K. (2010). *Artificial intelligence: Foundations of computational agents. Artificial Intelligence: Foundations of Computational Agents*. doi:10.1017/CBO9780511794797

Said Fathalla and Christoph Lange. (2018b). EVENTSKG: A Knowledge Graph Representation for Top-Prestigious Computer Science Events Metadata. In *International Conference on Computational Collective Intelligence* (Vol. 2, pp. 53-63).

Sánchez, D., & Batet, M. (2011). Semantic similarity estimation in the biomedical domain: An ontology-based information-theoretic perspective. *Journal of Biomedical Informatics*, *44*(5), 749–759. doi:10.1016/j.jbi.2011.03.013 PMID:21463704

Schriml, L. M., Arze, C., Nadendla, S., Chang, Y. W. W., Mazaitis, M., Felix, V., ... Kibbe, W. A. (2012). Disease ontology: A backbone for disease semantic integration. *Nucleic Acids Research*, *40*(D1), D940–D946. doi:10.1093/nar/gkr972 PMID:22080554

Shadbolt, N., Hall, W., & Berners-Lee, T. (2006). The semantic web revisited. *IEEE Intelligent Systems*, *21*(3), 96–101. doi:10.1109/MIS.2006.62

Shvaiko, P., & Euzenat, J. (2013). Ontology Matching: State of the Art and Future Challenges. *IEEE Transactions on Knowledge and Data Engineering*, *25*(1), 158–176. doi:10.1109/TKDE.2011.253

Smith, B., Ashburner, M., Rosse, C., Bard, J., Bug, W., & Ceusters, W. … Lewis, S. (2007). The OBO Foundry: Coordinated evolution of ontologies to support biomedical data integration. *Nature Biotechnology*. doi:10.1038/nbt1346

Spasić, I., & Ananiadou, S. (2005). A flexible measure of contextual similarity for biomedical terms. In *Pacific Symposium on Biocomputing. Pacific Symposium on Biocomputing*.

Trotman, B. W., Bernstein, S. E., Bove, K. E., & Wirth, G. D. (1980). Studies on the pathogenesis of pigment gallstones in hemolytic anemia. Description and characteristics of a mouse model. *The Journal of Clinical Investigation*, *65*(6), 1301–1308. doi:10.1172/JCI109793 PMID:7410545

Tsarkov, D., Riazanov, A., Bechhofer, S., & Horrocks, I. (2004, November). Using Vampire to reason with OWL. In International Semantic Web Conference (pp. 471-485). Springer. doi:10.1007/978-3-540-30475-3_33

Turgeon, M. L. (2015). *Linne & Ringsrud's Clinical Laboratory Science: The Basics and Routine Techniques*. Retrieved from https://books.google.com/books?id=D1umBgAAQBAJ&pgis=1

Zhao, M., Zhang, S., Li, W., & Chen, G. (2018). Matching biomedical ontologies based on formal concept analysis. *Journal of Biomedical Semantics*, *9*(1), 11. doi:10.118613326-018-0178-9 PMID:29554977

ENDNOTES

1 Disease Ontology: http://www.disease-ontology.org

2 Vaccine Ontology (VO): http://www.violinet.org/vaccineontology

3 Infectious Disease Ontology: http://infectiousdiseaseontology.org/page/Main_Page

4 Ontology for Biomedical Investigations: http://obi-ontology.org/

5 Ontology for General Medical Science: https://bioportal.bioontology.org/ontologies/OGMS

6 Adverse Event Reporting Ontology: https://github.com/mcourtot/adverse-event-reporting-ontology/tree/master/src/ontology

7 Blood Ontology (BLO): http://mba.eci.ufmg.br/BLO/

8 Beta Cell Genomics database: http://www.betacell.org/gbco/

9 Pubmed: http://www.ncbi.nlm.nih.gov/pubmed

10 MeSH: https://www.ncbi.nlm.nih.gov/mesh

11 RxNorm: https://www.nlm.nih.gov/research/umls/rxnorm/

12 https://creativecommons.org/publicdomain/zero/1.0/

13 https://github.com/DiseaseOntology/HumanDiseaseOntology/releases

Chapter 8
Mental Health Clinical Decision Support Exploiting Big Data

Jan Kalina
The Czech Academy of Sciences, Czech Republic

ABSTRACT

The complexity of clinical decision-making is immensely increasing with the advent of big data with a clinical relevance. Clinical decision systems represent useful e-health tools applicable to various tasks within the clinical decision-making process. This chapter is devoted to basic principles of clinical decision support systems and their benefits for healthcare and patient safety. Big data is crucial input for clinical decision support systems and is helpful in the task to find the diagnosis, prognosis, and therapy. Statistical challenges of analyzing big data in psychiatry are overviewed, with a particular interest for psychiatry. Various barriers preventing telemedicine tools from expanding to the field of mental health are discussed. The development of decision support systems is claimed here to play a key role in the development of information-based medicine, particularly in psychiatry. Information technology will be ultimately able to combine various information sources including big data to present and enforce a holistic information-based approach to psychiatric care.

INTRODUCTION

The objective of this chapter is to discuss clinical decision support systems, their benefits, the importance of big data for clinical decision making, and their analysis within clinical decision support. Particular attention is paid here to psychiatry, namely

DOI: 10.4018/978-1-5225-8244-1.ch008

to its specific features preventing telemedicine tools to become more widely spread or to specifics of statistical analysis of psychiatric data.

First, general principles of decision support systems together with their potential and limitations will be described. Recommendations for the design, implementation and validation stages are given, stressing that clinical decision support systems may bring new unexpected sources of errors which must be anticipated. While modern technology undergoing a dynamic progress allows a more effective diagnosis and therapy, the increase in effectiveness does not necessarily imply higher safety of patients and thus the criteria of effectiveness and safety must be considered jointly.

The interest in clinical decision support for the particular field of psychiatry penetrates throughout this chapter. While decision support systems are generally acknowledged to have potential for increasing the quality of healthcare, they have not apparently penetrated to a routine usage in psychiatry yet. Therefore, distinctive challenges for the development of telemental healthcare tools are discussed based on literature research on recent references. Decision support systems contribute to the shift of clinical practice to the ideals described as information-based medicine, which will include the analysis of big data as its integral part. Within psychiatry, there will be a need to overcome specific and rather serious barriers before the mental healthcare can reach the ideals of the information-based psychiatry.

CLINICAL DECISION SUPPORT SYSTEMS WITHIN CURRENT HEALTHCARE

Medical decision making can be described as a process of selecting an activity or series of activities among several alternatives integrating uncertainty as one of its intrinsic aspects with an influence on healthcare (Zvárová & Zvára, 2011). The physician solves the medical decision-making task based on knowledge and data connected to the cognition and determination of diagnosis, therapy and prognosis (Berner, 2016). Decision support systems can be described as very complex systems with a potential to compare different possibilities in terms of their risk. Thus, they represent potentially very useful and powerful e-health tools for the clinical decision-making process, capable to solve a variety of tasks, to analyze different information components, to extract information of different types, and deduce conclusions from them. While the first systems based only on expert knowledge were not sufficiently successful, improved performance has been obtained with systems learning the knowledge from clinically relevant data.

Up to now, clinical decision support systems have established their place as inherent part of e-health with an indisputable ability to improve clinical decision making and with a facility to contribute to a further transformation of clinical medicine (Hanson & Levin, 2013; Lech et al., 2014). There are specialized decision support systems focused on finding the diagnosis within individual clinical fields or prescription of medicaments. However, the search for the appropriate therapy is more complex and depends on many factors and only a few decision support systems aiming at therapy have been sufficiently evaluated up to now. There has been even less attention paid to decision support systems for prognosis, while there are still obstacles to apply decision support systems in healthcare routinely, although everyday healthcare would greatly benefit from reliable interdisciplinary and multidisciplinary systems.

DEVELOPING CLINICAL DECISION SUPPORT SYSTEMS

Designing and implementing a decision support system is a very complex and demanding process. The usage of decision support systems is strongly dependent on factors of legal, social, technical, economical and ethical environment. If the systems should offer a truly unobtrusive and easy-to-use interface, they must meet the needs of the particular healthcare providers and therefore their introduction requires changing organizational and workflow issues of hospitals as well as their healthcare specialists. Also, it is important to realize that adopting a foreign decision support system typically requires translating the system to the local language together with accommodating all details to the local environment.

A clinical decision support system acquires data from a variety of input sources (manual input, interface with a different software, data import from electronic health record). Because the data may be massive, effective tools for storage are needed, as well as communication platforms allowing interoperability with other e-health devices. Particularly, a communication platform between the electronic health record and decision support system becomes a necessity, because there exist so many different versions of electronic health records (Moja et al., 2014).

The implementation of a decision support system should start with a pilot version, which can reveal some weaknesses of the first plan. In addition, the process of implementing a reliable decision support system requires an intensive and long-range validation. The system must also allow for an effective but sufficiently thoroughgoing configurability and parameter tuning. The system should be evaluated at different healthcare providers (e.g. in different hospitals as well as at different self-standing physicians) under a variety of different conditions. In a validation mode, the system should be repeatedly exposed to a cycle form formulating requirements, proceeding to proposing the design (or modifications of the last version), implementation of modifications, and multi-level testing under artificial conditions, and ending with testing in real situations. The evaluation cannot be based entirely on statistical evaluation of the correctly classified diagnosis or prognosis, but also on patient safety and seriousness of misclassifications.

Each decision support system in real healthcare applications requires a permanent and laborious monitoring and maintenance. This is especially important immediately after introducing the system to real applications. Concurrently, the feedback from physicians is very important. The physician should immediately contact the supplier if having doubts about the precision of the recommendations of the decision support system. The supplier must remain open to proposals for improving the system and prepared to correct all mistakes quickly. This practice is opposite to hospital information systems, which are typically delivered as closed systems without a simple possibility of modifications.

In the course of operating the system, actualizations must be also implemented with the aim to adapt the system, taking into account possible errors, new results of medical research, availability of new technologies, or actualizations of the electronic health records. Also, medical guidelines become outdated quickly and it is necessary to follow their recent trends. Actualizations performed while the system keeps working also require consideration of patient safety issues. Big systems require more essential actualizations, especially if they were developed more spontaneously rather than as a result of well-considered preparations with a sophisticated design.

BENEFITS FROM CLINICAL DECISION SUPPORT SYSTEMS

A clinical decision support system improves the quality of the provided care. This section summarizes various positive effects of clinical decision support systems. At the point of care, they allow to exploit medical devices fully not only from the medical, but also from the technical point of view. They also allow an economic evaluation of any planned therapy or care and thus a significant reduction of financial costs. The ability of the systems to perform healthcare planning may be beneficial for health authorities. The systems may potentially incorporate patients' beliefs, which remain neglected across clinical disciplines but become increasingly interesting in the subjective health with cognitive and emotional components (Ortendahl, 2007).

The system brings benefits also to the physician, ensuring more comfort, a higher effectiveness and more time for the patient, and also a reduction of errors. It may be especially favorable during stress (e.g. at an emergency ward) or for treating complicated patients. Particularly (but not only) a less experienced physician may benefit from using a decision support system, which exploits the level of knowledge reflecting the latest developments even in a narrow domain of medicine (Kalina et al., 2013). The system may save human resources or reduce the implicit bias of healthcare professionals (FitzGerald & Hurst, 2017). The available data allow to remind the physician important aspects of family and personal history or diagnostic examinations, to warn about side effects or possible addictivity (e.g. of painkillers), to propose new alternatives not immediately apparent to the physician, or to prevent mistaking different samples. Still, it is the physician who remains to carry the responsibility for the medical decision-making processes in combination of scientific and empirical knowledge to infer the interpretation in all steps of healthcare provision. It is also only the physician, who can exploit non-quantified knowledge obtained through education, experience and intuition.

The medicament management can be greatly improved by a decision support system, which computes the amount of medicament or transmits an alert or warning signal about an incorrect prescription. It can evaluate critical situations and offer notifications and reminders with the ability to react quickly in life-threatening situations. It can warn the physician that a particular patient requires an alternate medicament dosing, e.g. because of higher age and/or a joint usage of other medicaments. It can identify patients with the risk of medication overdose, misuse (in patients with dementia) or abuse (in patients with schizophrenia). The decision support system is also helpful at transfers from one medicament to another. It reminds possible contraindications or avoid superfluous operations in the process of therapy planning or evaluate risk assessment.

From the data management point of view, clinical decision support systems can connect and aggregate various data types and search for their associations (e.g. between genetic information and fMRI brain images) for an individual patient. They can also screen over very large databases of medical images, which can be subsequently evaluated by an expert. A major advantage is the ability to visualize the available data chronologically, presenting a nice and well-arranged graphical output. The systems also have the ability to handle measurements performed by different medical devices, which measure in different units or on different scales.

The systems may access rigorous scientific knowledge by searching references in external information sources. If connected to a web search machine for extracting clinically valid information in large bibliographic databases of research articles, they save the physician also a time-consuming search for knowledge across free text. Decision support systems also have a potential to search automatically for previously performed clinical trials on a given topic in databases.

CLINICAL DECISION SUPPORT SYSTEMS AND PATIENT SAFETY

Improving healthcare quality requires to integrate a correctly and effectively determined diagnosis together with patient safety, where the latter is not automatically guaranteed by medical procedures, even if they reflect the most recent scientific knowledge. On the other hand, defensive healthcare with a sole focus on safety cannot ensure effective results. While the concept of patient safety is not primarily concerned with improving the effectiveness of healthcare, a correct diagnosis is crucial for achieving a higher level of patient safety. The ability of clinical decision support systems to improve patient safety by removing adverse effects of healthcare was appraised e.g. in the review by Gebru et al. (2015).

It is possible to distinguish between two different basic types of errors in healthcare. The first type is caused by limitations of current technologies or level of medical knowledge. These errors can be eliminated only in the future after discovering new scientific facts. The second type of errors are adverse effects of healthcare caused by human factors or system failures. A wrong diagnosis determination can fall into any of the two categories. An example of a wrong diagnosis resulting from an error of the second type is a physician's failure to carry out important clinical examinations of a particular patient, causing a superfluous time in the hospital or even death of the patient.

Patient safety as a field within healthcare considers only the second type of errors: preventable medical errors under the current level of technologies and medical research. Patient safety can be understood as a freedom for the patient from unnecessary harm or potential harm associated with healthcare. It studies not only diverse effect of healthcare, but also proposes ways for preventing or reducing medication-related errors or errors in diagnosis and allows to save also human and financial resources as a consequence. All this means that e.g. an ineffective therapy of a rare disease or even a lack of available therapy for severe rare diseases (e.g. Huntington's chorea) does not represent an issue for the area of patient safety.

Clinical decision support systems prevent medical errors and reduce the risk of treatment complications or redundant deaths of patients. They would not expose patients to redundant clinical studies, but rather save them from an unnecessary burden. By increasing the speed of the decision making the physician obtains more time and the probability of medical error decreases. The systems also look for inconsistencies, errors and omissions in the treatment plan. There exist even small decision support systems designed primarily for improving patient safety or healthcare quality control, which can yield patient-specific, evidence-based recommendations. However, the future seems not to be in specialized self-standing decision support systems designed only for patient safety, but primarily in multifunctional decision support systems covering the patient safety as one of their areas. In the current fast pace of development, big and reliable systems can be created only by large suppliers.

Patient safety may be threatened by any new technology and decision support systems do not represent an exception, as they may contribute to new (possibly unexpected) opportunities of errors or accidents. The sources of errors include a computer collapse, data overload, automated actions without the knowledge of the physician, the change of the system or software update, latent or system errors, entering the data incorrectly, misusing or losing sensitive data, or data protection violations. In case of collapse of the decision support system, the physician is not removed from ethical and legal responsibilities. The human factor is another source of problems, and the correct usage of the decision support system requires a well-educated physicians or healthcare professionals with a proper level of statistical literacy as well as computer literacy, who are free from fear of being limited by computers in the decision making process.

CLINICAL DECISION SUPPORT SYSTEMS IN PSYCHIATRIC CARE

Combining Various Types of Psychiatric Data

Like in other clinical fields, the amount of data relevant for psychiatric care rises enormously. Massive data of various sources and types represent a valuable capital for bringing new psychiatric knowledge, so far underutilized with a potential for a dramatic change of current practices of healthcare. This was documented by the review paper by Stewart & Davis (2016), who cited 198 references on applications of big data in mental health research. So far, big data in the psychiatric context are measured primarily for research purposes, while they also have potential to contribute to improving both the efficiency of clinical decision making as well as patient safety (Monteith et al., 2015).

The knowledge used by decision support systems may be integrated from an expert system created by top-class experts, but this knowledge should be validated on real data. Medical guidelines that describe recommended procedures for diagnosing specific diseases and/or their treatment represent an additional source of knowledge. A list of examples of various data types, which are relevant in psychiatry, together with particular examples includes:

- Numerical data, e.g. data on family and personal history, results of clinical and laboratory examinations in various forms (including gene expression measurements)
- Data measured by e-health tools for patient monitoring, e.g. non-stop wearable sensors
- Signals, e.g. analysis of EEG
- Voice records, e.g. detection of schizophrenia relapse in smartphones applications or detection of depression due to voice changes in a speech record
- 2D, 3D or 4D brain images, e.g. diagnosis of schizophrenia from facial images
- Using fMRI images, e.g. study of irreversible physical changes in the brain due to Alzheimer's disease
- Text in natural language, e.g. description of symptoms and signs, unstructured medical reports in the electronic health record, or analysis of computerized databases
- Molecular genetic data, e.g. study of genetic predisposition to bipolar disorder or mood disorders, genetic networks, or corresponding epigenetic mechanisms (Mahgoub & Monteggia, 2013)
- Social networks, e.g. diagnosis of a depression relapse or automatic mood detection of a facebook user (Appelbaum & Kopelman, 2014)
- Biochemical or biophysical brain models using differential equations (Anticevic et al., 2015)
- Time series, e.g. pharmacokinetic models for ethanol in the brain of an alcoholic, or drug efficacy models

From the statistical point of view, clinical decision support systems learn and apply classification rules allowing to assign a given (new) patient to one of given groups. It is a complex task to learn this classification rule from various input sources. The analysis of psychiatric data is difficult not only because of the plethora of various data types listed above, but also complicated by other common data properties:

- Different data types, including numerical data (continuous or categorical), together with other data types (text, images, videos, graphs)
- High dimensionality of data, i.e. a high number of variables (features), while its adverse effect is denoted as curse of dimensionality
- Different formats of the output as the cause of using a proprietary software by various suppliers
- Different units or different scale of different variables
- Small number of samples (patients)

Telemedicine in Mental Health: Potential and Barriers

This section describes the beneficial impact of decision support systems in the field of mental healthcare. In general, all positive effects of decision support systems described above are valid in psychiatry as well, but other specific benefits will be analyzed in this section. Numerous telemedicine tools are currently under development for psychiatry for remote decision making on diagnosis, therapy and prognosis, but also for psychiatric management or care. Until recently, clinical decision support systems seemed not to be extensively used in psychiatry, although their potential becomes already more acknowledged (Koposov et al., 2017). Various attempts for diagnostic decision support systems have produced frustrations (Bergman & Fors, 2008). This is true also for the rare examples of decision support systems proposed for finding the correct therapy for psychiatric diseases. Nevertheless, telepsychiatric or telemental health services become popular in developed countries, where they contribute to transforming the psychiatric care (Deslich et al., 2013) and help to increase access to mental healthcare.

Particularly, telepsychiatry enables to offer the psychiatric care also to patients with substance abuse problems, who would otherwise dare to search for a clinical intervention, or to highly sensitive individuals. Thus, telemedicine contributes to destigmatization of the psychiatric care (Maulik et al., 2015). Further potential can be found in reducing medication-related expenditures or providing intensive attention. Examples include online monitoring of biochemistry results, managing suicide attempts, video-consultations between a psychiatrist and patient, or mobile smartphone apps for schizophrenic patients. A promising area for decision support systems can be described as management of depression care (Fortney et al., 2010).

Only realizing the barriers for decision support systems in the psychiatric context will allow to overcome them. Sometimes it is claimed that the main limitation of clinical decision support systems is the health information technology itself (Deslich et al., 2013), without acknowledging limitations also in the clinical dimension of the task. However, also intrinsic limitations of psychiatry must be kept in mind. Therefore, it is possible to divide possible barriers of clinical decision support systems in psychiatry to four clusters:

Intrinsic barriers

- Decrease of work productivity (i.e. a need for additional time)
- System not fully automatic
- Insufficient technical support
- Inferior results (e.g. results on diagnosing mental disorders compared to an experienced psychiatrist)

- Negative effects on patient safety

Environmental barriers

- System not adapted for a particular physician/hospital
- System not able to obtain important data (e.g. not integrated with a particular hospital information system)
- The current status of the legislation worldwide still remains to be a big obstacle of a wider usage of decision support systems, particularly the requirement of paper-based healthcare record keeping

Barriers in the psychiatrist-system interaction

- Unrealistic expectations of the psychiatrist (e.g. no tolerance to software errors) or distrust of the system
- Often, the psychiatrist hesitates to change opinion due to prejudices
- Possible aversion of the psychiatrist to ideas of personalized healthcare, preference of one-size-fits-all approaches
- Complicated interpretation of the classification rule (i.e. if etiology of the disease is immensely complex, but the physician expects a fast, simple, comprehensible and justified answer)
- Subjective interpretation of the system instructions, which may depend on text understanding
- The success is also determined by the personality of the psychiatrist (mainly his/her age, sex, sociocultural background and experience), experience with psychiatric diagnosis making and with the system itself, while the performance of the system is improved if the physician is trained (Bergman & Fors, 2008)

Barriers due to specific aspects of psychiatry

- Unclear or unknown cause of the most common psychiatric illnesses
- Controversy concerning the classification of psychiatric diseases (Thornton, 2013)
- Various shapes and forms of the same disease (e.g. dementia), with a multitude of complex and heterogeneous symptoms and signs
- Current models based on genetic information fail to exploit the potential of epigenetics, while the activation of gene functions or their silencing plays

a crucial role in the pathophysiology of psychiatric diseases (Mahgoub & Monteggia, 2013)

- Too many factors are relevant for diagnosis making
- A purely biological perspective may ignore environmental stimuli (stress, hectic lifestyle, sleep deprivation, anxiety causes, somatic symptoms, non-clinical factors with cognitive and emotional components, risk, worries, some other unexpected issues), which play a major role in the development of civilization diseases (Ortendahl, 2007)
- Subjective health dimensions (beliefs or quality of life of psychiatric patients) may not be realiable due to disrupted boundaries between imagination and reality
- Psychiatric guidelines suffer from vagueness or indeterminacy in formulations (e.g. level of cognitive impairment, delusion);
- Complete lack of guidelines for specific tasks, e.g. for work ability evaluation for a mental health patient (Kemppinen et al., 2014)
- Determining the diagnosis based on objective checking a list of individual and conceptually independent symptoms and signs, while a skilled diagnostic judgment may be an exercise of tacit knowledge

STATISTICAL ASPECTS OF CLINICAL DECISION SUPPORT

Statistics vs. Machine Learning or Data Mining

Solving the classification task of clinical decision support systems is commonly performed by exploiting multivariate statistical methodology. This is able to capture the multivariate structure (i.e. correlation structure) of biomedical data, but at the cost of technical and often strong assumptions. Nevertheless, data analysis practitioners often adhere to machine learning tools or heuristic data mining approaches. In this respect, the methods or heuristic tools are commonly used without verifying the statistical assumptions. When these are fulfilled, statistical methods are more powerful compared to machine learning or data mining tools. This section has the aim to explain their differences and to discuss advantages of the (bio)statistical methodology.

In contrary to (multivariate) statistics, machine learning is commonly believed to contain universal (or universally valid) methods. Although often neglected, its methods including artificial neural networks or support vector machines do require certain (at least implicit) statistical (i.e. probabilistic) assumptions in order to solve classification tasks. On the other hand, machine learning methods do not commonly require a specific probabilistic distribution, which makes them more flexible tools compared to statistical methods.

Data mining can be characterized as a process of information or knowledge extraction from a dataset, revealing and investigating systematic associations among individual variables in a much more heuristic way compared to traditional statistics (Dziuda, 2010). It combines established methods for exploratory data analysis (EDA), descriptive modeling, classification and regression with heuristic principles, while classification together with regression are commonly denoted as predictive data mining. The concept of data mining can be described as the analytical part of the overall process of extracting useful information from empirical data, which is traditionally called knowledge discovery.

There are various advantages of statistical methods in comparison to machine learning approaches. Unique properties of parametric estimation in the multivariate normal model compared to machine learning techniques include:

- Comprehensibility
- Available diagnostic tools (together with remedies for the situation with violated assumptions)
- Efficient computation
- Available modifications for high-dimensional data (e.g. lasso-type regularization);
- Possible modifications robust to outliers (Kalina & Schlenker, 2015)
- Available hypothesis tests
- Less tendency to overfitting
- Confidence interval for parameter estimates
- Confidence band (region, ellipsoid) for the whole set of parameters

On the whole, statistical methods can be rather easily accompanied by additional tools for verifying the assumptions or for modifying the methods for non-standard situations.

Principles of Biomedical Big Data Analysis

Learning the classification rule for clinical decision support systems requires to pre-process the available biomedical data, i.e. cleaning and preparing for subsequent analyses. If the data are big, this pre-processing may actually represent the most time-consuming part of their analysis. The exploratory analysis includes primarily visualization tools (histograms, box plots or quantile-quantile plots for individual variables, or scatter plots for pairs of variables). If individual variables are measured in different groups, then descriptive statistics (quantiles, means and variances) or test statistics (of the F-test or chi-square test) are useful to evaluate the difference among the groups.

Recently, specific statistical and machine learning methods have been proposed for the analysis of big data, which is often denoted as big data analytics. This is true also for data with the number of variables p exceeding the number of observations n, which are commonly denoted as high-dimensional. Traditional statistical methods seem improperly used for big data, while on the other hand, principles of EDA seem still undervalued. Particularly, hypothesis tests are unsuitable as they have a too large power for a large number of observations (Terwisscha van Scheltinga et al., 2013).

Dimensionality reduction (variable selection, feature selection) methods are generally recommended to simplify subsequent analysis of big data. It can (perhaps surprisingly) improve the result of a consequent analysis in spite of losing some relevant information. On the other hand, it would be too strict to reduce the set of variables to a too small number of relevant ones.

Therefore, intrinsic variable selection ensuring sparsity (ignoring redundant variables) seems as the most promising approach, optimized for the supervised task (Matloff, 2017). It is recommended to ensure sparsity by regularization tailor-made for the classification task, so the analysis does not require any variable selection prior to the classification task itself.

Even recent biostatistical research papers continue to critically discuss statistical and data mining methods for big data or high-dimensional data (Matloff, 2017). Experience of researchers is critical mainly to neural networks or support vector machines for not being as good as presented in theoretical papers on simulated data. A list of such aspects of high-dimensional data, which are continuously debated by experts and their opinions seem dramatically different from one paper to another, will be now presented:

- Suitability of particular methods (and method selection) for the particular data, because no data analysis method is uniformly optimal for all available datasets
- Model choice (i.e. reduction of a model to a suitable sub-model)
- Quantifying model performance (standard concepts of reliability or validity have a tendency to a false optimism for big data due to overfitting, i.e. models can appear predictive even if the data are completely random)
- Assumptions of individual methods
- Recommended sample sizes

- Suitability of standard classifiers for data observed under matched case-control studies (standard approaches completely ignoring the paired structure of the data are suboptimal, e.g. in the study of features obtained in brain images by Balasubramanian et al. (2014))
- Efficient algorithms for computation (some of the methods, although theoretically suitable for data with a large *n*, are implemented in commercial software in a computationally inefficient or numerically unstable way)
- Comprehensibility of the results, which must be clearly interpretable from the point of view of the medical research topic; otherwise the methods are not suitable e.g. for patient critically ill or at highest suicide risk

There are numerous open problems concerning the analysis of big and high-dimensional data. Especially methods combining effectiveness with reliability are highly desirable (He & Petoukhov, 2011). Intensive attention has been also paid to sensitivity of existing methods to the presence of outlying or wrongly measured observations in the data (Kalina, 2014).

Specific Statistical Challenges of Analyzing Psychiatric Data

Statistics represents an essential aspect of medical informatics (Scotch et al., 2010) and a standing service for achieving its tasks. Apart from data quality issues, specific analytical challenges characteristic for psychiatric data will be considered in this section. Possible challenges in the analysis of psychiatric data mostly follow directly from the discussion of various sources of data presented above.

- No clear interpretation of the methods, while a clinical interpretation is crucial in psychiatry (Terwisscha van Scheltinga et al., 2013)
- The data structure is often complex, e.g. longitudinal or repeated measures data are very common (Gueorguieva, 2017)
- The data show trends or more complicated patterns across time
- Specific properties of magnetic resonance images of the brain (small effectiveness, non-homogeneous signal-to-noise ratio, spatial autocorrelation) or other medical imaging devices
- Noisy images contaminated by outliers (Kalina, 2018)
- No systematic comparisons of performance of various data mining methods across various biomedical applications
- Difficulty to combine measured data with tacit knowledge, which can be described as context-dependent practical knowledge based on a complex evaluation of the patient's psychological whole (Thornton, 2013)

The most common tasks of analyzing data in psychiatry seem to be classification or clustering. Most researchers in psychiatry or neuroimaging are unaware of recent methods for the analysis of big or high-dimensional data and the arsenal of these methods only starts to penetrate to these research fields. This may be explained by unreliability of newly proposed methods implemented in commercial statistical software, or delay with their implementation.

THE DAWN OF INFORMATION-BASED MEDICINE

The concept of evidence-based medicine (EBM) is nowadays widely accepted as a unifying idea describing the ideal practice of medicine. In this section, it is explained that the clinical practice is gradually undergoing improvements towards more advanced ideals which may be denoted as information-based medicine. This vision of future medicine emerges from the established principles of EBM and goes far beyond it.

The pioneering approach to EBM originally proposed by Guyatt et al. (1992) spread out quickly as a progressive idea during 1990s. The concept of evidence had primarily the meaning of current best evidence in making decisions about the care of individual patients (Sackett et al., 1996) and was later refined as a thorough, unique, and critical use of the best objective and most topical proofs in the process of decision making about the diagnosis, therapy, and prognosis for individual patients. The practice of evidence-based medicine integrates clinical expertise of individual physicians with these proofs, i.e. clinical evidence acquired within systematically performed clinical research.

The cornerstones of EBM require that physicians demonstrate their capability to use up-to-date research results and exploit them in their everyday clinical practice. This includes e.g. searching and systematic critical evaluation of clinical research publications, analysis of activities, risk analysis, or analysis of ethical and legal consequences of using a given approach. By considering economic analysis of costs (Kemppinen et al, 2014), EBM contributes also to healthcare effectiveness.

Clinical trials remain to be the main source of medical knowledge within EBM. This is true in spite of their serious disadvantages, which include artificial conditions or averaged results obtained by statistical methods for an averaged (virtual) patient, without reflecting his/her individual situation. From the statistical point of view, principles of personalized care require to consider clusters of patients or quantiles (even multivariate quantiles) instead of averaging the results. The entire dataset in a clinical trial is also typically forbidding to draw more precise conclusions for an atypical (statistically outlying, extreme) patient. Decision support systems may help to decide whether a new clinical study should be performed. While each clinical study must undergo an ethical review process, many of current clinical studies are superfluous. The same studies are namely carried out repeatedly or have an inappropriate design, which does not allow to generalize the results to be valid also under different conditions.

Criticism of current practice of clinical trials includes the data collection or risk of unintentional avoiding some important variables (James et al., 2015). Besides, proponents of personalized healthcare promote clinical trials with small sample sizes, i.e. performed on small groups of specific patients. In reality, there is however a tendency for clinical trials to be ceaselessly bigger and more expensive. In addition, the behavior of patients is known to be influenced by their sole presence in a clinical trial.

While numerous e-health tools are appealing primarily as commercial products, their dynamic development can be accelerated only after new results of basic research become available. This is true e.g. for the whole segment of m-health. The market of available applications has been denoted as selective without a clear roadmap of the m-health domain and a first systematic ontology for the field was proposed only recently (Cameron et al., 2017).

Current clinical practice is constantly enriched by quickly emerging new results of basic (i.e. not only clinical) research obtained by the analysis of large datasets measured by new biomedical technology. Beyond the EBM, the clinical practice is hoped to gradually converge to an ideal state characterized by the model of information-based medicine (Borangíu & Purcarea, 2008), connecting basic biomedical research with patient-specific information. The role of tools of medical informatics is to perform the integration of knowledge from various sources, primarily from basic research (i.e. understanding diseases on a molecular level), epidemiological studies, and examinations of an individual patient. At the same time, basic research together with information technology and big data analysis extend the possibilities for a targeted healthcare solution beyond the current concept of EBM and allow to overcome its limitations.

The concept of information-based medicine as a recent and perspective medicine paradigm describes the effort to transform the evidence for the (imaginary) averaged patient towards a real individual participative patient based on his/her individual data with clinical as well genetic or metabolic parameters. The concept starts to find first applications, such as the study of Senders et al. (2018) exploiting artificial intelligence in clinical decision making.

INFORMATION-BASED PSYCHIATRY

The current paradigm of evidence-based medicine in the specialty field of psychiatry has been called by various synonyms, including evidence-based medicine in psychiatry, evidence-based clinical practice in psychiatry, evidence-based mental health, or evidence-based practices for mental health (Hanson & Levin, 2013; Lech et al., 2014).

Clinical decision support systems together with other e-health tools and with results of the basic research (e.g. in neuroscience or molecular genetics) strongly contribute to bringing new sources of medical knowledge (and thus the decision-making process) closer to an individual patient, improving the effectiveness of therapy and patient safety. The availability of big data together with a new biomedical knowledge, as described in the visionary paper by Monteith et al. (2015), may allow to make the therapy efficient, compared to the current state when the therapy of common diseases aims only at easing the suffering of patients. Integration of molecular medicine with clinical psychiatry will be of course a demeaning task due to a large gap between the two fields and a transform of psychiatry will be able only by means of a paradigm shift (Demkow & Wolanczyk, 2017).

Currently, an on-going transform of psychiatry can be anticipated, which is enabled by a vast number of technological tools recently introduced for psychiatric care. The fast improvement of technology and rise of big data of various types and formats from unthinkable sources have a potential to contribute to clinical usage. For all these reasons, the paradigm of evidence-based psychiatry should be replaced by deeper ideas going more beyond and the information-based medicine can be expected to develop also in the area of psychiatry. Thus, it is possible to introduce the concept of information-based psychiatry (IBP) intended for the ideals of information-based medicine within psychiatric practice. Some emerging directions of psychiatry have been already described under different concepts in available literature:

- Predictive, preventive, personalized and participatory medicine (Auffray et al., 2010), where predictive healthcare is often denoted as predictive analytics, i.e. stands on big data and their analysis for prediction for an individual patient;
- Evidence-based pragmatic psychiatry (Paulus, 2017), which exploits an empirically based decision making;

- Computational psychiatry, which has been introduced as a concept for computationally demanding approaches to analyzing data measured for psychiatric patients (Maia, 2015; Demkow & Wolanczyk, 2017);
- Precision care (Stein & Smoller, 2018).

Decision support systems may also contribute to shared (collaborative) decision making in routine mental healthcare (Fortney et al., 2010). As a by-product, the transform of healthcare will go hand in hand with the transform of nursing towards information-based nursing. A particular evidence of the drift of psychiatry towards participative healthcare is also the current international transition of mental health services towards community-based services (Slade, 2017), applying patient (client)-centered approaches in healthcare.

One might have the feeling that information technology restricts the physician by limitations of hardware and software. However, it is exactly the information technology, which offers to capture a human body and subsequent healthcare in a holistic approach, because it has the capacity (if correctly organized) to store all available data (including big data) and information, to analyze them, and search for associations. In this way, information technology performing a holistic approach to information (Zvárová, 2014) encompassing the subjective data, especially useful in psychiatry, may capture the full bio-psycho-socio-spiritual model of health. This has the potential to incorporate a high quality of diagnostics with principles of patient safety.

Contribution of the Work

The amount of clinical data relevant for clinical decision making rises enormously and so does the amount of biomedical knowledge obtained as result of basic research. This naturally complicates the process of clinical decision making. This chapter discusses general principles of clinical decision support systems mainly for diagnostics and therapy, together with specifics in the field of psychiatry. Numerous benefits of decision support systems for physicians and for an individual patient at all levels of care are characterized in the chapter. If appropriately implemented, the systems reduce the burden for patients and also reduce costs, which is important not only in psychiatry, where the number of patients as well as the financial demands have increased remarkably world-wide.

Clinical decision support systems can be characterized as prospective e-health tools with a unique ability to extract information from various sources of (big) data. Their importance increases, as the systems unlock tremendous potential to improve both the healthcare quality and patient safety and also may combine objective and patient-subjective data with expert knowledge. They may successfully exploit also the most recently proposed tools for big data analytics, even in spite of high computational demands.

The vision of information-based psychiatry together with discussing its assumptions or barriers preventing its development represent also a contribution of this chapter. The development of telemedicine tools in psychiatry is currently slowed down or complicated mainly by unrealistic expectations and barriers, including general barriers or barriers in the interaction between e-health tool and the psychiatrist. Specific barriers typical for the field of psychiatry have obtained the least attention so far. Reliable statistical or data mining procedures for learning a reliable classification rule for the decision support system are highly desirable. Again, for the particular context of psychiatry, tailor-made methods for the data analysis (e.g. in the form of brain images) are required for extracting relevant information from big data coming from various sources in various formats.

Big data as a still underutilized capital for clinical decision making represent a key accelerator of improving the efficiency of clinical decision making as well as patient safety. Reflecting the dawn of big data in clinical medicine and their analysis, the popular concept of evidence-based medicine is surmounted by the vision of information-based medicine formulated in this chapter. The most recently initiated transforms of psychiatry towards information-based principles are described here as perspective and progressive, although limited by various specifics of psychiatry and thus incessantly slowed down compared to the higher pace of development acquired within other clinical fields. E-health tools contribute to psychiatry transformation and development of information-based psychiatry, i.e. psychiatric care based on information-based principles. However, its ideals assume also a fundamental progress of basic research in molecular genetics and particularly in neurosciences in order to perform an individualized healthcare based on individual clinical, genetic or structural brain imaging parameters.

PROJECT DESCRIPTION

A large portion of the presented work in the field of clinical decision support stems from the project Robust analysis of high-dimensional data in the years 2014-2016. The project was financed by the Neuron Fund for Support of Science, a private fund in the Czech Republic.

The cross-disciplinary part of the project focused on applying methods to particular high-dimensional data. An important research direction was the research of modifications of resting-state brain networks of schizophrenic patients (Kalina & Hlinka, 2017). The spontaneous brain activity of patients was measured and compared with that of healthy individuals. The analysis of the high-dimensional fMRI measurements was performed by robust classification methods. The final robust classification rule is able to find the diagnosis of a new individual very reliably.

Within the project, a cardiovascular genetic study was also analyzed, extending the results of Kalina et al. (2013). The very aim was to find a relatively small set of genes responsible for the development of cardiovascular disease. Diagnostic tests were investigated, which are based entirely on gene expression measurements of individuals. Another practical result is a robust pre-processing procedure for images obtained by Illumina BeadChip microarrays (Kalina, 2018).

Theoretical interests of the project were devoted to such statistical procedures for the analysis of high-dimensional data, which are robust (resistant) to the presence of outlying measurements (outliers) in the data. The particular interests of the project were devoted to robust classification for clinical decision support (Kalina, 2014) or to robust dimensionality reduction by means of a minimum redundancy maximum relevance criterion (Kalina & Schlenker, 2015).

Jana Zvárová passed away in July 2017. After the end of the project, Jan Kalina continues the research focused on connecting classification and decision support with robustness. The methods are applied within in the field on machine learning, particularly (again) to fMRI measurements of patients with mental disorders.

ACKNOWLEDGMENT

The work was supported by the project 19-05704S of the Czech Science Foundation.

REFERENCES

Anticevic, A., Murray, J. D., & Barch, D. M. (2015). Bridging levels of understanding in schizophrenia through computational modeling. *Clinical Psychological Science*, *3*(3), 433–459. doi:10.1177/2167702614562041 PMID:25960938

Appelbaum, P. S., & Kopelman, A. (2014). Social media's challenges for psychiatry. *World Psychiatry; Official Journal of the World Psychiatric Association (WPA)*, *13*(1), 21–23. doi:10.1002/wps.20085 PMID:24497238

Auffray, C., Charron, D., & Hood, L. (2010). Predictive, preventive, personalized and participatory medicine: Back to the future. *Genome Medicine*, *2*(8), 57. doi:10.1186/gm178 PMID:20804580

Balasubramanian, R., Houseman, E. A., Coull, B. A., Lev, M. H., Schwamm, L. H., & Betensky, R. A. (2014). Variable importance in matched case-control studies in settings of high dimensional data. *Applied Statistics*, *63*(4), 639–655. doi:10.1111/rssc.12056

Bergman, L. G., & Fors, U. G. H. (2008). Decision support in psychiatry– A comparison between the diagnostic outcomes using a computerized decision support system versus manual diagnosis. *BMC Medical Informatics and Decision Making*, *8*(1), 9. doi:10.1186/1472-6947-8-9 PMID:18261222

Berner, E. S. (2016). *Clinical decision support systems. Theory and practice* (3rd ed.). Basel: Springer International Publishing.

Borangíu, T., & Purcarea, V. (2008). The future of healthcare-Information based medicine. *Journal of Medicine and Life*, *1*, 233–237. PMID:20108471

Cameron, J. D., Ramaprasad, A., & Syn, T. (2017). An ontology of and roadmap for mHealth research. *International Journal of Medical Informatics*, *100*, 16–25. doi:10.1016/j.ijmedinf.2017.01.007 PMID:28241934

Demkow, U., & Wolanczyk, T. (2017). Genetic tests in major psychiatric disorders–integrating molecular medicine with clinical psychiatry–why is it so difficult? *Translational Psychiatry*, *7*(6), e1151. doi:10.1038/tp.2017.106 PMID:28608853

Deslich, S., Stec, B., Tomblin, S., & Coustasse, A. (2013). Telepsychiatry in the 21st century: Transforming healthcare with technology. *Perspectives in Health Information Management, 10*, Article 1f.

Dziuda, D. M. (2010). *Data mining for genomics and proteomics: Analysis of gene and protein expression data.* New York, NY: Wiley. doi:10.1002/9780470593417

Guyatt, G., Cairns, J., Churchill, D., Cook, D., Haynes, B., Hirsh, J., ... Sackett, D. (1992). Evidence-based medicine. A new approach to teaching the practice of medicine. *Journal of the American Medical Association*, *268*(17), 2420–2425. doi:10.1001/jama.1992.03490170092032 PMID:1404801

FitzGerald, C., & Hurst, S. (2017). Implicit bias in healthcare professionals: A systematic review. *BMC Medical Ethics*, *18*(1), 19. doi:10.118612910-017-0179-8 PMID:28249596

Fortney, J. C., Pyne, J. M., Steven, C. A., Williams, J. S., Hedrick, R. G., Lunsford, A. K., ... Smith, J. L. (2010). A web-based clinical decision support system for depression care management. *The American Journal of Managed Care*, *16*, 849–854. PMID:21348556

Gebru, A. A., Yimam, Y., Nigussie, A. W., Kahsay, W. G., Gelaye, N. D., & Mengistie, Z. (2015). Clinical decision support system in nursing: A review of literature. *Indian Journal of Basic and Applied Medical Research*, *4*, 437–452.

Gueorguieva, R. (2017). *Statistical methods in psychiatry and related fields: Longitudinal, clustered, and other repeated measures data*. Boca Raton, FL: Chapman & Hall/CRC. doi:10.1201/9781315151526

Hanson, A., & Levin, B. L. (2013). *Mental health informatics*. Oxford: Oxford University Press.

He, M., & Petoukhov, S. (2011). *Mathematics of bioinformatics: Theory, methods and applications*. Hoboken, NJ: Wiley.

James, S., Rao, S. V., & Granger, C. B. (2015). Registry-based randomized clinical trials–A new clinical trial paradigm. *Nature Reviews. Cardiology*, *12*(5), 312–316. doi:10.1038/nrcardio.2015.33 PMID:25781411

Kalina, J. (2014). Classification methods for high-dimensional genetic data. *Biocybernetics and Biomedical Engineering*, *34*(1), 10–18. doi:10.1016/j.bbe.2013.09.007

Kalina, J. (2018). A robust pre-processing of BeadChip microarray images. *Biocybernetics and Biomedical Engineering*, *38*(3), 556–563. doi:10.1016/j.bbe.2018.04.005

Kalina, J., & Hlinka, J. (2017). Implicitly weighted robust classification applied to brain activity research. *Communications in Computer and Information Science*, *690*, 87–107. doi:10.1007/978-3-319-54717-6_6

Kalina, J., & Schlenker, A. (2015). A robust supervised variable selection for noisy high-dimensional data. *BioMed Research International, 2015*, 1–10.

Kalina, J., Seidl, L., Zvára, K., Grünfeldová, H., Slovák, D., & Zvárová, J. (2013). System for selecting relevant information for decision support. *Studies in Health Technology and Informatics*, *186*, 83–87. PMID:23542973

Kemppinen, J., Korpela, J., Elfvengren, K., Salmisaari, T., & Polkko, J. (2014). Decision support in evaluating the impacts of mental disorders on work ability. In *47th Hawaii International Conference on System Science* (pp. 2958-2966). Washington, DC: IEEE Computer Society. 10.1109/HICSS.2014.368

Koposov, R., Fossum, S., Frodl, T., Nytro, O., Leventhal, B., Sourander, A., ... Skokauskas, N. (2017). Clinical decision support systems in child and adolescent psychiatry: A systematic review. *European Child & Adolescent Psychiatry*, *26*(11), 1309–1317. doi:10.100700787-017-0992-0 PMID:28455596

Lech, M., Song, I., Yellowlees, P., & Diederich, J. (2014). *Mental health informatics*. New York: Springer. doi:10.1007/978-3-642-38550-6

Mahgoub, M., & Monteggia, L. M. (2013). Epigenetics and psychiatry. *Neurotherapeutics; the Journal of the American Society for Experimental NeuroTherapeutics*, *10*(4), 734–741. doi:10.100713311-013-0213-6 PMID:24092614

Maia, T. V. (2015). Introduction to the series on computational psychiatry. *Clinical Psychological Science*, *3*(3), 374–377. doi:10.1177/2167702614567350

Matloff, N. (2017). *Statistical regression and classification. From linear models to machine learning*. Boca Raton, FL: CRC Press. doi:10.1201/9781315119588

Maulik, P. K., Tewari, A., Devarapalli, S., Kallakuri, S., & Patel, A. (2015). The systematic medical appraisal, referral and treatment (SMART) mental health project: Development and testing of electronic decision support system and formative research to understand perceptions about mental health in rural India. *PLoS One*, *11*(10), e0164404. doi:10.1371/journal.pone.0164404 PMID:27732652

Moja, L., Kwag, K. H., Lytras, T., Bertizzolo, L., Brandt, L., Pecoraro, V., ... Bonovas, S. (2014). Effectiveness of computerized decision support systems linked to electronic health records: A systematic review and meta-analysis. *American Journal of Public Health*, *104*(12), e12–e22. doi:10.2105/AJPH.2014.302164 PMID:25322302

Monteith, S., Glenn, T., Geddes, J., & Bauer, M. (2015). Big data are coming to psychiatry: A general introduction. *International Journal of Bipolar Disorders*, *3*(1), 21. doi:10.118640345-015-0038-9 PMID:26440506

Ortendahl, M. (2007). The New Subjective Medicine: Understanding the Patient's Worry Improves Shared Decision Making and Increases Compliance. *Medical Principles and Practice*, *16*(1), 79–80. doi:10.1159/000096147 PMID:17159371

Paulus, M. P. (2017). Evidence-based pragmatic psychiatry– A call to action. *JAMA Psychiatry*, *74*(12), 1185–1186. doi:10.1001/jamapsychiatry.2017.2439 PMID:29094142

Sackett, D., Rosenberg, W. M. C., Gray, M. J. A., Haynes, B. R., & Richardson, W. S. (1996). Evidence based medicine: What it is and what it isn't. *BMJ (Clinical Research Ed.)*, *312*(7023), 71–72. doi:10.1136/bmj.312.7023.71 PMID:8555924

Scotch, M., Duggal, M., Brandt, C., Lin, Z., & Schiffman, R. (2010). Use of statistical analysis in the biomedical informatics literature. *Journal of the American Medical Informatics Association*, *17*(1), 3–5. doi:10.1197/jamia.M2853 PMID:20064794

Senders, J. T., Harary, M., Stopa, B. M., Staples, P., Broekman, M. L. D., Smith, T. R., ... Arnaout, O. (2018). Information-based medicine in glioma patients: A clinical perspective. *Computational and Mathematical Methods in Medicine*, *2018*, 8572058. doi:10.1155/2018/8572058 PMID:30008798

Slade, M. (2017). Implementing shared decision making in routine mental health care. *World Psychiatry; Official Journal of the World Psychiatric Association (WPA)*, *16*(2), 146–153. doi:10.1002/wps.20412 PMID:28498575

Stein, M. B., & Smoller, J. W. (2018). Precision psychiatry– Will genomic medicine lead the way? *JAMA Psychiatry*, *75*(7), 663–664. doi:10.1001/jamapsychiatry.2018.0375 PMID:29800947

Stewart, R., & Davis, K. (2016). 'Big Data' in mental health research: Current status and emerging possibilities. *Social Psychiatry and Psychiatric Epidemiology*, *51*(8), 1055–1072. doi:10.100700127-016-1266-8 PMID:27465245

Straus, S. E., Glasziou, P., Richardson, W. S., & Haynes, R. B. (2019). *Evidence-based medicine: How to practice and teach EBM* (5th ed.). Edinburgh: Elsevier.

Terwisscha van Scheltinga, A. F., Bakker, S. C., van Haren, N. E., Derks, E. M., Buizer-Voskamp, J. E., Cahn, W., & Ripke, S.Psychiatric Genome-Wide Association Study (GWAS) Consortium. (2013). Schizophrenia genetic variants are not associated with intelligence. *Psychological Medicine*, *43*(12), 2563–2570. doi:10.1017/S0033291713000196 PMID:23410598

Thornton, T. (2013). *Clinical judgment, tacit knowledge, and recognition in psychiatric diagnosis*. Oxford: Oxford Handbooks Online.

Zvárová, J. (2014). Information-based holistic electronic healthcare. *International Journal of Biomedicine and Healthcare*, *2*(2), 2–7.

Zvárová, J., & Zvára, K. (2011). e3Health: Three main features of modern healthcare. In A. Moumtzoglou & A. Kastania (Eds.), E-health systems quality and reliability. Models and standards (pp. 18-27). Hershey, PA: IGI Global.

Chapter 9
Glycemic Monitoring and Prediction With Response Improvement via Psyllium

Sally Shuk Han Pang
The University of Hong Kong, Hong Kong

Kwok Tai Chui
City University of Hong Kong, Hong Kong

Miltiadis D. Lytras
Deree – The American College of Greece, Greece

ABSTRACT

Fibers are proven to provide health benefits in preventing metabolic diseases. This chapter first presents the existing blood glucose monitoring sensors and a prediction model for blood glucose concentration. It also aims at analyzing the efficacy of a functional fiber, psyllium on the glycemic control function. Three studies included suggesting psyllium supplementation would significantly improve glycemic response while two studies included showed no effects. Advantages and limitations of each study were evaluated. Overall, it is generally believed that psyllium might give glycemic response improvement effect, especially in Type II Diabetes Mellitus patients.

INTRODUCTION

It has been well documented that fibers have beneficial effects on human health, with its action on preventing and acting as treatment of chronic diseases (Anderson et al., 2009). According to the Institute of Medicine, fiber can be categorized into 2

DOI: 10.4018/978-1-5225-8244-1.ch009

groups (Trumbo et al., 2002) (i) Dietary fiber, refers to non-digestible carbohydrates and lignin that are intrinsic and intact in plants; and (ii) Functional fiber, refers to isolated non-digestible carbohydrates which have beneficial physiological effects in humans. This chapter focuses on a commonly known functional fiber, psyllium.

Psyllium is one of the popular used functional fiber supplements in the world which has shown to have positive effects on weight management, constipation, diarrhea (McRorie Jr, 2015; Mcrorie and Fahey, 2013) and irritable bowel syndrome (Eswaran et al., 2013; Luther and Chey, 2010). It contains approximately 67% natural concentrated soluble fiber (Gelissen et al., 1994) and is derived from the husks of ripe seeds from Plantago ovate (Singh, 2007).

In addition, psyllium, with its viscous and gel-forming property of a soluble fiber, has long been believed to improve hypercholesterolemia (Dennison and Levine, 1993; Glassman et al., 1990; Taneja et al., 1989). Similarly, it has been suggested that these properties allow psyllium to act as a potential therapeutic treatment in lowering blood glucose level since the 1970s (Fagerberg, 1982; Gupta et al., 1994; Kenkins et al., 1978; Pastors et al., 1991).

However, some researchers (De Bock et al., 2012; Frost et al., 2003; Pal et al., 2011) doubted on the effectiveness of psyllium on prevention and treatment of diabetes mellitus and this topic is still controversial. Recent studies have been carried out on psyllium and blood glucose level among different population in different situations for further investigation (Abutair et al., 2016; De Bock et al., 2012; Feinglos et al., 2013; Karhunen et al., 2010; Pal et al., 2011).

Diabetes is one of the series epidemic diseases in the world. Over 400 million people in the world are living with diabetes (World Health Organization, 2016). Prevalence of diabetes among adults increases globally. It is expected that by 2035, the total number of adults with diabetes in the world would increase to 592 million (Guariguata et al., 2014). Its subsequent microvascular and macrovascular complications could be fetal. Enormous financial burden are putting on diabetes related area. Many patients have to rely on medication in their lifetimes to control diabetes. Therefore, interventions that help glycemic control are worth discussing and investigating. In this review, the effect of psyllium supplement on glycemic control will be evaluated.

BLOOD GLUCOSE MONITORING

Patients with diabetes are always being reminded to maintain their blood glucose level to an acceptable euglycemic range and try their best to minimize the fluctuation in blood glucose. The tools for blood glucose monitoring thus become crucial elements in doing so. Recently, blood glucose monitoring has been revolutionized by the advent of continuous glucose monitoring sensors, consisting of wearable subcutaneous needle-based and minimally-invasive devices that allow measuring the blood glucose concentration continuously, in minute interval (tradeoff between sampling rate and battery lifespan).

In general, blood glucose sensor is categorized into point sample test and continuous glucose monitor (Wang, & Lee, 2015). Table 1 summarizes the common sensors for blood glucose measurement.

Point sample tests rely on taking sample of patients' blood with needle a few times every day. It is limited by human activities like driving and sleeping. Besides, hypoglycaemia and hyperglycaemia are rarely detected.

There are four methods for invasive continuous glucose sensor research which are microneedles/micropores, intravenous implantable devices, microdialysis and subcutaneous amperometric electrodes. It is worth mentioning that only the last two have been commercialized. Typical products are FreeStyle by Abbott, Dexcon G4 Platinum by Dexcorn, MiniMed 530G with Enlite by Medtronic and Guardian Real-time by Medtronic which were approved by U.S. Food and Drug Administration (FDA) 10 years ago.

The availability of home-use glucometers has significantly improved quality of life for diabetes sufferers. Nevertheless, a new strip is needed for each test, as well as a blood draw from the finger pricks, with the latter causing pain and inconvenience. To overcome the short lifetime and calibration needs of the invasive continuous glucose system, and to increase patient compliance, non-invasive continuous glucose sensors represent an obvious solution. Numerous technologies pursued as non-invasive sensor systems can be classified as optical and transdermal sensors.

Authors in (Kim, Campbell, & Wang, 2018) have made a comparison on various epidermal wearable glucose devices which is shown in Table 2, comprising of the

Table 1. Common sensors for blood glucose measurement

Sensor Type	Measurement Type	Method
Blood glucose sensor	Point sample test	(i) Finger prick glucometer (ii) Urine dipstick
	Continuous (invasive)	(i) Microneedles/micropores (ii) Intravenous implantable devices (iii) Microdialysis (iv) Subcutaneous amperometric electrodes
	Continuous (non-invasive)	(i) Optical: Raman spectroscopy, infrared spectroscopy, and fluorescence (ii) Transdermal: Sonophoresis, and reverse iontophoresis

Table 2. Comparison of epidermal wearable glucose devices

Work	Wearable Glucose Sensor	Biofluid	Sampling Method	Pros	Next Steps
Bandodkar et al., 2014	Eyeglasses sensor	Sweat	Exercise	(i) Integrate customized wireless electronics (ii) Sweat glucose monitoring	(i) pH/Temperature compensation (ii) Study and validation
Emaminejad et al., 2017	Multimodal glucose sensor, wearable patch	Sweat	Exercise	(i) accuracy improvement (ii) Control the uptake of sweat	(i) Adopt conformal interface instead of commercial analyzer (ii) Continuous monitoring
Gao et al., 2016	Graphene-based stretchable patch	Sweat	Exercise	(i) soft materials incorporated for flexible/stretchable device (ii) nanomaterials-based sensitive glucose sensor (iii) accuracy improvement	(i) Scalability validation (ii) Adopt conformal interface instead of commercial analyzer (iii) Higher sampling frequency
Lee et al., 2016	Sensor array patch coupled with induced sweating	Sweat	Stimulated iontophoresis	(i) Integrate customized wireless electronics (ii) Integrate iontophoretic sweat generation with glucose sensing	(i) On-body monitoring
Lee et al., 2017	Multiplexed wearable, flexible array patch	Sweat	Exercise	(i) Characterize sweat (ii) Integrate customized wireless electronics (iii) Simultaneous multiplexed sweat sensing	(i) Large-scale validation (ii) Correlation analysis on blood glucose
Sempionatto et al., 2017	Temporary tattoo	Interstitial fluid	Reverse iontophoresis	(i) No skin irritation (ii) easy to wear (iii) cost effective	(i) Reproducibility and stability (ii) Single use
Tierney et al., 2001	GlucoWatch* biographer	Interstitial fluid	Reverse iontophoresis	(i) Combine data storage and electronics for measurement (ii) Continuous monitoring (iii) First commercialized product (iv) FDA approved	(i) Time lag (ii) Interference by sweat generation (iii) Shorter warming up period (iv) Minimize skin irritation

discussion in existing works (Bandodkar et al., 2014; Emaminejad et al., 2017; Gao et al., 2016; Lee et al., 2016; Lee et al., 2017; Sempionatto et al., 2017; Tierney et al., 2001).

The availability of blood glucose data forms the source for prediction model of blood glucose concentration. Thus, it allows patients to take therapeutic actions on the basis of predicted glycemic levels instead of the current glycemic status, possibly mitigating and avoiding imminent critical events (Svensson et al., 2017; Zecchin et al., 2013). Various algorithms have been proposed for the prediction of hyperglycemic and hypoglycaemic states, for instance multi-model system (Tkachenko et al., 2016), neural network (Zecchin et al., 2016), linear multi-step predictor (Cescon, Johansson,

& Renard, 2015), regression model (Georga et al., 2015), sparse kernel filtering (Yu et al., 2018), non-convex sparse and low-rank based robust subspace segmentation (Cheng et al., 2017) and support vector machine (Gadaleta et al., 2018).

DISCUSSION

This chapter includes five studies with three studies showing significant effects of psyllium supplement which improved glycemic response on either healthy or type 2 diabetes mellitus (T2DM) patients (Abutair et al., 2016; Feinglos et al., 2013; Karhunen et al., 2010). The other two studies did not show significant effect or showed no effect on psyllium supplement alone (De Bock et al., 2012; Pal et al., 2011). Characteristics of the above studies are shown in Table 3.

Positive Effects of Psyllium on Glycemic Control

(A) A randomized control study (Abutair et al., 2016) examined glycemic response after psyllium supplementation among 40 T2DM patients who aged more than 35. These subjects were newly diagnosed with diabetes for maximum 1 year and on antihyperglycemic medication. The subjects were divided into 2 groups; the experimental group took 10.5g daily psyllium whereas the control group continued their regular diet as prescribed before intervention.

After 8 weeks intervention, the experimental group was observed to have an improvement on glycemic response in six parameters. The changes of the parameters from baseline level were as follows; HbA1c (8.5 to 7.5%); fasting blood glucose level (FBG) (163 to 119 mg/dl); insulin level (27.9 to 19.7 μIU/ml); Homeostatic model assessment for insulin resistance (HOMA IR) (11.3 to 5.8); Homeostatic model assessment for β-cell function (HOMA-β) (103 to 141%) and C-peptide (5.8 to 3.8 ng/ml).

- **Strengths:** This study consisted of a dietary stabilization phase which subjects were restricted to follow a prescribed diet for 1 week just before the intervention. This ensured all the subjects having the same diet before the intervention and helped them to maintain the regular diet throughout the study.

In addition, six different parameters for assessing glycemic response were included in this study. It gave a comprehensive assessment on the glycemic effect.

Table 3. Characteristics of studies examining the effect of psyllium supplementation on glycemic control

Study	Study Design	Subjects	n (F, %); Mean Age	Study Country	Treatment Duration	Dose, Meal/ Day, g	Psyllium Dose Form	Glycemic Response Improvement
Positive Effect on Glycemic Control								
Karhunen et al., 2010	R, SB, CX, NC	Healthy adults	16 (81)	Finland	Postpandial	23	Psyllium	Postprandial glucose and insulin level were blunted
Feinglos et al., 2013	R, DB, PG, PC	T2DM patients	37 (32); 36-80	United States	12 weeks	3.4/6.8 & 6.8/13.6	Metamucil	FBG compared to placebo at week 4 (-35.2 & -43.2 mg/dL for 3.4g & 6.8g psyllium), week 8 (-26.1 & -30.9 mg/dL for 3.4g & 6.8g psyllium) and week 12 (-30.6 & -40.7 mg/dL for 3.4g & 6.8g psyllium); HbAlc compared to placebo at week 12 (0.53 & 0.65 for 3.4g & 6.8g psyllium)
Abutair et al., 2016	R, NC	T2DM patients	40 (50); >35	Gaza Strip	8 weeks	7&3.5/ 10.5	Psyllium	Parameters compared to baseline: HbA1c (8.5 to 7.5%); fasting blood glucose level (FBG) (163 to 119 mg/dl); insulin level (27.9 to 19.7 μIU/ml); HOMA IR (11.3 to 5.8); HOMA-β (103 to 141%) and C-peptide (5.8 to 3.8 ng/ml)
No Positive Effect on Glycemic Control								
Pal et al., 2010	R, SB, PG, PC	Over-weight	72 (49)	Australia	12 weeks	12/36	Metamucil	Glucose and insulin of psyllium group do not significantly change compared to baseline (p-value>0.05)
de Bock et al., 2012	R, SB, CX, PC	Healthy	45 (0); 15-16	New Zealand	6 weeks	Flexible/6	Encapsulated psyllium	Glycemic response parameters of psyllium group compared placebo group is not significant: Plasma glucose level (p-value: 0.19); Insulin (p-value: 0.51); Insulin sensitivity (p-value: 0.9)

CX, crossover; DB, double blind; NC, negative controlled (meal alone without added psyllium) PC, placebo controlled; PG, parallel group; R, randomized; SB, single blind

Also, β-cell function and insulin sensitivity accessed by the HOMA model could help to detect the pathophysiology of individuals with glucose intolerance. Thus, HOMA could be a widely used epidemiological and clinical tool for analyzing the effectiveness of the treatment (Wallace et al., 2004).

(B) The study by Feinglos et al. included a total of 37 T2DM patients aged 62 in average (Feinglos et al., 2013). They were assigned into 3 groups i) placebo; ii) 3.4g psyllium twice a day and iii) 6.8g psyllium twice a day, in order to assess the dose response effect of psyllium on glycemic control. In this study, subjects were only allowed to have the restricted diet for 8 weeks before treatment and 12 weeks during treatment period.

After the intervention period, both doses of psyllium in the treatment groups showed significant decrease in FBG compared to placebo at week 4 (-35.2 & -43.2 mg/dL for 3.4g & 6.8g psyllium), week 8 (-26.1 & -30.9 mg/dL for 3.4g & 6.8g psyllium) and week 12 (-30.6 & -40.7 mg/dL for 3.4g & 6.8g psyllium), but not at week 2. Also, HbAlc in these dose groups significantly reduced compared to placebo at week 12 (-0.53% & -0.65%), while only significantly lower in the 6.8g psyllium group (-0.58%) at week 8, but no observable reduction at week 4.

The results suggested psyllium would provide long term positive effect as well as supporting the dose-response hypothesis where higher dose of psyllium would lead to a greater effect. This helps to provide evidence for further studies related to individualizing psyllium therapies for different diabetes stage patients.

- **Strengths:** Both of the above 2 studies adopted a restricted diet for subjects to follow before as well as during the intervention period. In Abutair's study (Abutair et al., 2016), even though the diet in dietary stabilization phase was not designed for any glucose-lowering effect, it would be considered as rather healthy than the usual diet the subjects were having attributable to ethnic issues. Therefore, the results showed in these 2 studies suggested that the beneficial effect of psyllium in glycemic control would be remarkable than just a healthy diet (Abutair et al., 2016) and a regular anti-diabetic medication sulfonylurea (Feinglos et al., 2013) alone.

(C) In a study, 16 healthy young adults were randomized to consume one of the following isoenergetic meals: i) low protein (2.8g) and fiber (7.6g); ii) low protein (2.6g) and high soluble fiber (23g psyllium); iii) high protein (19.7g soy) and low fiber (6.2g); iv) high protein (18.4g) and high soluble fiber (23g psyllium); and v) white wheat bread to investigate the postprandial glucose response (Karhunen et al., 2010).

Plasma glucose and serum insulin concentrations were assessed before and 20, 40, 60, 90 and 120 minutes after the test meal. For subjects having psyllium-enriched diet (group ii and iv), their postprandial glucose and insulin level were blunted for the 120 minutes testing period compared to those having low fiber meals (group i, iii and v).

- **Limitations:** One of the limitations of this study is the representativeness of using insulin as a glycemic response assessing parameter. It is proved that insulin secretion would be stimulated by incretins, like GLP-1 (Holst and Gromada, 2004). However, previous studies have reported inconsistent result on postprandial GLP-1 response, including enhanced (Adam and Westerterp-Plantenga, 2005), reduced (Juntunen et al., 2002), and no effects (Frost et al., 2003; Raben et al., 1994), after a fiber-enriched meal. A study has also shown that diet rich in soy protein would stimulate GLP-1 release compared to a diet rich in carbohydrate (Bowen et al., 2006). The meals prescribed to individuals in this study consist of certain amount of soy protein and this might deviate the result from actual condition.

In addition, it has mentioned that subjects would enjoy a buffet-like meal 2 hours after the test meal, i.e. after the completion of all the assessments, in order to investigate the effect of appetite and subsequent food consumption after the test meals. However, since the subjects knew there would be a feast afterwards, it was possible to have some psychological factors leading to physiological changes in glucose metabolism. This may affect the plasma glucose and serum insulin results.

Moreover, the psyllium dose in this study was rather large, 23g, and it was not practical to have this large amount of psyllium supplementation in daily life. Karhunen stated a study showed no significant effect on insulin or glucose metabolism after consuming 1.7g psyllium-enriched pasta compared to the control pasta (Frost et al., 2003). More recent studies against the proposed effect of psyllium would be discussed in next subsection.

Null Effects of Psyllium on Glycemic Control

(A) A randomized, controlled study that was designed to examined 94 overweight and obese adults concluded that psyllium alone did not provide beneficial effects on glucose control (Pal et al., 2011). Subjects are assigned to consume 4 different treatments including: i) Placebo with their usual diet (as control); ii) 12g psyllium with their usual diet; iii) Placebo with healthy eating regime; and iv) 12g psyllium with healthy eating regime. It is noted that the healthy eating regime was designed by a registered dietitian. Placebo or psyllium was provided 3 times a day before breakfast, lunch and dinner.

After 6 weeks and 12 weeks intervention, there was no significant change of fasting serum glucose between groups. The significant decreases in fasting insulin level were only observed in the group having placebo with healthy eating regime and the group having psyllium with healthy eating regime when compared to the control group and the psyllium with usual diet group at week 6 and week 12, as well as comparing with baseline. The result showed that psyllium supplementation without healthy eating did not alter fasting serum glucose and insulin level after 12 weeks, even the dose is 36g/day.

- **Strength:** Including a healthy diet in this study is advantageous on comparing the degree of efficacy on glycemic control of psyllium and healthy eating regime. Both were commonly thought to be very effective on improving glucose response. Form this study, healthy eating seems to be more effective than psyllium among overweight and obese individuals.
- **Limitation:** The limitation is measuring fasting insulin level as glycemic response. Since the insulin level is highly associated with the degree of obesity and the metabolic syndrome of an individual (Heinonen et al. 2007), there might be factors, which attributed to the physiology of the overweight and obese subjects, affecting insulin level other than the psyllium content of meal solely.

(B) In addition, a recent randomized, single blinded, placebo-controlled study among 47 healthy adolescent showed no significant effects after examination the effect of psyllium on plasma glucose, plasma insulin and insulin sensitivity (De Bock et al., 2012).

Dose of 6g/day psyllium was prescribed to individuals for 6 weeks, followed by 6 week potato starch placebo, or vice versa, with a 2 weeks washout period in between.

- **Strength:** One advantage of this study is a washout period was included. This reduced the variability between subjects since comparison of the intervention was made on the same subject (Jones and Kenward, 2014).
- **Limitations:** Unlike the aforementioned studies (Abutair et al., 2016; Feinglos et al., 2013; Karhunen et al., 2010) that subjects followed a diet restriction, they were advised to continue their ordinary diet in this study. The food intake was recorded by 3-day dietary record, and the physical activity was assessed by Physical Activity Questionnaire. Although the researchers

could closely monitor the diet intake of the individuals, theirs dietary habit might vary and affect the results.

Among the 5 studies mentioned, only this study assessed insulin sensitivity solely. However, insulin sensitivity is not a good parameter on assessing glycemic response since its changes depending on various factors, for instance, the production of short-chain fatty acid (Weickert and Pfeiffer, 2008). Therefore, no effect showed in this study may result from the use of psyllium which is poorly fermented into fatty acid (Bourquin et al., 1993; Campbell and Fahey, 1997).

Furthermore, the way to measure insulin sensitivity is a potential limitation. In this study, an oral glucose tolerance test is used instead of the gold standard method hyperinsulinemic-euglycemic clamp (Tam et al., 2012).

Mechanism of Action

From the above studies, it is possible that psyllium provides beneficial effect on glycemic control, especially in patients with T2DM (Abutair et al., 2016). Numerous studies investigating the effects of psyllium on glycemic control were trying to propose the action of psyllium to human health. One of the possible mechanisms, like other soluble fiber, is it forms a viscous gel-like substance in the intestine, so that it delays the intestinal transit time and helps retard glucose from entering the bloodstream (Bergmann et al., 1992; Braaten et al., 1994; Dikeman and Fahey Jr, 2006).

Advantages of Summarizing Studies

This chapter provides latest scientific evidence on the efficacy of psyllium on glycemic control. From the above studies, psyllium might provide therapeutic effects of diabetes (Abutair et al., 2016). The effect observed in a short period of time with this inexpensive natural food source. This beneficial effect seems to be more significant than healthy diet (Abutair et al., 2016) or anti-diabetic medication sulfonylurea (Feinglos et al., 2013) alone.

Also, it is important to point out that there was no observable adverse effect, especially hypoglycemia, caused by psyllium in these studies, whereas they are common in anti-hyperglycemic agents treatment (Gross et al., 2011). However, further studies have to be done on risk of hypoglycemia when oral anti-hyperglycemic agents and psyllium are taking simultaneously.

Moreover, psyllium provides extra health benefits to diabetes patients, like promoting weight loss and reducing the risk of suffering from cardiovascular disease

(Anderson et al., 2009). Psyllium could be an additional remedy to diabetes patients. This review provides future prospect to public health promotion sectors and food producers on developing effective health food products.

Limitations of Summarizing Studies

As this review included only five studies, the analysis may not be comprehensive enough. Also, it is expected the sample size of each study can be increased in order to obtain more reliable results and conclusions.

These studies worked on different population in different settings. The demography of the subjects was different, like amount of physical activities, the type of diabetes treatment and medication, as well as the weight change of the subjects would influence the result. The duration of intervention was not unified. Also, the assessment parameters of glucose response were not the same, for instance, some studies measured postprandial glucose (Karhunen et al., 2010) and some measured fasting blood glucose (Abutair et al., 2016; Feinglos et al., 2013). Moreover, the measurement methods differed, for example, in de Bock's study, insulin sensitivity was based on Matsuda method (De Bock et al., 2012), while in Abutair's study, insulin sensitivity was represented by HOMA model (Abutair et al., 2016). These variations in different studies cannot draw a comprehensive conclusion based on the above 5 studies.

In addition, there were differences in the carbohydrates compositions of the intervention and control diets in some studies, for example the amount, glycemic index and source of the carbohydrates would affect the results (De Bock et al., 2012; Karhunen et al., 2010; Pal et al., 2011). Another possible limitation is many negative studies were not published (Post et al., 2012). Most of the studies found showed positive effects and it may affect the perception of the author on the effectiveness of psyllium on diabetes.

CONCLUSION

Glycemic monitoring, prediction and control are essential to diabetes sufferers. In conclusion, based on the above five studies, it is believed psyllium might possibly give glycemic response improvement effect, and the effect is greater among T2DM patients. Psyllium before meal has been shown to be a beneficial addition to medications and lifestyle modification on diabetes control (Abutair et al., 2016). Therefore, soluble fiber from psyllium is worth to develop into potential natural dietary supplements or even therapeutic use for T2DM patients. It is possible that food producers could take part in public health promotion via fortification of food with psyllium, in order to slow down the rise of prevalence of diabetes. It is believed that this would also be a breakthrough in food and nutritional aspects that benefits over 350 million T2DM patients worldwide. It is important that more studies should be kept on doing to provide supportive evidence on effect of glycemic control of psyllium. Further studies on dose-effect relationship of psyllium on diabetes could be also done for the development of therapeutic use. Authors agree that disease diagnosis via smart healthcare (Chui et al., 2017) and advanced algorithm techniques (Jotsov, Chui, & Zhu, 2017) and will be the only way to improve quality of life.

REFERENCES

Abutair, A. S., Naser, I. A., & Hamed, A. T. (2016). Soluble fibers from psyllium improve glycemic response and body weight among diabetes type 2 patients (randomized control trial). *Nutrition Journal, 15*(1), 86. doi:10.118612937-016-0207-4 PMID:27733151

Adam, T., & Westerterp-Plantenga, M. (2005). Nutrient-stimulated GLP-1 release in normal-weight men and women. *Hormone and Metabolic Research. Hormon- und Stoffwechselforschung. Hormones et Metabolisme, 37*(2), 111–117. doi:10.1055-2005-861160 PMID:15778929

Anderson, J. W., Baird, P., Davis, R. H. Jr, Ferreri, S., Knudtson, M., Koraym, A., ... Williams, C. L. (2009). Health benefits of dietary fiber. *Nutrition Reviews, 67*(4), 188–205. doi:10.1111/j.1753-4887.2009.00189.x PMID:19335713

Bandodkar, A. J., Jia, W., Yardımcı, C., Wang, X., Ramirez, J., & Wang, J. (2014). Tattoo-based noninvasive glucose monitoring: A proof-of-concept study. *Analytical Chemistry, 87*(1), 394–398. doi:10.1021/ac504300n PMID:25496376

Bergmann, J., Chassany, O., Petit, A., Triki, R., Caulin, C., & Segrestaa, J. (1992). Correlation between echographic gastric emptying and appetite: Influence of psyllium. *Gut, 33*(8), 1042–1043. doi:10.1136/gut.33.8.1042 PMID:1398229

Bourquin, L., Titgemeyer, E., Fahey, G., & Garleb, K. (1993). Fermentation of dietary fibre by human colonic bacteria: Disappearance of, short-chain fatty acid production from, and potential water-holding capacity of, various substrates. *Scandinavian Journal of Gastroenterology, 28*(3), 249–255. doi:10.3109/00365529309096081 PMID:8383353

Bowen, J., Noakes, M., & Clifton, P. M. (2006). Appetite regulatory hormone responses to various dietary proteins differ by body mass index status despite similar reductions in ad libitum energy intake. *The Journal of Clinical Endocrinology and Metabolism*, *91*(8), 2913–2919. doi:10.1210/jc.2006-0609 PMID:16735482

Braaten, J., Scott, F., Wood, P., Riedel, K., Wolynetz, M., Brule, D., & Collins, M. (1994). High β-Glucan Oat Bran and Oat Gum Reduce Postprandial Blood Glucose and Insulin in Subjects With and Without Type 2 Diabetes. *Diabetic Medicine*, *11*(3), 312–318. doi:10.1111/j.1464-5491.1994.tb00277.x PMID:8033532

Campbell, J. M., & Fahey, G. C. Jr. (1997). Psyllium and methylcellulose fermentation properties in relation to insoluble and soluble fiber standards. *Nutrition Research (New York, N.Y.)*, *17*(4), 619–629. doi:10.1016/S0271-5317(97)00034-1

Cescon, M., Johansson, R., & Renard, E. (2015). Subspace-based linear multi-step predictors in type 1 diabetes mellitus. *Biomedical Signal Processing and Control*, *22*, 99–110. doi:10.1016/j.bspc.2014.09.012

Cheng, W., Zhao, M., Xiong, N., & Chui, K. T. (2017). Non-convex sparse and low-rank based robust subspace segmentation for data mining. *Sensors (Basel)*, *17*(7), 1633. doi:10.339017071633 PMID:28714886

Chui, K. T., Alhalabi, W., Pang, S. S. H., Pablos, P. O. D., Liu, R. W., & Zhao, M. (2017). Disease Diagnosis in Smart Healthcare: Innovation, Technologies and Applications. *Sustainability*, *9*(12), 2309. doi:10.3390u9122309

De Bock, M., Derraik, J. G., Brennan, C. M., Biggs, J. B., Smith, G. C., Cameron-Smith, D., ... Cutfield, W. S. (2012). Psyllium supplementation in adolescents improves fat distribution & lipid profile: A randomized, participant-blinded, placebo-controlled, crossover trial. *PLoS One*, *7*(7), e41735. doi:10.1371/journal.pone.0041735 PMID:22848584

Dennison, B. A., & Levine, D. M. (1993). Randomized, double-blind, placebo-controlled, two-period crossover clinical trial of psyllium fiber in children with hypercholesterolemia. *The Journal of Pediatrics*, *123*(1), 24–29. doi:10.1016/S0022-3476(05)81532-X PMID:8391569

Dikeman, C. L., & Fahey, G. C. Jr. (2006). Viscosity as related to dietary fiber: A review. *Critical Reviews in Food Science and Nutrition*, *46*(8), 649–663. doi:10.1080/10408390500511862 PMID:17092830

Emaminejad, S., Gao, W., Wu, E., Davies, Z. A., Nyein, H. Y. Y., Challa, S., ... Talebi, S. (2017). Autonomous sweat extraction and analysis applied to cystic fibrosis and glucose monitoring using a fully integrated wearable platform. *Proceedings of the National Academy of Sciences of the United States of America*, *114*(18), 4625–4630. doi:10.1073/pnas.1701740114 PMID:28416667

Eswaran, S., Muir, J., & Chey, W. D. (2013). Fiber and functional gastrointestinal disorders. *The American Journal of Gastroenterology*, *108*(5), 718–727. doi:10.1038/ajg.2013.63 PMID:23545709

Fagerberg, S. (1982). The Effects of a bulk laxative (Metamucil) on fasting blood-glucose, serum-lipids and other variables in constipated patients with non-insulin dependent adult diabetes. *Current Therapeutic Research, Clinical and Experimental*, *31*, 166–172.

Feinglos, M. N., Gibb, R. D., Ramsey, D. L., Surwit, R. S., & Mcrorie, J. W. (2013). Psyllium improves glycemic control in patients with type-2 diabetes mellitus. *Bioactive Carbohydrates and Dietary Fibre*, *1*(2), 156–161. doi:10.1016/j.bcdf.2013.02.003

Frost, G., Brynes, A., Dhillo, W., Bloom, S., & Mcburney, M. (2003). The effects of fiber enrichment of pasta and fat content on gastric emptying, GLP-1, glucose, and insulin responses to a meal. *European Journal of Clinical Nutrition*, *57*(2), 293–298. doi:10.1038j.ejcn.1601520 PMID:12571662

Gadaleta, M., Facchinetti, A., Grisan, E., & Rossi, M. (2018). Prediction of Adverse Glycemic Events from Continuous Glucose Monitoring Signal. *IEEE Journal of Biomedical and Health Informatics*, 1. doi:10.1109/JBHI.2018.2823763 PMID:29993992

Gao, W., Emaminejad, S., Nyein, H. Y. Y., Challa, S., Chen, K., Peck, A., ... Lien, D. H. (2016). Fully integrated wearable sensor arrays for multiplexed in situ perspiration analysis. *Nature*, *529*(7587), 509–514. doi:10.1038/nature16521 PMID:26819044

Gelissen, I. C., Brodie, B., & Eastwood, M. A. (1994). Effect of Plantago ovata (psyllium) husk and seeds on sterol metabolism: Studies in normal and ileostomy subjects. *The American Journal of Clinical Nutrition*, *59*(2), 395–400. doi:10.1093/ajcn/59.2.395 PMID:8310991

Georga, E. I., Protopappas, V. C., Polyzos, D., & Fotiadis, D. I. (2015). Evaluation of short-term predictors of glucose concentration in type 1 diabetes combining feature ranking with regression models. *Medical & Biological Engineering & Computing*, *53*(12), 1305–1318. doi:10.100711517-015-1263-1 PMID:25773366

Glassman, M., Spark, A., Berezin, S., Schwarz, S., Medow, M., & Newman, L. J. (1990). Treatment of type IIa hyperlipidemia in childhood by a simplified American Heart Association diet and fiber supplementation. *American Journal of Diseases of Children, 144*, 973–976. PMID:2168676

Gross, J., Kramer, C., Leitão, C., Hawkins, N., Viana, L., Schaan, B., ... Azevedo, M. (2011). Diabetes and Endocrinology Meta-analysis Group (DEMA). Effect of antihyperglycemic agents added to metformin and a sulfonylurea on glycemic control and weight gain in type 2 diabetes: A network metaanalysis. *Annals of Internal Medicine, 154*, 672–679. doi:10.7326/0003-4819-154-10-201105170-00007 PMID:21576535

Guariguata, L., Whiting, D., Hambleton, I., Beagley, J., Linnenkamp, U., & Shaw, J. (2014). Global estimates of diabetes prevalence for 2013 and projections for 2035. *Diabetes Research and Clinical Practice, 103*(2), 137–149. doi:10.1016/j.diabres.2013.11.002 PMID:24630390

Gupta, R., Agrawal, C., Singh, G., & Ghatak, A. (1994). Lipid-lowering efficacy of psyllium hydrophilic mucilloid in non insulin dependent diabetes mellitus with hyperlipidaemia. *The Indian Journal of Medical Research, 100*, 237–241. PMID:7829159

Heinonen, M. V., Karhunen, L. J., Chabot, E. D., Toppinen, L. K., Juntunen, K. S., Laaksonen, D. E., ... Niskanen, L. K. (2007). Plasma ghrelin levels after two high-carbohydrate meals producing different insulin responses in patients with metabolic syndrome. *Regulatory Peptides, 138*(2-3), 118–125. doi:10.1016/j.regpep.2006.08.011 PMID:17030069

Holst, J. J., & Gromada, J. (2004). Role of incretin hormones in the regulation of insulin secretion in diabetic and nondiabetic humans. *American Journal of Physiology. Endocrinology and Metabolism, 287*(2), E199–E206. doi:10.1152/ajpendo.00545.2003 PMID:15271645

Jenkins, D., Wolever, T., Leeds, A. R., Gassull, M. A., Haisman, P., Dilawari, J., ... Alberti, K. (1978). Dietary fibres, fibre analogues, and glucose tolerance: Importance of viscosity. *British Medical Journal, 1*(6124), 1392–1394. doi:10.1136/bmj.1.6124.1392 PMID:647304

Jones, B., & Kenward, M. G. (2014). *Design and analysis of cross-over trials*. CRC Press.

Jotsov, V., Chui, K. T., & Zhu, H. (2017). Guest Editorial: Advanced Algorithms and Techniques for Engineering Applications. *Journal of Internet Technology*, *18*, 645–646.

Juntunen, K. S., Niskanen, L. K., Liukkonen, K. H., Poutanen, K. S., Holst, J. J., & Mykkänen, H. M. (2002). Postprandial glucose, insulin, and incretin responses to grain products in healthy subjects. *The American Journal of Clinical Nutrition*, *75*(2), 254–262. doi:10.1093/ajcn/75.2.254 PMID:11815315

Karhunen, L. J., Juvonen, K. R., Flander, S. M., Liukkonen, K.-H., Lähteenmäki, L., Siloaho, M., ... Poutanen, K. S. (2010). A psyllium fiber-enriched meal strongly attenuates postprandial gastrointestinal peptide release in healthy young adults. *The Journal of Nutrition*, *140*(4), 737–744. doi:10.3945/jn.109.115436 PMID:20147463

Kim, J., Campbell, A. S., & Wang, J. (2018). Wearable non-invasive epidermal glucose sensors: A review. *Talanta*, *177*, 163–170. doi:10.1016/j.talanta.2017.08.077 PMID:29108571

Lee, H., Choi, T. K., Lee, Y. B., Cho, H. R., Ghaffari, R., Wang, L., ... Choi, S. H. (2016). A graphene-based electrochemical device with thermoresponsive microneedles for diabetes monitoring and therapy. *Nature Nanotechnology*, *11*(6), 566–572. doi:10.1038/nnano.2016.38 PMID:26999482

Lee, H., Song, C., Hong, Y. S., Kim, M. S., Cho, H. R., Kang, T., ... Kim, D. H. (2017). Wearable/disposable sweat-based glucose monitoring device with multistage transdermal drug delivery module. *Science Advances*, *3*(3), e1601314. doi:10.1126ciadv.1601314 PMID:28345030

Luther, J., & Chey, W. D. (2010). Psyllium increased symptom relief in patients with the irritable bowel syndrome more than bran or placebo. *Annals of Internal Medicine*, 152. PMID:20083814

Mcrorie, J. W. Jr. (2015). Evidence-based approach to fiber supplements and clinically meaningful health benefits, part 2: What to look for and how to recommend an effective fiber therapy. *Nutrition Today*, *50*(2), 90–97. doi:10.1097/NT.0000000000000089 PMID:25972619

Mcrorie, J. W., & Fahey, G. C. (2013). A review of gastrointestinal physiology and the mechanisms underlying the health benefits of dietary fiber: Matching an effective fiber with specific patient needs. *Clinical Nursing Studies*, *1*(4), 82. doi:10.5430/cns.v1n4p82

Pal, S., Khossousi, A., Binns, C., Dhaliwal, S., & Ellis, V. (2011). The effect of a fibre supplement compared to a healthy diet on body composition, lipids, glucose, insulin and other metabolic syndrome risk factors in overweight and obese individuals. *British Journal of Nutrition*, *105*(01), 90–100. doi:10.1017/S0007114510003132 PMID:20727237

Pastors, J. G., Blaisdell, P. W., Balm, T. K., Asplin, C. M., & Pohl, S. L. (1991). Psyllium fiber reduces rise in postprandial glucose and insulin concentrations in patients with non-insulin-dependent diabetes. *The American Journal of Clinical Nutrition*, *53*(6), 1431–1435. doi:10.1093/ajcn/53.6.1431 PMID:1852093

Post, R. E., Mainous, A. G., King, D. E., & Simpson, K. N. (2012). Dietary fiber for the treatment of type 2 diabetes mellitus: A meta-analysis. *Journal of the American Board of Family Medicine*, *25*(1), 16–23. doi:10.3122/jabfm.2012.01.110148 PMID:22218620

Raben, A., Christensen, N. J., Madsen, J., Holst, J. J., & Astrup, A. (1994). Decreased postprandial thermogenesis and fat oxidation but increased fullness after a high-fiber meal compared with a low-fiber meal. *The American Journal of Clinical Nutrition*, *59*(6), 1386–1394. doi:10.1093/ajcn/59.6.1386 PMID:8198065

Sempionatto, J. R., Nakagawa, T., Pavinatto, A., Mensah, S. T., Imani, S., Mercier, P., & Wang, J. (2017). Eyeglasses based wireless electrolyte and metabolite sensor platform. *Lab on a Chip*, *17*(10), 1834–1842. doi:10.1039/C7LC00192D PMID:28470263

Singh, B. (2007). Psyllium as therapeutic and drug delivery agent. *International Journal of Pharmaceutics*, *334*(1-2), 1–14. doi:10.1016/j.ijpharm.2007.01.028 PMID:17329047

Svensson, E., Baggesen, L. M., Johnsen, S. P., Pedersen, L., Nørrelund, H., Buhl, E. S., ... Thomsen, R. W. (2017). Early glycemic control and magnitude of HbA1c reduction predict cardiovascular events and mortality: Population-based cohort study of 24,752 metformin initiators. *Diabetes Care*. PMID:28404659

Tam, C. S., Xie, W., Johnson, W. D., Cefalu, W. T., Redman, L. M., & Ravussin, E. (2012). Defining insulin resistance from hyperinsulinemic-euglycemic clamps. *Diabetes Care*, *35*(7), 1605–1610. doi:10.2337/dc11-2339 PMID:22511259

Taneja, A., Bhat, C., Arora, A., & Kaur, A. (1989). Effect of incorporation of isabgol husk in a low fibre diet on faecal excretion and serum levels of lipids in adolescent girls. *European Journal of Clinical Nutrition*, *43*, 197. PMID:2543555

Tierney, M. J., Tamada, J. A., Potts, R. O., Jovanovic, L., & Garg, S. (2001). Clinical evaluation of the GlucoWatch® biographer: A continual, non-invasive glucose monitor for patients with diabetes. *Biosensors & Bioelectronics*, *16*(9-12), 621–629. doi:10.1016/S0956-5663(01)00189-0 PMID:11679237

Tkachenko, P., Kriukova, G., Aleksandrova, M., Chertov, O., Renard, E., & Pereverzyev, S. V. (2016). Prediction of nocturnal hypoglycemia by an aggregation of previously known prediction approaches: Proof of concept for clinical application. *Computer Methods and Programs in Biomedicine*, *134*, 179–186. doi:10.1016/j.cmpb.2016.07.003 PMID:27480742

Trumbo, P., Schlicker, S., Yates, A. A., & Poos, M. (2002). Dietary reference intakes for energy, carbohydrate, fiber, fat, fatty acids, cholesterol, protein and amino acids. *Journal of the American Dietetic Association*, *102*(11), 1621–1630. doi:10.1016/S0002-8223(02)90346-9 PMID:12449285

Wallace, T. M., Levy, J. C., & Matthews, D. R. (2004). Use and abuse of HOMA modeling. *Diabetes Care*, *27*(6), 1487–1495. doi:10.2337/diacare.27.6.1487 PMID:15161807

Wang, H. C., & Lee, A. R. (2015). Recent developments in blood glucose sensors. *Journal of Food and Drug Analysis*, *23*(2), 191–200. doi:10.1016/j.jfda.2014.12.001 PMID:28911373

Weickert, M. O., & Pfeiffer, A. F. (2008). Metabolic effects of dietary fiber consumption and prevention of diabetes. *The Journal of Nutrition*, *138*(3), 439–442. doi:10.1093/jn/138.3.439 PMID:18287346

World Health Organization. (2016). Global report on diabetes.

Yu, X., Rashid, M., Feng, J., Hobbs, N., Hajizadeh, I., Samadi, S., ... Quinn, L. (2018). Online Glucose Prediction Using Computationally Efficient Sparse Kernel Filtering Algorithms in Type-1 Diabetes. *IEEE Transactions on Control Systems Technology*, *99*, 1–13.

Zecchin, C., Facchinetti, A., Sparacino, G., & Cobelli, C. (2013). Reduction of number and duration of hypoglycemic events by glucose prediction methods: A proof-of-concept in silico study. *Diabetes Technology & Therapeutics*, *15*(1), 66–77. doi:10.1089/dia.2012.0208 PMID:23297671

Zecchin, C., Facchinetti, A., Sparacino, G., & Cobelli, C. (2016). How much is short-term glucose prediction in type 1 diabetes improved by adding insulin delivery and meal content information to CGM data? A proof-of-concept study. *Journal of Diabetes Science and Technology*, *10*(5), 1149–1160. doi:10.1177/1932296816654161 PMID:27381030

Compilation of References

Aasman, J., Mulder, J., & Mulder, L. J. M. (1987). Operator effort and the measurement of heartrate variability. *Human Factors*, *29*(2), 161–170. doi:10.1177/001872088702900204 PMID:3610181

Abramson, E. L., Patel, V., Malhotra, S., Pfoh, E. R., Osorio, S. N., Cheriff, A., ... Kaushal, R. (2012). Physician experiences transitioning between an older versus newer electronic health record for electronic prescribing. *International Journal of Medical Informatics*, *81*(8), 539–548. doi:10.1016/j.ijmedinf.2012.02.010 PMID:22465355

Abutair, A. S., Naser, I. A., & Hamed, A. T. (2016). Soluble fibers from psyllium improve glycemic response and body weight among diabetes type 2 patients (randomized control trial). *Nutrition Journal*, *15*(1), 86. doi:10.118612937-016-0207-4 PMID:27733151

Adam, T., & Westerterp-Plantenga, M. (2005). Nutrient-stimulated GLP-1 release in normal-weight men and women. *Hormone and Metabolic Research. Hormon- und Stoffwechselforschung. Hormones et Metabolisme*, *37*(2), 111–117. doi:10.1055-2005-861160 PMID:15778929

Adebayo, K., & Edward, O. (2014). Issues on E-health Adoption in Nigeria. *International Journal of Modern Education and Computer Science*, *6*(9), 36–46. doi:10.5815/ijmecs.2014.09.06

Adeyemi, A., & Ayegboyin, M. (2004). A study on the use of information systems to prevent HIV/AIDS in Lagos state, Nigeria. *Paper presented at 3rd Virtual Congress in Internet Informedica: Information and Communication Technologies in Healthcare Development.*

Adler-Milstein, J., DesRoches, C. M., Kravolec, P., Foster, G., Worzala, C., Charles, D., ... Jha, A. K. (2015). Electronic health record adoption in US hospitals: Progress continues, but challenges persist. *Health Affairs*, *34*(11). doi:10.1377/hlthaff.2015.0992 PMID:26561387

Afolayan, A., & Oyekunle, S. (2014). Availability, Accessibility and Frequency of Use of ICT Tools by Health Professionals in Ilorin Metropolis. *Covenant Journal of Informatics and Communication Technology*, *2*(1), 1–15.

Ajuwon, G. (2006). Use of the Internet for health information by physicians for patient care in a teaching hospital in Ibadan, Nigeria. *Biomedical Digital Libraries*, *3*(12), 1–9. PMID:17163991

Akadiri, O.A., Olusanya, A.A., & Omitola, O.O. (2009). Impact of Improved Telecommunication Services on Health Care Delivery in Nigerian Teaching Hospitals – A Survey of Opinions. *Journal of Information Technology Impact*, *9*(3), 125–134.

Alexander, A. G., & Ballou, K. A. (2018). Work-Life Balance, Burnout, and the Electronic Health Record. *The American Journal of Medicine*, *131*(8), 857–858. doi:10.1016/j.amjmed.2018.02.033 PMID:29608876

Anderson, D. M., Asher, L. M., Whitler, E. T., & Wilson, E. A. (2007). Physician computer skills: A prerequisite to the future in healthcare services. *The Journal of the Kentucky Medical Association*, *105*, 67–71. PMID:17390734

Anderson, J. W., Baird, P., Davis, R. H. Jr, Ferreri, S., Knudtson, M., Koraym, A., ... Williams, C. L. (2009). Health benefits of dietary fiber. *Nutrition Reviews*, *67*(4), 188–205. doi:10.1111/j.1753-4887.2009.00189.x PMID:19335713

Antel, S. B., Li, L. M., Cendes, F., Collins, D. L., Kearney, R. E., Shinghal, R., & Arnold, D. L. (2002). Predicting surgical outcome in temporal lobe epilepsy patients using MRI and MRSI. *Neurology*, *58*(10), 1505–1512. doi:10.1212/WNL.58.10.1505 PMID:12034787

Anticevic, A., Murray, J. D., & Barch, D. M. (2015). Bridging levels of understanding in schizophrenia through computational modeling. *Clinical Psychological Science*, *3*(3), 433–459. doi:10.1177/2167702614562041 PMID:25960938

Antoniou, G., & van Harmelen, F. (2004). *Semantic Web Primer*. The MIT Press.

Appelbaum, P. S., & Kopelman, A. (2014). Social media's challenges for psychiatry. *World Psychiatry; Official Journal of the World Psychiatric Association (WPA)*, *13*(1), 21–23. doi:10.1002/wps.20085 PMID:24497238

Applebaum, A. (2001). The constant customer. *Gallup Management Journal*, *17*, 1–5.

Armañanzas, R., Alonso-Nanclares, L., DeFelipe-Oroquieta, J., Kastanauskaite, A., de Sola, R. G., DeFelipe, J., ... Larrañaga, P. (2013). Machine learning approach for the outcome prediction of temporal lobe epilepsy surgery. *PLoS One*, *8*(4), e62819. doi:10.1371/journal.pone.0062819 PMID:23646148

Armon, C., Radtke, R. A., Friedman, A. H., & Dawson, D. V. (1996). Predictors of outcome of epilepsy surgery: Multivariate analysis with validation. *Epilepsia*, *37*(9), 814–821. doi:10.1111/j.1528-1157.1996.tb00033.x PMID:8814093

Arndt, B. G., Beasley, J. W., Watkinson, M. D., Temte, J. L., Tuan, W. J., Sinsky, C. A., & Gilchrist, V. J. (2017). Tethered to the EHR: Primary care physician workload assessment using EHR event log data and time-motion observations. *Annals of Family Medicine*, *15*(5), 419–426. doi:10.1370/afm.2121 PMID:28893811

Arrieux, J. P., Cole, W. R., & Ahrens, A. P. (2017). A review of the validity of computerized neurocognitive assessment tools in mild traumatic brain injury assessment. *Concussion*, *2*(1). doi:10.2217/cnc-2016-0021 PMID:30202572

Arudino. (2005). Arudino. http://www.arduino.cc/

Asanganasi, I. A. (2008, January). Computer use among doctors in Africa: Survey of trainees in a Nigerian teaching hospital. *Journal of Health Informatics in Developing Countries*, *2*(1), 10–14.

Asaro, P. V., & Boxerman, S. B. (2008). Effects of computerized provider order entry and nursing documentation on workflow. *Academic Emergency Medicine*, *15*(10), 908–915. doi:10.1111/j.1553-2712.2008.00235.x PMID:18785946

Ash, J. S., & Bates, D. W. (2005). Factors and forces affecting EHR system adoption: Report of a 2004 ACMI discussion. *Journal of the American Informatics Association*, *12*(1), 8–12. doi:10.1197/jamia.M1684 PMID:15492027

Atherton, J. S. (2003). *Competence, proficiency and beyond*. Retrieved from http://www.doceo.co.uk/background/expertise.htm

Audet, A., Doty, M. M., Peugh, J., Shamasdin, J., Zapert, K., & Schoenbaum, S. (2004). Information technology: When will they make it into physicians' black bags? *Medscape General Medicine*, *6*(4), 2–16. PMID:15775829

Auffray, C., Charron, D., & Hood, L. (2010). Predictive, preventive, personalized and participatory medicine: Back to the future. *Genome Medicine*, *2*(8), 57. doi:10.1186/gm178 PMID:20804580

Balasubramanian, R., Houseman, E. A., Coull, B. A., Lev, M. H., Schwamm, L. H., & Betensky, R. A. (2014). Variable importance in matched case-control studies in settings of high dimensional data. *Applied Statistics*, *63*(4), 639–655. doi:10.1111/rssc.12056

Baltagi, B. H., Lagravinese, R., Moscone, F., & Tosetti, E. (2017). Health care expenditure and income: A global perspective. *Health Economics*, *26*(7), 863–874. doi:10.1002/hec.3424 PMID:27679983

Bandodkar, A. J., Jia, W., Yardımcı, C., Wang, X., Ramirez, J., & Wang, J. (2014). Tattoo-based noninvasive glucose monitoring: A proof-of-concept study. *Analytical Chemistry*, *87*(1), 394–398. doi:10.1021/ac504300n PMID:25496376

Bandrowski, A., Brinkman, R., Brochhausen, M., Brush, M. H., Bug, B., & Chibucos, M. C. … Zheng, J. (2016). The Ontology for Biomedical Investigations. *PLoS One*. doi:10.1371/journal.pone.0154556

Bauer, R. M., Iverson, G. I., Cernich, A. N., Binder, L. M., Ruff, R. M., & Naugle, R. I. (2012). Computerized Neuropsychological Assessment Devices: Joint Position Paper of the American Academy of Clinical Neuropsychology and the National Academy of Neuropsychology. *Archives of Clinical Neuropsychology*, *27*(3), 362–373. doi:10.1093/arclin/acs027 PMID:22382386

Bello, S. M., Shimoyama, M., Mitraka, E., Laulederkind, S. J. F., Smith, C. L., Eppig, J. T., & Schriml, L. M. (2018). Disease Ontology: Improving and unifying disease annotations across species. *Disease Models & Mechanisms*, *11*(3), dmm032839. doi:10.1242/dmm.032839 PMID:29590633

Benner, P. (2004). Using the Dreyfus model of skill acquisition to describe and interpret skill acquisition and clinical judgment in nursing practice and education. *Bulletin of Science, Technology & Society*, *24*(3), 188–199. doi:10.1177/0270467604265061

Berg, A. T., Walczak, T., Hirsch, L. J., & Spencer, S. S. (1998). Multivariable prediction of seizure outcome one year after resective epilepsy surgery: Development of a model with independent validation. *Epilepsy Research*, *29*(3), 185–194. doi:10.1016/S0920-1211(97)00083-1 PMID:9551780

Berg, M. (2001). Implementing information systems in health care organizations: Myths and challenges. *International Journal of Medical Informatics*, *64*(2), 143–156. doi:10.1016/S1386-5056(01)00200-3 PMID:11734382

Bergman, L. G., & Fors, U. G. H. (2008). Decision support in psychiatry– A comparison between the diagnostic outcomes using a computerized decision support system versus manual diagnosis. *BMC Medical Informatics and Decision Making*, *8*(1), 9. doi:10.1186/1472-6947-8-9 PMID:18261222

Bergmann, J., Chassany, O., Petit, A., Triki, R., Caulin, C., & Segrestaa, J. (1992). Correlation between echographic gastric emptying and appetite: Influence of psyllium. *Gut*, *33*(8), 1042–1043. doi:10.1136/gut.33.8.1042 PMID:1398229

Berner, E. S. (2016). *Clinical decision support systems. Theory and practice* (3rd ed.). Basel: Springer International Publishing.

Berner, E. S., Detmer, D. E., & Simborg, D. (2005). Will the wave finally break? A brief view of the adoption of electronic medical records in the United States. *Journal of the American Medical Informatics Association*, *12*(1), 3–7. doi:10.1197/jamia.M1664 PMID:15492029

Berners-Lee, T., Hendler, J., & Lassila, O. (2001). The Semantic Web. *Scientific American*, *284*(5), 34–43. doi:10.1038cientificamerican0501-34 PMID:11323639

Blumenthal, D. (2009). Stimulating the adoption of health information technology. *The New England Journal of Medicine*, *360*(15), 1477–1479. doi:10.1056/NEJMp0901592 PMID:19321856

Blumenthal, D. (2011a). Wiring the health system – Origins and provisions of a new federal program (Part One of Two). *The New England Journal of Medicine*, *365*(24), 2323–2329. doi:10.1056/NEJMsr1110507 PMID:22168647

Blumenthal, D. (2011b). Implementation of the federal health information technology initiative (Part Two of Two). *The New England Journal of Medicine*, *365*(54), 2426–2431. doi:10.1056/NEJMsr1112158 PMID:22187990

Blumenthal, D. (2017). Realizing the value (and profitability) of digital health data. *Annals of Internal Medicine*, *166*(11), 842–843. doi:10.7326/M17-0511 PMID:28462419

Borangíu, T., & Purcarea, V. (2008). The future of healthcare-Information based medicine. *Journal of Medicine and Life*, *1*, 233–237. PMID:20108471

Bourquin, L., Titgemeyer, E., Fahey, G., & Garleb, K. (1993). Fermentation of dietary fibre by human colonic bacteria: Disappearance of, short-chain fatty acid production from, and potential water-holding capacity of, various substrates. *Scandinavian Journal of Gastroenterology*, *28*(3), 249–255. doi:10.3109/00365529309096081 PMID:8383353

Bovier, P. A., & Perneger, T. V. (2003). Predictors of work satisfaction among physicians. *European Journal of Public Health*, *13*(4), 299–305. doi:10.1093/eurpub/13.4.299 PMID:14703315

Bowen, J., Noakes, M., & Clifton, P. M. (2006). Appetite regulatory hormone responses to various dietary proteins differ by body mass index status despite similar reductions in ad libitum energy intake. *The Journal of Clinical Endocrinology and Metabolism*, *91*(8), 2913–2919. doi:10.1210/jc.2006-0609 PMID:16735482

Braaten, J., Scott, F., Wood, P., Riedel, K., Wolynetz, M., Brule, D., & Collins, M. (1994). High β-Glucan Oat Bran and Oat Gum Reduce Postprandial Blood Glucose and Insulin in Subjects With and Without Type 2 Diabetes. *Diabetic Medicine*, *11*(3), 312–318. doi:10.1111/j.1464-5491.1994.tb00277.x PMID:8033532

Brennan, M. G., & Coles, C. (2003). Developing professional skills. *Lancet*, *362*(9394), 1506. doi:10.1016/S0140-6736(03)14716-2 PMID:14602462

Buntin, M. B., Jain, S. H., & Blumenthal, D. (2010). Health information technology: Laying the infrastructure for national health reform. *Health Affairs*, *29*(6), 1214–1219. doi:10.1377/hlthaff.2010.0503 PMID:20530358

Burez, J., & Van den Poel, D. (2009). Handling class imbalance in customer churn prediction. *Expert Systems with Applications*, *36*(3), 4626–4636. doi:10.1016/j.eswa.2008.05.027

Cameron, J. D., Ramaprasad, A., & Syn, T. (2017). An ontology of and roadmap for mHealth research. *International Journal of Medical Informatics*, *100*, 16–25. doi:10.1016/j.ijmedinf.2017.01.007 PMID:28241934

Campbell, J. M., & Fahey, G. C. Jr. (1997). Psyllium and methylcellulose fermentation properties in relation to insoluble and soluble fiber standards. *Nutrition Research (New York, N.Y.)*, *17*(4), 619–629. doi:10.1016/S0271-5317(97)00034-1

Carlton, E. L., Holsinger, J. W. Jr, & Anunobi, N. (2016). Physician engagement with health information technology: Implications for practice and professionalism. *International Journal of Computers in Clinical Practice*, *1*(2), 51–73. doi:10.4018/IJCCP.2016070103

Cescon, M., Johansson, R., & Renard, E. (2015). Subspace-based linear multi-step predictors in type 1 diabetes mellitus. *Biomedical Signal Processing and Control*, *22*, 99–110. doi:10.1016/j.bspc.2014.09.012

Chan, J. Y. C., Kwong, J. S. W., Wong, A., Kwok, T. C. Y., & Tsoi, K. K. F. (2018). Comparison of Computerized and Paper-and-Pencil Memory Tests in Detection of Mild Cognitive Impairment and Dementia: A Systematic Review and Meta-analysis of Diagnostic Studies. *Journal of the American Medical Directors Association*, *19*(9), 748–756. doi:10.1016/j.jamda.2018.05.010 PMID:29921507

Cheng, W., Zhao, M., Xiong, N., & Chui, K. T. (2017). Non-convex sparse and low-rank based robust subspace segmentation for data mining. *Sensors (Basel)*, *17*(7), 1633. doi:10.339017071633 PMID:28714886

Chowdhury, G. G. (2003). Natural language processing. *Annual Review of Information Science & Technology*, *37*(1), 51–89. doi:10.1002/aris.1440370103

Chui, K. T., Alhalabi, W., Pang, S. S. H., Pablos, P. O. D., Liu, R. W., & Zhao, M. (2017). Disease Diagnosis in Smart Healthcare: Innovation, Technologies and Applications. *Sustainability*, *9*(12), 2309. doi:10.3390u9122309

Chui, M., Löffler, M., & Roberts, R. (2010). The internet of things. *The McKinsey Quarterly*, *2*, 1–9.

Clusmann, H., Schramm, J., Kral, T., Helmstaedter, C., Ostertun, B., Fimmers, R., ... Elger, C. E. (2002). Prognostic factors and outcome after different types of resection for temporal lobe epilepsy. *Journal of Neurosurgery*, *97*(5), 1131–1141. doi:10.3171/jns.2002.97.5.1131 PMID:12450036

Cohen, R., Aviram, I., Elhadad, M., & Elhadad, N. (2014). Redundancy-aware topic modeling for patient record notes. *PLoS One*, *9*(2), e87555. doi:10.1371/journal.pone.0087555 PMID:24551060

Collerton, J., Barrass, K., Bond, J., Eccles, M., Jagger, C., James, O., ... Kirkwood, T. (2007). The Newcastle 85+ study: biological, clinical and psychosocial factors associated with healthy ageing: Study protocol. *BMC Geriatrics*, *7*(1), 14. doi:10.1186/1471-2318-7-14 PMID:17594470

Collie, A., Maruff, P., Makdissi, M., McCrory, P., McStephen, M., & Darby, D. (2003). CogSport: Reliability and correlation with conventional cognitive tests used in postconcussion medical evaluations. *Clinical Journal of Sport Medicine*, *13*(1), 28–32. doi:10.1097/00042752-200301000-00006 PMID:12544161

Collins, A. M., & Loftus, E. F. (1975). A spreading-activation theory of semantic processing. *Psychological Review*, *82*(6), 407–428. doi:10.1037/0033-295X.82.6.407

Cook, A., Cotteleer, M., & Holdowsky, J. (2018). *Digital reality – A technical primer*. Deloitte Insights.

Coussement, K., Lessmann, S., & Verstraeten, G. (2017). A comparative analysis of data preparation algorithms for customer churn prediction: A case study in the telecommunication industry. *Decision Support Systems*, *95*, 27–36. doi:10.1016/j.dss.2016.11.007

Coussement, K., & Van den Poel, D. (2008). Churn prediction in subscription services: An application of support vector machines while comparing two parameter-selection techniques. *Expert Systems with Applications*, *34*(1), 313–327. doi:10.1016/j.eswa.2006.09.038

Cox, J., King, J., Hutchinson, A., & McAvoy, P. (2006). *Understanding doctors' performance*. Oxford: Radcliffe Publishing.

Cybulski, G. R. (2014). Engaging Doctors in the Health Care Revolution. *Harvard Business Review*, *92*(10), 20–20. Retrieved from https://hbr.org/2014/06/engaging-doctors-in-the-health-care-revolution PMID:25051859

Davey, S., & Davey, A. (2014). Assessment of smartphone addiction in Indian adolescents: A mixed method study by systematic review and metaanalysis approach. *International Journal of Preventive Medicine*, *5*(12), 1500–1511. PMID:25709785

De Bock, M., Derraik, J. G., Brennan, C. M., Biggs, J. B., Smith, G. C., Cameron-Smith, D., ... Cutfield, W. S. (2012). Psyllium supplementation in adolescents improves fat distribution & lipid profile: A randomized, participant-blinded, placebo-controlled, crossover trial. *PLoS One*, *7*(7), e41735. doi:10.1371/journal.pone.0041735 PMID:22848584

De Maio, C., Loia, V., Fenza, G., Gallo, M., Linciano, R., & Morrone, A. (2011). Fuzzy knowledge approach to automatic disease diagnosis. In *IEEE International Conference on Fuzzy Systems*. 10.1109/FUZZY.2011.6007498

Dechant, A., Spann, M., & Becker, J. U. (2018). Positive Customer Churn: An Application to Online Dating. *Journal of Service Research.*

Demkow, U., & Wolanczyk, T. (2017). Genetic tests in major psychiatric disorders–integrating molecular medicine with clinical psychiatry–why is it so difficult? *Translational Psychiatry*, *7*(6), e1151. doi:10.1038/tp.2017.106 PMID:28608853

Dennison, B. A., & Levine, D. M. (1993). Randomized, double-blind, placebo-controlled, two-period crossover clinical trial of psyllium fiber in children with hypercholesterolemia. *The Journal of Pediatrics*, *123*(1), 24–29. doi:10.1016/S0022-3476(05)81532-X PMID:8391569

Deslich, S., Stec, B., Tomblin, S., & Coustasse, A. (2013). Telepsychiatry in the 21st century: Transforming healthcare with technology. *Perspectives in Health Information Management, 10*, Article 1f.

DesRoches, C. M., Campbell, E. G., Rao, S. R., Donelan, K., Ferris, T. G., Jha, A., ... Blumenthal, D. (2008). Electronic health records in ambulatory care: A national survey of physicians. *The New England Journal of Medicine*, *359*(1), 50–60. doi:10.1056/NEJMsa0802005 PMID:18565855

Dhamankar, R., Lee, Y., Doan, A., Halevy, A., & Domingos, P. (2004). iMAP: discovering complex semantic matches between database schemas. In *Proceedings of the 2004 ACM SIGMOD International Conference on Management of Data - SIGMOD '04* (pp. 383–394). 10.1145/1007568.1007612

Dikeman, C. L., & Fahey, G. C. Jr. (2006). Viscosity as related to dietary fiber: A review. *Critical Reviews in Food Science and Nutrition*, *46*(8), 649–663. doi:10.1080/10408390500511862 PMID:17092830

Dimick, M., Hall, M. A., Madison, K., Painter, M., Rodwin, M., Rosenbaum, S., & Tomes, N. J. (2010). *Medical professionalism in the new information age*. Rutgers University Press.

Doebbeling, B. N., Vaughn, T. E., McCoy, K. D., & Glassman, P. (2006). Informatics implementation in the Veterans Health Administration (VHA) Healthcare System to improve quality of care. In *AMIA 2006 Symposium Proceedings* (pp. 204-208). Bethesda: AMIA.

Do, H.-H., & Rahm, E. (2002). COMA: a system for flexible combination of schema matching approaches. In *Proceedings of the 28th international conference on Very Large Data Bases* (pp. 610–621). 10.1016/B978-155860869-6/50060-3

Doyle, R. J., Wang, N., Anthony, D., Borkan, J., Shield, R. R., & Goldman, R. E. (2012). Computers in the examination room and the electronic health record: Physicians' perceived impact on clinical encounters before and after full installation and implementation. *Family Practice*, *29*(5), 601–608. doi:10.1093/fampra/cms015 PMID:22379185

Dreyfus, H. L. (manuscript). *A phenomenology of skill acquisition as the basis for a Merleau-Pontian non-representationalist cognitive science*. Retrieved from http://socrates.berkeley.edu/~hdreyfus/pdf.MerieauPontySkillCogSci.pdf

Dreyfus, H. L. (2002). Intelligence without representation – Merleau-Ponty's critique of mental representation. *Phenomenology and the Cognitive Sciences*, *1*(4), 367–383. doi:10.1023/A:1021351606209

Dreyfus, H. L., & Dreyfus, S. E. (1986). *Mind over machine: The power of human intuition and expertise in the era of the computer*. New York: Free Press.

Duffield, C. M., Roche, M. A., Dimitrelis, S., Homer, C., & Buchan, J. (2015). Instability in patient and nurse characteristics, unit complexity and patient and system outcomes. *Journal of Advanced Nursing*, *71*(6), 1288–1298. doi:10.1111/jan.12597 PMID:25511970

Duffield, C., Diers, D., Aisbett, C., & Roche, M. (2009). Churn: Patient turnover and case mix. *Nursing Economics*, *27*(3), 185. PMID:19558079

Duffield, C., Diers, D., O'Brien-Pallas, L., Aisbett, C., Roche, M., King, M., & Aisbett, K. (2011). Nursing staffing, nursing workload, the work environment and patient outcomes. *Applied Nursing Research*, *24*(4), 244–255. doi:10.1016/j.apnr.2009.12.004 PMID:20974086

Duffield, C., Roche, M., Diers, D., Catling-Paull, C., & Blay, N. (2010). Staffing, skill mix and the model of care. *Journal of Clinical Nursing*, *19*(15-16), 2242–2251. doi:10.1111/j.1365-2702.2010.03225.x PMID:20659202

Dumontier, M., Baker, C. J. O., Baran, J., Callahan, A., Chepelev, L., & Cruz-Toledo, J. … Hoehndorf, R. (2014). The semanticscience integrated ontology (SIO) for biomedical research and knowledge discovery. *Journal of Biomedical Semantics*. doi:10.1186/2041-1480-5-14

Duncan, J., Bundesen, C., Olson, A., Humphreys, G., Chavda, S., & Shibuya, H. (1999). Systematic analysis of deficits in visual attention. *Journal of Experimental Psychology. General*, *128*(4), 450–478. doi:10.1037/0096-3445.128.4.450 PMID:10650583

Dziuda, D. M. (2010). *Data mining for genomics and proteomics: Analysis of gene and protein expression data*. New York, NY: Wiley. doi:10.1002/9780470593417

Ekene, E. A. (2014). ICT adoption in logistics operations: An emerging trend for sustainable development and human capacity building in South-Eastern Nigeria. *Journal of Emerging Trends in Engineering and Applied Sciences*, *5*(7), 24–28.

Elisevich, K., Kasunic, K., Hathaway, S. J., Smith, B. J., Stewart, R. W., & Barkley, G. L. (1996). Clinical Care Pathways in a Surgical Epilepsy Program: A Comparison of Costs by Diagnostic Related Groups for Program and Nonprogram Admissions. *Epilepsy Research*, *9*(4), 282–290. doi:10.1016/S0896-6974(96)00021-7

Elkind, J. S., Rubin, E., Rosenthal, S., Skoff, B., & Prather, P. (2001). A simulated reality scenario compared with the computerized Wisconsin card sorting test: An analysis of preliminary results. *Cyberpsychology & Behavior*, *4*(4), 489–496. doi:10.1089/109493101750527042 PMID:11708728

Emaminejad, S., Gao, W., Wu, E., Davies, Z. A., Nyein, H. Y. Y., Challa, S., ... Talebi, S. (2017). Autonomous sweat extraction and analysis applied to cystic fibrosis and glucose monitoring using a fully integrated wearable platform. *Proceedings of the National Academy of Sciences of the United States of America*, *114*(18), 4625–4630. doi:10.1073/pnas.1701740114 PMID:28416667

Epstein, R. M., & Hundert, E. M. (2002). Defining and assessing professional competence. *Journal of the American Medical Association*, *287*(2), 226–235. doi:10.1001/jama.287.2.226 PMID:11779266

Eswaran, S., Muir, J., & Chey, W. D. (2013). Fiber and functional gastrointestinal disorders. *The American Journal of Gastroenterology*, *108*(5), 718–727. doi:10.1038/ajg.2013.63 PMID:23545709

Euzenat, J., Meilicke, C., Stuckenschmidt, H., Shvaiko, P., & Trojahn, C. (2011). Ontology Alignment Evaluation Initiative: Six Years of Experience. *Journal on Data Semantics*, *XV*, 158–192. doi:10.1007/978-3-642-22630-4_6

Fagerberg, S. (1982). The Effects of a bulk laxative (Metamucil) on fasting blood-glucose, serum-lipids and other variables in constipated patients with non-insulin dependent adult diabetes. *Current Therapeutic Research, Clinical and Experimental*, *31*, 166–172.

Fathalla, S. (2018). Detecting Human Diseases Relatedness: A Spreading Activation Approach Over Ontologies. *International Journal on Semantic Web and Information Systems, 14*(3), 120–133. doi:10.4018/IJSWIS.2018070106

Fathalla, S., Hassan, Y., & El-Sayed, M. (2012). A hybrid method for user query reformation and classification. In *22nd International Conference on Computer Theory and Applications, ICCTA 2012* (pp. 132–138). 10.1109/ICCTA.2012.6523559

Fathalla, S., & Kannot, Y. (2017a). A Bidirectional-Based Spreading Activation Method for Human Diseases Relatedness Detection Using Disease Ontology. In *Conference on Computational Collective Intelligence Technologies and Applications* (pp. 14–23). Springer. 10.1007/978-3-319-67074-4_2

Fathalla, S., & Kannot, Y. (2017b). A Bidirectional-Based Spreading Activation Method for Human Diseases Relatedness Detection Using Disease Ontology. *International Journal of Computers in Clinical Practice, 2*(1), 14–23. doi:10.4018/IJCCP.2017010104

Fathalla, S., & Lange, C. (2018a). EVENTSKG: A Knowledge Graph Representation for Top-Prestigious Computer Science Events Metadata. In *International Conference on Computational Collective Intelligence*. Springer. 10.1007/978-3-319-98443-8_6

Fathalla, S., Vahdati, S., Auer, S., & Lange, C. (2017). Towards a knowledge graph representing research findings by semantifying survey articles. In *International Conference on Theory and Practice of Digital Libraries,* LNCS (Vol. 10450, pp. 315–327). Springer. 10.1007/978-3-319-67008-9_25

Feigenbaum, L., Herman, I., Hongsermeier, T., Neumann, E., & Stephens, S. (2007). The semantic web in action. *Scientific American, 297*(6), 90–97. doi:10.1038cient ificamerican1207-90 PMID:18237102

Feinglos, M. N., Gibb, R. D., Ramsey, D. L., Surwit, R. S., & Mcrorie, J. W. (2013). Psyllium improves glycemic control in patients with type-2 diabetes mellitus. *Bioactive Carbohydrates and Dietary Fibre, 1*(2), 156–161. doi:10.1016/j.bcdf.2013.02.003

Feis, D. L., Schoene-Bake, J. C., Elger, C., Wagner, J., Tittgemeyer, M., & Weber, B. (2013). Prediction of post-surgical seizure outcome in left mesial temporal lobe epilepsy. *NeuroImage. Clinical, 2*, 903–911. doi:10.1016/j.nicl.2013.06.010 PMID:24179841

Finke, K., Myers, N., Bublak, P., & Sorg, C. (2013). A biased competition account of attention and memory in Alzheimer's disease. *Philosophical Transactions of the Royal Society of London. Series B, Biological Sciences*, *368*(1628), 1–11. doi:10.1098/rstb.2013.0062 PMID:24018724

Finkel, D., Reynolds, C. A., McArdle, J. J., & Pedersen, N. L. (2007). Age changes in processing speed as a leading indicator of cognitive aging. *Psychology and Aging*, *22*(3), 558–568. doi:10.1037/0882-7974.22.3.558 PMID:17874954

Firth-Cozens, J. (2006). Leadership and the quality of healthcare. In J. Cox, J. King, A. Hutchinson, & P. McAvoy (Eds.), *Understanding doctors' performance* (pp. 123–133). Oxford: Radcliffe Publishing.

Firth-Cozens, J., & King, J. (2006). Are psychological factors linked to performance? In J. Cox, J. King, A. Hutchinson, & P. McAvoy (Eds.), *Understanding doctors' performance* (pp. 61–77). Oxford: Radcliffe Publishing.

Fisher, D. H. (1987). Knowledge acquisition via incremental conceptual clustering. *Machine Learning*, *2*(2), 139–172. doi:10.1007/BF00114265

FitzGerald, C., & Hurst, S. (2017). Implicit bias in healthcare professionals: A systematic review. *BMC Medical Ethics*, *18*(1), 19. doi:10.118612910-017-0179-8 PMID:28249596

Foerster, R. M., Poth, C. H., Behler, C., Botsch, M., & Schneider, W. X. (2016). Using the virtual reality device Oculus rift for neuropsychological assessment of visual processing capabilities. *Scientific Reports*, *6*(1), 37016. doi:10.1038rep37016 PMID:27869220

Fogel, P., Young, S. S., Hawkins, D. M., & Ledirac, N. (2007). Inferential, robust non-negative matrix factorization analysis of microarray data. *Bioinformatics (Oxford, England)*, *23*(1), 44–49. doi:10.1093/bioinformatics/btl550 PMID:17092989

Fonseca, F., Davis, C., & Câmara, G. (2003). Bridging ontologies and conceptual schemas in geographic information integration. *GeoInformatica*, *7*(4), 355–378. doi:10.1023/A:1025573406389

Fortney, J. C., Pyne, J. M., Steven, C. A., Williams, J. S., Hedrick, R. G., Lunsford, A. K., ... Smith, J. L. (2010). A web-based clinical decision support system for depression care management. *The American Journal of Managed Care*, *16*, 849–854. PMID:21348556

Franzen, M. D., & Wilhelm, K. L. (1996). Conceptual foundations of ecological validity in neuropsychological assessment. In R.J. Sbordone & C.J. Long (Eds.), Ecological validity of neuropsychological testing (pp. 91-112). Delray Beach, FL: Gr Press/St Lucie Press, Inc.

Fromkin, V., Rodman, R., & Hyams, N. (2013). *An introduction to language*. Cengage Learning.

Frost, G., Brynes, A., Dhillo, W., Bloom, S., & Mcburney, M. (2003). The effects of fiber enrichment of pasta and fat content on gastric emptying, GLP-1, glucose, and insulin responses to a meal. *European Journal of Clinical Nutrition*, *57*(2), 293–298. doi:10.1038j.ejcn.1601520 PMID:12571662

Fujita, E., Ogura, Y., Ochiai, N., Miao, T., Shimizu, T., Kamei, T., . . . Kaneko, S. (2004). Development of simplified appraisal method of fatigue on sitting for extended periods by the data of finger plethysmogram. Japan Ergonomics Society, 40(5), 254-263.

Fujita, E., Ogura, Y., Ochiai, N., Yasuda, E., Doi, S., Murata, K., . . . Kaneko, S. (2005). Development of the measurement method of the prediction of sleep by finger plethysmogram data. Japan Ergonomics Society, 41(4), 203-212.

Gadaleta, M., Facchinetti, A., Grisan, E., & Rossi, M. (2018). Prediction of Adverse Glycemic Events from Continuous Glucose Monitoring Signal. *IEEE Journal of Biomedical and Health Informatics*, 1. doi:10.1109/JBHI.2018.2823763 PMID:29993992

Gao, W., Emaminejad, S., Nyein, H. Y. Y., Challa, S., Chen, K., Peck, A., ... Lien, D. H. (2016). Fully integrated wearable sensor arrays for multiplexed in situ perspiration analysis. *Nature*, *529*(7587), 509–514. doi:10.1038/nature16521 PMID:26819044

Gavali, M. Y., Khismatrao, D. S., Gavali, Y. V., & Patil, K. B. (2017). Smartphone, the new learning aid amongst medical students. *Journal of Clinical and Diagnostic Research*, *11*(5), JC05–JC08. doi:10.7860/JCDR/2017/20948.9826 PMID:28658804

Gebru, A. A., Yimam, Y., Nigussie, A. W., Kahsay, W. G., Gelaye, N. D., & Mengistie, Z. (2015). Clinical decision support system in nursing: A review of literature. *Indian Journal of Basic and Applied Medical Research*, *4*, 437–452.

Gelissen, I. C., Brodie, B., & Eastwood, M. A. (1994). Effect of Plantago ovata (psyllium) husk and seeds on sterol metabolism: Studies in normal and ileostomy subjects. *The American Journal of Clinical Nutrition, 59*(2), 395–400. doi:10.1093/ajcn/59.2.395 PMID:8310991

Georga, E. I., Protopappas, V. C., Polyzos, D., & Fotiadis, D. I. (2015). Evaluation of short-term predictors of glucose concentration in type 1 diabetes combining feature ranking with regression models. *Medical & Biological Engineering & Computing, 53*(12), 1305–1318. doi:10.100711517-015-1263-1 PMID:25773366

Geyman, J. P. (2015). A five-year assessment of the Affordable Care Act: Market forces still trump the common good in US health care. *International Journal of Health Services, 45*(2), 209–225. doi:10.1177/0020731414568505 PMID:25674797

Gibson, K., Kartsounis, L., & Kopelman, M. (2006). Cognitive impairment and performance. In J. Cox, J. King, A. Hutchinson, & P. McAvoy (Eds.), *Understanding doctors' performance* (pp. 48–60). Oxford: Radcliffe Publishing.

Gill, M., & Krentz, H. (2009). Unappreciated epidemiology: The churn effect in a regional HIV care programme. *International Journal of STD & AIDS, 20*(8), 540–544. doi:10.1258/ijsa.2008.008422 PMID:19625584

Giunchiglia, F., Yatskevich, M., & Shvaiko, P. (2007). Semantic Matching : Algorithms and Implementation. *Journal on Data Semantics*. doi:10.1007/978-3-540-74987-5_1

Glassman, M., Spark, A., Berezin, S., Schwarz, S., Medow, M., & Newman, L. J. (1990). Treatment of type IIa hyperlipidemia in childhood by a simplified American Heart Association diet and fiber supplementation. *American Journal of Diseases of Children, 144*, 973–976. PMID:2168676

Glei, D. A., Goldman, N., Chuang, Y. L., & Weinstein, M. (2007). Do chronic stressors lead to physiological dysregulation? Testing the theory of allostatic load. *Psychosomatic Medicine, 69*(8), 769–776. doi:10.1097/PSY.0b013e318157cba6 PMID:17942833

Goble, C., & Stevens, R. (2008). State of the nation in data integration for bioinformatics. *Journal of Biomedical Informatics, 41*(5), 687–693. doi:10.1016/j.jbi.2008.01.008 PMID:18358788

Gough, F., Budhrani, S., Cohn, E., Dappen, A., Leenknecht, C., Lewis, B., ... Bernard, J. (2015). ATA practice guidelines for live, on-demand primary and urgent care. *Telemedicine Journal and e-Health, 21*(3), 233–241. doi:10.1089/tmj.2015.0008 PMID:25658882

Gregory, R. J. (2015). *Psychological testing: History, principles, and applications* (7th ed.). Boston: Allyn and Bacon.

Griffiths, F., Lindenmeyer, A., Powell, J., Lowe, P., & Thorogood, M. (2006). Why are health care interventions delivered over the internet? A systematic review of the published literature. *Journal of Medical Internet Research, 8*(2), 10–17. doi:10.2196/jmir.8.2.e10 PMID:16867965

Gross, J., Kramer, C., Leitão, C., Hawkins, N., Viana, L., Schaan, B., ... Azevedo, M. (2011). Diabetes and Endocrinology Meta-analysis Group (DEMA). Effect of antihyperglycemic agents added to metformin and a sulfonylurea on glycemic control and weight gain in type 2 diabetes: A network metaanalysis. *Annals of Internal Medicine, 154*, 672–679. doi:10.7326/0003-4819-154-10-201105170-00007 PMID:21576535

Grover, V., & Davenport, T. H. (2001). General perspectives on knowledge management: Fostering a research agenda. *Journal of Management Information Systems, 18*(1), 5–22. doi:10.1080/07421222.2001.11045672

Guariguata, L., Whiting, D., Hambleton, I., Beagley, J., Linnenkamp, U., & Shaw, J. (2014). Global estimates of diabetes prevalence for 2013 and projections for 2035. *Diabetes Research and Clinical Practice, 103*(2), 137–149. doi:10.1016/j.diabres.2013.11.002 PMID:24630390

Gueorguieva, R. (2017). *Statistical methods in psychiatry and related fields: Longitudinal, clustered, and other repeated measures data*. Boca Raton, FL: Chapman & Hall/CRC. doi:10.1201/9781315151526

Guo, J., Fan, Y., Ai, Q., & Croft, W. B. (2016). Semantic Matching by Non-Linear Word Transportation for Information Retrieval. In *Proceedings of the 25th ACM International on Conference on Information and Knowledge Management - CIKM '16* (pp. 701–710). ACM. 10.1145/2983323.2983768

Gupta, R., Agrawal, C., Singh, G., & Ghatak, A. (1994). Lipid-lowering efficacy of psyllium hydrophilic mucilloid in non insulin dependent diabetes mellitus with hyperlipidaemia. *The Indian Journal of Medical Research, 100*, 237–241. PMID:7829159

Gupta, V., & Lehal, G. S. (2009). A survey of text mining techniques and applications. *Journal of Emerging Technologies in Web Intelligence, 1*(1), 60–76. doi:10.4304/jetwi.1.1.60-76

Gustafsson, A., Johnson, M. D., & Roos, I. (2005). The effects of customer satisfaction, relationship commitment dimensions, and triggers on customer retention. *Journal of Marketing, 69*(4), 210–218. doi:10.1509/jmkg.2005.69.4.210

Guyatt, G., Cairns, J., Churchill, D., Cook, D., Haynes, B., Hirsh, J., ... Sackett, D. (1992). Evidence-based medicine. A new approach to teaching the practice of medicine. *Journal of the American Medical Association, 268*(17), 2420–2425. doi:10.1001/jama.1992.03490170092032 PMID:1404801

Haas, R. W. (1979). Reducing stress and depression with exercise. *Bulletin - American Protestant Hospital Association, 43*, 24–25. PMID:10246574

Hadden, J., Tiwari, A., Roy, R., & Ruta, D. (2006). Churn prediction using complaints data. *Paper presented at the Proceedings Of World Academy Of Science, Engineering and Technology.*

Hadden, J., Tiwari, A., Roy, R., & Ruta, D. (2006). Churn prediction: Does technology matter. *International Journal of Intelligent Technology, 1*(1), 104–110.

Hadden, J., Tiwari, A., Roy, R., & Ruta, D. (2007). Computer assisted customer churn management: State-of-the-art and future trends. *Computers & Operations Research, 34*(10), 2902–2917. doi:10.1016/j.cor.2005.11.007

Hall, M. A. (2000). Correlation-based feature selection for discrete and numeric class machine learning. *Paper presented at the Proc Seventeenth International Conference on Machine Learning.*

Hamanaka, Y., Nomura, R., Nakazono, Y., & Mizusawa, J. (2006). Development and Evaluation of stress measuring mouse. *IEICE, 106*(253), 69–72.

Hanson, A., & Levin, B. L. (2013). *Mental health informatics*. Oxford: Oxford University Press.

Hanson, E. K., Godaert, G. L., Maas, C. J., & Meijman, T. F. (2001). Vagal cardiac control throughout the day: The relative importance of effort-reward imbalance and within day measurements of mood, demand and satisfaction. *Biological Psychology*, *56*(1), 23–44. doi:10.1016/S0301-0511(01)00066-7 PMID:11240313

Haugh, R. (2004). Wiring docs. *Hospitals & Health Networks*, *78*(11), 44–46, 55. PMID:15597697

Hayes, P. (2004). RDF Semantics. *W3C Recommendation.*

He, Y., Cowell, L., Diehl, A. D., Mobley, H. L., Peters, B., & Ruttenberg, A. … others. (2009). VO: vaccine ontology. In *The 1st International Conference on Biomedical Ontology (ICBO 2009) Nature Proceedings* (Vol. 2009).

Health Information Technology for Economic and Clinical Health (HITECH) Act, Title XIII of Division A and Title IV of Division B of the American Recovery and Reinvestment Act of 2009 (ARRA), Pub. L. No. 111-5, 123 Stat. 226 (Feb. 17, 2009), *codified at* 42 U.S.C. §§300jj *et seq.*; §§17901 *et seq.* (2009).

Health Insurance Portability and Accountability Act (HIPAA). Pub. L. No. 104-191, § 264, 110 Stat.1936. (1996).

Heinonen, M. V., Karhunen, L. J., Chabot, E. D., Toppinen, L. K., Juntunen, K. S., Laaksonen, D. E., ... Niskanen, L. K. (2007). Plasma ghrelin levels after two high-carbohydrate meals producing different insulin responses in patients with metabolic syndrome. *Regulatory Peptides*, *138*(2-3), 118–125. doi:10.1016/j.regpep.2006.08.011 PMID:17030069

Heisey-Grove, D., & Patel, V. (2014) Physician Motivations for Adoption of Electronic Health Records. ONC Data Brief, no. 21. Office of the National Coordinator for Health Information Technology: Washington DC. Retrieved from https://www.healthit.gov/sites/default/files/oncdatabrief-physician-ehr-adoption-motivators-2014.pdf

He, M., & Petoukhov, S. (2011). *Mathematics of bioinformatics: Theory, methods and applications*. Hoboken, NJ: Wiley.

Hennessy, M. J., Elwes, R. D., Honavar, M., Rabe-Hesketh, S., Binnie, C. D., & Polkey, C. E. (2001). Predictors of outcome and pathological considerations in the surgical treatment of intractable epilepsy associated with temporal lobe lesions. *Journal of Neurology, Neurosurgery, and Psychiatry*, *70*(4), 450–458. doi:10.1136/jnnp.70.4.450 PMID:11254766

Hilty, D., Chan, S., Torous, J., Mahautmr, J., & Mucic, D. (2015). New frontiers in healthcare and technology: Internet- and web-based mental options emerge to complement in-person and telepsychiatric care options. *Journal of Health and Medical Informatics*, *6*(4), 1–14.

Hintsanen, M., Elovainio, M., Puttonen, S., Kivimäki, M., Koskinen, T., Raitakari, O. T., & Keltinkangas-Järvinen, L. (2007). Effort-reward imbalance, heart rate and heart rate variability: The cardiovascular risk in young Finns study. *International Journal of Behavioral Medicine*, *14*(4), 202–212. doi:10.1007/BF03002994 PMID:18001235

Hitzler, P., Parsia, B., Patel-schneider, P. F., & Rudolph, S. (2009). OWL 2 Web Ontology Language Primer. *W3C Recommendation*. Retrieved from http://www.w3.org/TR/owl2-primer/

Hoehndorf, R., Dumontier, M., & Gkoutos, G. V. (2013). Evaluation of research in biomedical ontologies. *Briefings in Bioinformatics*, *14*(6), 696–712. doi:10.1093/bib/bbs053 PMID:22962340

Hoehndorf, R., Schofield, P. N., & Gkoutos, G. V. (2015). The role of ontologies in biological and biomedical research: A functional perspective. *Briefings in Bioinformatics*, *16*(6), 1069–1080. doi:10.1093/bib/bbv011 PMID:25863278

Hoffman, M., Arnoldi, C., & Chuang, I. (2005). The clinical bioinformatics ontology: A curated semantic network utilizing RefSeq information. *Pacific Symposium on Biocomputing*. PMID:15759621

Hoff, T., Young, G., Xiang, E., & Raver, E. (2015). Understanding U.S. physician satisfaction: State of the evidence and future directions. *Journal of Healthcare Management*, *60*(6), 409–427. doi:10.1097/00115514-201511000-00007 PMID:26720985

Holsinger, J. W., & Beaton, B. (2006). Physician professionalism for a new century. *Clinical Anatomy (New York, N.Y.)*, *19*(5), 473–479. doi:10.1002/ca.20274 PMID:16506233

Holst, J. J., & Gromada, J. (2004). Role of incretin hormones in the regulation of insulin secretion in diabetic and nondiabetic humans. *American Journal of Physiology. Endocrinology and Metabolism*, *287*(2), E199–E206. doi:10.1152/ajpendo.00545.2003 PMID:15271645

Horrocks, I., Patel-schneider, P. F., Boley, H., Tabet, S., Grosof, B., & Dean, M. (2004). SWRL : A Semantic Web Rule Language Combining OWL and RuleML. *W3C*.

Hsiao, C. J., Hing, E., Socey, T. C., & Cai, B. (2011). Electronic health record systems and intent to apply for meaningful use incentives among office-based phsycian practices: United States, 2001-2011. NCHS data brief, No. 79. Hyattsville, MD: National Center for Health Statistics. Retrieved from http://www.cdc.gov/nchs/data/databriefs/db79.htm

Hughes, C. (2013). Executive function: development, individual differences, and clinical insights. In J. L. R. Rubenstein & P. Rakic (Eds.), *Neural Circuit Development and Function in the Brain, - Comprehensive Developmental Neuroscience* (pp. 429–445). Amsterdam: Academic Press. doi:10.1016/B978-0-12-397267-5.00062-5

Idowu, P. A., Adagunodo, E. R., & Adedoyin, R. (2006). Information technology infusion model for health sector in a developing country: Nigeria as a case. *Technology and Health Care*, *14*, 69–77. PMID:16720950

Idowu, P. A., Eyitope, O., & Idowu, B. (2003). Information and Communications Technology in Nigeria - The Health Sector Experience. *Journal of Information Technology Impact*, *3*(2), 69–73.

Idowu, P. A., Oyetunji, M. O., Oladeji, F. A., & Balogun, J. A. (2017). An ICT Infusion Model for Nigerian Transport Sector. *Computing, Information Systems. Development Informatics and Allied Research Journal*, *8*(1), 103–120.

Idowu, P., Cornford, D., & Bastin, L. (2008). Health informatics development in Nigeria. *Journal of Health Informatics in Developing Countries*, *2*(1), 15–23.

Ikonomakis, M., Kotsiantis, S., & Tampakas, V. (2005). Text classification using machine learning techniques. *WSEAS Transactions on Computers*, *4*(8), 966–974.

Jafari-Khouzani, K., Siadat, M. R., Soltanian-Zadeh, H., & Elisevich, K. (2003, May). Texture analysis of hippocampus for epilepsy. In Medical Imaging 2003: Physiology and Function: Methods, Systems, and Applications (Vol. 5031, pp. 279-289). International Society for Optics and Photonics. doi:10.1117/12.480697

Jahromi, A. T., Stakhovych, S., & Ewing, M. (2014). Managing B2B customer churn, retention and profitability. *Industrial Marketing Management*, *43*(7), 1258–1268. doi:10.1016/j.indmarman.2014.06.016

James, S., Rao, S. V., & Granger, C. B. (2015). Registry-based randomized clinical trials–A new clinical trial paradigm. *Nature Reviews. Cardiology*, *12*(5), 312–316. doi:10.1038/nrcardio.2015.33 PMID:25781411

Janszky, J., Janszky, I., Schulz, R., Hoppe, M., Behne, F., Pannek, H. W., & .... (2005). Temporal lobe epilepsy with hippocampal sclerosis: Predictors for long-term surgical outcome. *Brain*, *128*(Pt 2), 395–404. doi:10.1093/brain/awh358 PMID:15634733

Janszky, J., Pannek, H. W., Fogarasi, A., Bone, B., Schulz, R., Behne, F., & Ebner, A. (2006). Prognostic factors for surgery of neocortical temporal lobe epilepsy. *Seizure*, *15*(2), 125–132. doi:10.1016/j.seizure.2005.12.002 PMID:16414290

Jeha, L. E., Najm, I. M., Bingaman, W. E., Khandwala, F., Widdess-Walsh, P., Morris, H. H., ... Luders, H. O. (2006). Predictors of outcome after temporal lobectomy for the treatment of intractable epilepsy. *Neurology*, *66*(12), 1938–1940. doi:10.1212/01.wnl.0000219810.71010.9b PMID:16801667

Jenkins, D., Wolever, T., Leeds, A. R., Gassull, M. A., Haisman, P., Dilawari, J., ... Alberti, K. (1978). Dietary fibres, fibre analogues, and glucose tolerance: Importance of viscosity. *British Medical Journal*, *1*(6124), 1392–1394. doi:10.1136/bmj.1.6124.1392 PMID:647304

Jha, A., DesRoches, C. M., Campbell, E. G., Donelan, K., Rao, S. R., Ferris, T. G., ... Blumenthal, D. (2009). Use of electronic health records in U.S. hospitals. *The New England Journal of Medicine*, *360*(16), 1628–1638. doi:10.1056/NEJMsa0900592 PMID:19321858

Jiayin, Q., Yangming, Z., Yingying, Z., & Shuang, S. (2006, December 12-15). TreeLogit Model for Customer Churn Prediction. *Paper presented at the IEEE Asia-Pacific Conference on Services Computing APSCC '06.*

Joachims, T. (1999). Transductive inference for text classification using support vector machines. *Paper presented at the machine learning-international workshop then conference.*

Johnes, M., Mothersbaugh, D. L., & Betty, S. E. (2000). Switching barriers and repurchase intentions in service. *Journal of Retailing*, *76*(2), 259–274. doi:10.1016/S0022-4359(00)00024-5

Johnson, B. (2006). Hospitals, physicians, and information technology. *Trustee*, *59*(5), 23, 27.

Jones, B., & Kenward, M. G. (2014). *Design and analysis of cross-over trials*. CRC Press.

Jotsov, V., Chui, K. T., & Zhu, H. (2017). Guest Editorial: Advanced Algorithms and Techniques for Engineering Applications. *Journal of Internet Technology, 18*, 645–646.

Juntunen, K. S., Niskanen, L. K., Liukkonen, K. H., Poutanen, K. S., Holst, J. J., & Mykkänen, H. M. (2002). Postprandial glucose, insulin, and incretin responses to grain products in healthy subjects. *The American Journal of Clinical Nutrition, 75*(2), 254–262. doi:10.1093/ajcn/75.2.254 PMID:11815315

Kaiser Family Foundation. (2002). *National survey of physicians part III: doctors' opinions about their profession, March, 2002*. Retrieved from https://kaiserfamilyfoundation.files.wordpress.com/2013/01/highlights-and-chart-pack-2.pdf

Kalina, J. (2014). Classification methods for high-dimensional genetic data. *Biocybernetics and Biomedical Engineering, 34*(1), 10–18. doi:10.1016/j.bbe.2013.09.007

Kalina, J. (2018). A robust pre-processing of BeadChip microarray images. *Biocybernetics and Biomedical Engineering, 38*(3), 556–563. doi:10.1016/j.bbe.2018.04.005

Kalina, J., & Hlinka, J. (2017). Implicitly weighted robust classification applied to brain activity research. *Communications in Computer and Information Science, 690*, 87–107. doi:10.1007/978-3-319-54717-6_6

Kalina, J., & Schlenker, A. (2015). A robust supervised variable selection for noisy high-dimensional data. *BioMed Research International, 2015*, 1–10.

Kalina, J., Seidl, L., Zvára, K., Grünfeldová, H., Slovák, D., & Zvárová, J. (2013). System for selecting relevant information for decision support. *Studies in Health Technology and Informatics, 186*, 83–87. PMID:23542973

Kanavos, A., Theodoridis, E., & Tsakalidis, A. (2014). A PubMed Meta search engine based on biomedical entity mining. In *Proceedings - International Workshop on Database and Expert Systems Applications, DEXA*. 10.1109/DEXA.2014.32

Karasek, R. (1979). Job demands, job decision latitude, and mental strain: Implications for job redesign. *Administrative Science Quarterly, 24*(2), 285–305. doi:10.2307/2392498

Karhunen, L. J., Juvonen, K. R., Flander, S. M., Liukkonen, K.-H., Lähteenmäki, L., Siloaho, M., ... Poutanen, K. S. (2010). A psyllium fiber-enriched meal strongly attenuates postprandial gastrointestinal peptide release in healthy young adults. *The Journal of Nutrition*, *140*(4), 737–744. doi:10.3945/jn.109.115436 PMID:20147463

Kawakami, N., & Haratani, T. (1999). Epidemiology of job stress and health in Japan: Review of current evidence and future direction. *Industrial Health*, *37*(2), 174–186. doi:10.2486/indhealth.37.174 PMID:10319566

Kemppinen, J., Korpela, J., Elfvengren, K., Salmisaari, T., & Polkko, J. (2014). Decision support in evaluating the impacts of mental disorders on work ability. In *47th Hawaii International Conference on System Science* (pp. 2958-2966). Washington, DC: IEEE Computer Society. 10.1109/HICSS.2014.368

Kibbe, W. A., Arze, C., Felix, V., Mitraka, E., Bolton, E., Fu, G., ... Schriml, L. M. (2015). Disease Ontology 2015 update: An expanded and updated database of Human diseases for linking biomedical knowledge through disease data. *Nucleic Acids Research*, *43*(D1), D1071–D1078. doi:10.1093/nar/gku1011 PMID:25348409

Kim, J., Campbell, A. S., & Wang, J. (2018). Wearable non-invasive epidermal glucose sensors: A review. *Talanta*, *177*, 163–170. doi:10.1016/j.talanta.2017.08.077 PMID:29108571

King, J., Patel, V., Jamoom, E. W., & Furukawa, M. F. (2014). Clinical benefits of electronic health record use: National findings. *Health Services Research*, *49*(1pt2), 392–404. doi:10.1111/1475-6773.12135 PMID:24359580

Knight, R., & Titov, N. (2009). Use of Virtual Reality Tasks to Assess Prospective Memory: Applicability and Evidence. *Brain Impairment*, *10*(1), 3–13. doi:10.1375/brim.10.1.3

Kocher, R., Emanuel, E. J., & DeParle, N. M. (2010). The Affordable Care Act and the future of clinical medicine: The opportunities and challenges. *Annals of Internal Medicine*, *153*(8), 536–539. doi:10.7326/0003-4819-153-8-201010190-00274 PMID:20733178

Köhler, S., Doelken, S. C., Mungall, C. J., Bauer, S., Firth, H. V., Bailleul-Forestier, I., ... Robinson, P. N. (2014). The Human Phenotype Ontology project: Linking molecular biology and disease through phenotype data. *Nucleic Acids Research*, *42*(D1), D966–D974. doi:10.1093/nar/gkt1026 PMID:24217912

Kohn, L. T., Corrigan, J. M., & Donaldson, M. S. (Eds.). (1999). *To err is human: Building a safer health system*. Washington: National Academy Press.

Kononenko, I. (1994). Estimating Attributes: Analysis and Extensions of RELIEF. *Paper presented at the European Conference on Machine Learning*. 10.1007/3-540-57868-4_57

Kontio, E., Airola, A., Pahikkala, T., Lundgren-Laine, H., Junttila, K., Korvenranta, H., ... Salanterä, S. (2014). Predicting patient acuity from electronic patient records. *Journal of Biomedical Informatics*, *51*, 35–40. doi:10.1016/j.jbi.2014.04.001 PMID:24726853

Koposov, R., Fossum, S., Frodl, T., Nytro, O., Leventhal, B., Sourander, A., ... Skokauskas, N. (2017). Clinical decision support systems in child and adolescent psychiatry: A systematic review. *European Child & Adolescent Psychiatry*, *26*(11), 1309–1317. doi:10.100700787-017-0992-0 PMID:28455596

KORESS. (2010). A.P.Sheild 05: Arduino corresponding Heart Rate sensor (Pulse sensor) shield. Retrieved from http://koress.jp/2010/05/arduinoap_shield.html

Kundi, G. M., Shah, B., Qureshi, A., Nawaz, A., Miankhel, A. K., Chishti, K. A., & Qureshi, N. A. (2013). Infrastructural Barriers to e-Health Implementation in Developing Countries. *European Journal of Sustainable Development*, *2*(1), 163–170.

Kvedar, J., Coye, M. J., & Everett, W. (2014). Connected health: A review of technologies and strategies to improve patient care with telemedicine and telehealth. *Health Affairs*, *33*(2), 194–199. doi:10.1377/hlthaff.2013.0992 PMID:24493760

Lapointe, L., & Rivard, S. (2006). Getting physicians to accept new information technology: Insights from case studies. *Canadian Medical Association Journal*, *174*(11), 1572–1578. doi:10.1503/cmaj.050281 PMID:16717265

Lazarus, R. S., & Folkman, S. (1984). *Stress, appraisal, and coping*. New York: Springer Publishing.

Leach, D. C. (2002). Competence is a habit. *Journal of the American Medical Association*, *287*(2), 243–244. doi:10.1001/jama.287.2.243 PMID:11779269

Leach, D. C. (2004). Professionalism: The formation of physicians. *The American Journal of Bioethics*, *4*(2), 11–12. doi:10.1162/152651604323097619 PMID:15186669

Lee, D. D., & Seung, H. (1999). Learning the parts of objects by non-negative matrix factorization. *Nature*, *401*(6755), 788–791. doi:10.1038/44565 PMID:10548103

Lee, H., Choi, T. K., Lee, Y. B., Cho, H. R., Ghaffari, R., Wang, L., ... Choi, S. H. (2016). A graphene-based electrochemical device with thermoresponsive microneedles for diabetes monitoring and therapy. *Nature Nanotechnology*, *11*(6), 566–572. doi:10.1038/nnano.2016.38 PMID:26999482

Lee, H., Song, C., Hong, Y. S., Kim, M. S., Cho, H. R., Kang, T., ... Kim, D. H. (2017). Wearable/disposable sweat-based glucose monitoring device with multistage transdermal drug delivery module. *Science Advances*, *3*(3), e1601314. doi:10.1126ciadv.1601314 PMID:28345030

Lemmens, A., & Croux, C. (2006). Bagging and boosting classification trees to predict churn. *JMR, Journal of Marketing Research*, *43*(2), 276–286. doi:10.1509/jmkr.43.2.276

Lemmens, A., & Gupta, S. (2017). *Managing churn to maximize profits*. Cambridge, MA: Harvard Business School. doi:10.2139srn.2964906

Lezak, M. D., Howieson, D. B., Bigler, E. D., & Tranel, D. (2012). *Neuropsychological assessment* (5th ed.). New York, NY: Oxford University Press.

Li, H., & Xu, J. (2014). Semantic Matching in Search. *Foundations and Trends® in Information Retrieval, 7*(5), 343–469. doi:10.1561/1500000035

Lima, E., Mues, C., & Baesens, B. (2009). Domain knowledge integration in data mining using decision tables: Case studies in churn prediction. *The Journal of the Operational Research Society*, *60*(8), 1096–1106. doi:10.1057/jors.2008.161

Lin, C., Chung, I., Ko, L., Chen, Y., Liang, S., & Duann, J. (2007). EEG-based assessment of driver cognitive responses in a dynamic virtual reality driving environment. *IEEE Transactions on Biomedical Engineering*, *54*(7), 1349–1352. doi:10.1109/TBME.2007.891164 PMID:17605367

Lin, C.-S., Tzeng, G.-H., & Chin, Y.-C. (2011). Combined rough set theory and flow network graph to predict customer churn in credit card accounts. *Expert Systems with Applications*, *38*(1), 8–15. doi:10.1016/j.eswa.2010.05.039

Liu, B. (2010). Sentiment analysis and subjectivity. In Handbook of Natural Language Processing (pp. 627-666).

Liu, J. X., Goryakin, Y., Maeda, A., Bruckner, T., & Scheffler, R. (2017). Global health workforce labor market projections for 2030. *Human Resources for Health*, *15*(1). doi:10.118612960-017-0187-2

Li, Y., Algarni, A., Albathan, M., Shen, Y., & Bijaksana, M. A. (2015). Relevance feature discovery for text mining. *IEEE Transactions on Knowledge and Data Engineering*, *27*(6), 1656–1669. doi:10.1109/TKDE.2014.2373357

Loomis, G. A., Ries, J. S., Saywell, R. M., & Thakker, N. R. (2002). If electronic medical records are so great, why aren't family physicians using them? *Journal of Family Medicine*, *51*, 636–641. PMID:12160503

Lu, N., Lin, H., Lu, J., & Zhang, G. (2014). A customer churn prediction model in telecom industry using boosting. *IEEE Transactions on Industrial Informatics*, *10*(2), 1659–1665. doi:10.1109/TII.2012.2224355

Luther, J., & Chey, W. D. (2010). Psyllium increased symptom relief in patients with the irritable bowel syndrome more than bran or placebo. *Annals of Internal Medicine*, 152. PMID:20083814

Madden, G., Savage, S. J., & Coble-Neal, G. (1999). Subscriber churn in the Australian ISP market. *Information Economics and Policy*, *11*(2), 195–207. doi:10.1016/S0167-6245(99)00015-3

Mahgoub, M., & Monteggia, L. M. (2013). Epigenetics and psychiatry. *Neurotherapeutics; the Journal of the American Society for Experimental NeuroTherapeutics*, *10*(4), 734–741. doi:10.100713311-013-0213-6 PMID:24092614

Maia, T. V. (2015). Introduction to the series on computational psychiatry. *Clinical Psychological Science*, *3*(3), 374–377. doi:10.1177/2167702614567350

Makam, A. N., Lanham, H. J., Batchelor, K., Moran, B., Howell-Stampley, T., Kirk, L., ... Halm, E. A. (2014). The good, the bad and the early adopters: Providers' attitudes about a common, commercial EHR. *Journal of Evaluation in Clinical Practice*, *20*(1), 36–42. doi:10.1111/jep.12076 PMID:23962319

Mann, M. Y., Lloyd-Puryear, M. A., & Linzer, D. (2006). Enhancing communication in the 21st century. *Pediatrics*, *117*(Supplement 3), S315–S319. doi:10.1542/peds.2005-2633K PMID:16735258

Marshall, B., Su, H., McDonald, D., Eggers, S., & Chen, H. (2006). Aggregating automatically extracted regulatory pathway relations. *IEEE Transactions on Information Technology in Biomedicine*, *10*(1), 100–108. doi:10.1109/TITB.2005.856857 PMID:16445255

Matloff, N. (2017). *Statistical regression and classification. From linear models to machine learning*. Boca Raton, FL: CRC Press. doi:10.1201/9781315119588

Maulik, P. K., Tewari, A., Devarapalli, S., Kallakuri, S., & Patel, A. (2015). The systematic medical appraisal, referral and treatment (SMART) mental health project: Development and testing of electronic decision support system and formative research to understand perceptions about mental health in rural India. *PLoS One*, *11*(10), e0164404. doi:10.1371/journal.pone.0164404 PMID:27732652

McAlearney, A. S., Chisolm, D. J., Schweikhart, S., Medow, M. A., & Kelleher, K. (2007). The story behind the story: Physician skepticism about relying on clinical information technologies to reduce medical errors. *International Journal of Medical Informatics*, *76*(11-12), 836–842. doi:10.1016/j.ijmedinf.2006.09.021 PMID:17112779

McEwen, B., & Lasley, E. N. (2003). Allostatic load: When protection gives way to damage. *Advances in Mind-Body Medicine*, *19*, 28–33. PMID:12825411

Mcrorie, J. W., & Fahey, G. C. (2013). A review of gastrointestinal physiology and the mechanisms underlying the health benefits of dietary fiber: Matching an effective fiber with specific patient needs. *Clinical Nursing Studies*, *1*(4), 82. doi:10.5430/cns.v1n4p82

Mcrorie, J. W. Jr. (2015). Evidence-based approach to fiber supplements and clinically meaningful health benefits, part 2: What to look for and how to recommend an effective fiber therapy. *Nutrition Today*, *50*(2), 90–97. doi:10.1097/NT.0000000000000089 PMID:25972619

Meijman, T. F., & Mulder, G. (1998). Psychological aspects of workload. In P. J. D. Drenth, H. Thierry, & C. J. de Wolff (Eds.), *New handbook of work and organizational psychology.2 Work Psychology* (pp. 5–33). Hove, UK: Psychology Press.

Meilke, M. M., Machulda, M. M., Hagen, C. E., Edwards, K. K., Roberts, R. O., Pankratz, V. S., ... Petersen, R. C. (2015). Performance of the CogState computerized battery in the Mayo clinic study on aging. *Alzheimer's & Dementia*, *11*(11), 1367–1376. doi:10.1016/j.jalz.2015.01.008 PMID:25858683

Melville, N. K., Kraemer, & Gurbaxani. (2004). Review: Information technology and organizational performance: An integartive model of IT business value. *Management Information Systems Quarterly*, *28*(2), 283–322. doi:10.2307/25148636

MHLW. (2018). Patients survey. Retrieved from http://www.mhlw.go.jp/toukei/list/10-20.html

Middleton, B., Bloomrosen, M., Dente, M. A., Hashmat, B., Koppel, R., Overhage, J. M., ... Zhang, J. (2013). Enhancing patient safety and quality of care by improving the usability of electronic health record systems: Recommendations from AMIA. *Journal of the American Medical Informatics Association*, *20*(e1), e2–e8. doi:10.1136/amiajnl-2012-001458 PMID:23355463

Miettinen, M., & Korhonen, M. (2008, June 17-19). Information Quality in Healthcare: Coherence of Data Compared between Organization's Electronic Patient Records. *Paper presented at the 21st IEEE International Symposium on Computer-Based Medical Systems CBMS '08.*

Miguéis, V. L., Van den Poel, D., Camanho, A. S., & Cunha, J. F. (2012). Modeling partial customer churn: On the value of first product-category purchase sequences. *Expert Systems with Applications*, *39*(12), 11250–11256. doi:10.1016/j.eswa.2012.03.073

Milošević, M., Živić, N., & Andjelković, I. (2017). Early churn prediction with personalized targeting in mobile social games. *Expert Systems with Applications*, *83*, 326–332. doi:10.1016/j.eswa.2017.04.056

Minamitani, H., Hayashi, S., & Nagata, T. (1999). Heart rate variability related with mental stress and cumulative fatigue: Assessment of the autonomic nervous functions by using neural networks. *IEICE*, *98*(672), 115–122.

Mittman, R., & Cain, M. (1999). *The Future of the Internet in Health Care: Five Year Forecast.* California Healthcare Foundation.

Moja, L., Kwag, K. H., Lytras, T., Bertizzolo, L., Brandt, L., Pecoraro, V., ... Bonovas, S. (2014). Effectiveness of computerized decision support systems linked to electronic health records: A systematic review and meta-analysis. *American Journal of Public Health*, *104*(12), e12–e22. doi:10.2105/AJPH.2014.302164 PMID:25322302

Monteith, S., Glenn, T., Geddes, J., & Bauer, M. (2015). Big data are coming to psychiatry: A general introduction. *International Journal of Bipolar Disorders*, *3*(1), 21. doi:10.118640345-015-0038-9 PMID:26440506

Morid, M. A., Sheng, O. R., & Abdelrahman, S. (2017). Leveraging Time Series Data in Similarity Based Healthcare Predictive Models: The Case of Early ICU Mortality Prediction. Retrieved from https://arxiv.org/ftp/arxiv/papers/1704/1704.07499.pdf

Muris, P., & Petrocchi, N. (2017). Protection or vulnerability? A meta-analysis of the relations between the positive and negative components of self-compassion and psychopathology. *Clinical Psychology & Psychotherapy*, *24*(2), 373–383. doi:10.1002/cpp.2005 PMID:26891943

Murphy, D. R., Laxmisan, A., Reis, B. A., Thomas, E. J., Esquivel, A., Forjuoh, S. N., ... & Singh, H. (2013). Electronic health record-based triggers to detect potential delays in cancer diagnosis. *BMJ Qual Saf.*

Mutanen, T., Ahola, J., & Nousiainen, S. (2006). Customer churn prediction-a case study in retail banking. *Practical Data Mining: Applications, Experiences and Challenges*, *13*.

Nassirtoussi, A. K., Aghabozorgi, S., Wah, T. Y., & Ngo, D. C. L. (2014). Text mining for market prediction: A systematic review. *Expert Systems with Applications*, *41*(16), 7653–7670. doi:10.1016/j.eswa.2014.06.009

Needleman, J., Buerhaus, P. I., Stewart, M., Zelevinsky, K., & Mattke, S. (2006). Nurse staffing in hospitals: Is there a business case for quality? *Health Affairs*, *25*(1), 204–211. doi:10.1377/hlthaff.25.1.204 PMID:16403755

Needleman, J., Buerhaus, P., Mattke, S., Stewart, M., & Zelevinsky, K. (2002). Nurse-staffing levels and the quality of care in hospitals. *The New England Journal of Medicine*, *346*(22), 1715–1722. doi:10.1056/NEJMsa012247 PMID:12037152

Needleman, J., Buerhaus, P., Pankratz, V. S., Leibson, C. L., Stevens, S. R., & Harris, M. (2011). Nurse staffing and inpatient hospital mortality. *The New England Journal of Medicine*, *364*(11), 1037–1045. doi:10.1056/NEJMsa1001025 PMID:21410372

Neff, K. D. (2016). Does self-compassion entail reduced self-judgment, isolation, and over-identification? A Response to Muris, Otgaar, and Petrocchi (2016). *Mindfulness*, *7*(3), 791–797. doi:10.100712671-016-0531-y

Negash, S. (2004). Business Intelligence. *Communications of the Association for Information Systems*, *13*, 177–195. doi:10.17705/1CAIS.01315

Neguț, A., Matu, S., Sava, F. A., & David, D. (2016). Virtual reality measures in neuropsychological assessment: A meta-analytic review. *The Clinical Neuropsychologist*, *30*(2), 165–184. doi:10.1080/13854046.2016.1144793 PMID:26923937

Neslin, S., Gupta, S., Kamakura, W., Lu, J., & Mason, C. (2006). Defection detection: Measuring and understanding the predictive accuracy of customer churn models. *JMR, Journal of Marketing Research*, *XLIII*(May), 204–211. doi:10.1509/jmkr.43.2.204

Ngai, E. W., Xiu, L., & Chau, D. (2009). Application of data mining techniques in customer relationship management: A literature review and classification. *Expert Systems with Applications*, *36*(2), 2592–2602. doi:10.1016/j.eswa.2008.02.021

Ngo, V. M., Cao, T. H., & Le, T. M. V. (2010). Combining named entities with WordNet and using query-oriented spreading activation for semantic text search. In *2010 IEEE-RIVF International Conference on Computing and Communication Technologies: Research, Innovation and Vision for the Future, RIVF 2010*. 10.1109/RIVF.2010.5633401

Nigam, K., McCallum, A. K., Thrun, S., & Mitchell, T. (2000). Text classification from labeled and unlabeled documents using EM. *Machine Learning*, *39*(2), 103–134. doi:10.1023/A:1007692713085

O'Malley, A. S., Reschovsky, J. D., & Saiontz-Martinez, C. (2015). Interspecialty communication supported by health information technology associated with lower hospitalization rates for ambulatory care–sensitive conditions. *Journal of the American Board of Family Medicine*, *28*(3), 404–417. doi:10.3122/jabfm.2015.03.130325 PMID:25957373

Oberle, D. (2014). How ontologies benefit enterprise applications. *Semantic Web*, *5*(6), 473–491. doi:10.3233/SW-130114

Ohno-Machado, L., Sansone, S. A., Alter, G., Fore, I., Grethe, J., & Xu, H. … Kim, H. E. (2017). Finding useful data across multiple biomedical data repositories using DataMed. *Nature Genetics*. doi:10.1038/ng.3864

Okundaye, K. E. (2016). Adoption of Information and Communication Technology in Nigerian Small – to – Medium size Enterprises [PhD Thesis]. College of Management and Technology. Walden University, USA.

Olatokun, W. M., & Adeboyejo, O. C. (2009). Information and Communication Technology use by Reproductive Health Workers in Nigeria: State of the art, issues and challenges. *Human Technology*, *5*(2), 181–207. doi:10.17011/ht/urn.200911234470

Onoda, K., & Yamaguchi, S. (2014). Revision of the cognitive assessment for dementia, iPad version (CADi2). *PLoS ONE*, *9*(10), e109931. doi:.pone.0109931 doi:10.1371/journal

Onoda, K., Hamano, T., Nabika, Y., Aoyama, A., Takayoshi, H., Nakagawa, T., ... Yamaguchi, S. (2013). Validation of new mass screening tool for cognitive impairment: Cognitive assessment for dementia, iPad version. *Clinical Interventions in Aging*, *8*, 353–360. doi:10.2147/CIA.S42342 PMID:23569368

Ortendahl, M. (2007). The New Subjective Medicine: Understanding the Patient's Worry Improves Shared Decision Making and Increases Compliance. *Medical Principles and Practice*, *16*(1), 79–80. doi:10.1159/000096147 PMID:17159371

Paice, E. (2006). The role of education and training. In J. Cox, J. King, A. Hutchinson, & P. McAvoy (Eds.), *Understanding doctors' performance* (pp. 78–90). Oxford: Radcliffe Publishing.

Pal, S., Khossousi, A., Binns, C., Dhaliwal, S., & Ellis, V. (2011). The effect of a fibre supplement compared to a healthy diet on body composition, lipids, glucose, insulin and other metabolic syndrome risk factors in overweight and obese individuals. *British Journal of Nutrition*, *105*(01), 90–100. doi:10.1017/S0007114510003132 PMID:20727237

Panagioti, M., Panagopoulou, E., Bower, P., Lewith, G., Kontopantelis, E., Chew-Graham, C., ... Esmail, A. (2017). Controlled interventions to reduce burnout in physicians: A systematic review and meta-analysis. *JAMA Internal Medicine*, *177*(2), 195–205. doi:10.1001/jamainternmed.2016.7674 PMID:27918798

Pang, B., & Lee, L. (2008). Opinion Mining and Sentiment Analysis. *Foundations and Trends in Information Retrieval*, *2*(1-2), 1–135.

Park, D.-H., Lee, J., & Han, I. (2007). The effect of on-line consumer reviews on consumer purchasing intention: The moderating role of involvement. *International Journal of Electronic Commerce*, *11*(4), 125–148. doi:10.2753/JEC1086-4415110405

Park, S. H., Blegen, M. A., Spetz, J., Chapman, S. A., & De Groot, H. (2012). Patient turnover and the relationship between nurse staffing and patient outcomes. *Research in Nursing & Health*, *35*(3), 277–288. doi:10.1002/nur.21474 PMID:22457013

Parsons, T. D. (2015). Ecological Validity in Virtual Reality-Based Neuropsychological Assessment. In M. Khosrow-Pour, D.B.A. (Ed.), Encyclopedia of Information Science and Technology (3rd ed., pp. 1006-1015). Hershey, PA: IGI Global. doi:10.4018/978-1-4666-5888-2.ch095

Parsons, T. D., McPherson, S., & Interrante, V. (2013). Enhancing neurocognitive assessment using immersive virtual reality. In *2013 1st Workshop on Virtual and Augmented Assistive Technology, VAAT 2013; Co-located with the 2013 Virtual Reality Conference - Proceedings* (pp. 27-34). IEEE Computer Society. 10.1109/VAAT.2013.6786190

Parsons, T. D., Courtney, C. G., Arizmendi, B., & Dawson, M. (2011). Virtual reality stroop task for neurocognitive assessment. *Studies in Health Technology and Informatics*, *163*, 433–439. PMID:21335835

Pastors, J. G., Blaisdell, P. W., Balm, T. K., Asplin, C. M., & Pohl, S. L. (1991). Psyllium fiber reduces rise in postprandial glucose and insulin concentrations in patients with non-insulin-dependent diabetes. *The American Journal of Clinical Nutrition*, *53*(6), 1431–1435. doi:10.1093/ajcn/53.6.1431 PMID:1852093

Patient Protection and Affordable Care Act (PPACA), 42 U.S.C. § 18001. (2010).

Paulus, M. P. (2017). Evidence-based pragmatic psychiatry– A call to action. *JAMA Psychiatry*, *74*(12), 1185–1186. doi:10.1001/jamapsychiatry.2017.2439 PMID:29094142

Payne, T. R., & Lassila, O. (2004). Semantic Web Services. *IEEE Intelligent Systems*, *19*(4), 14–15. doi:10.1109/MIS.2004.29

Pedersen, C. A., Schneider, P. J., & Scheckelhoff, D. J. (2017). ASHP national survey of pharmacy practice in hospital settings: Prescribing and transcribing—2016. *American Journal of Health-System Pharmacy*, *74*(17), 1336–1352. doi:10.2146/ajhp170228 PMID:28743758

Peers, P., & Dutre, P. (2006). *Update Rules for a Weighted Non-negative FH*G Factorization*. Heverlee, Belgium: Katholieke Universiteit Leuven.

Pendharkar, P. C. (2009). Genetic algorithm based neural network approaches for predicting churn in cellular wireless network services. *Expert Systems with Applications*, *36*(3, Part 2), 6714–6720. doi:10.1016/j.eswa.2008.08.050

Petersen, R. C. (2016). Mild cognitive impairment. Continuum, 22(2), 404 – 418.

Pletscher-Frankild, S., Palleјà, A., Tsafou, K., Binder, J. X., & Jensen, L. J. (2015). Diseases: Text mining and data integration of disease–gene associations. *Methods (San Diego, Calif.)*, *74*, 83–89. doi:10.1016/j.ymeth.2014.11.020 PMID:25484339

Poole, D. L., & Mackworth, A. K. (2010). *Artificial intelligence: Foundations of computational agents. Artificial Intelligence: Foundations of Computational Agents*. doi:10.1017/CBO9780511794797

Poon, E. G., Blumenthal, D., Jaggi, T., Houour, M. M., Bates, D. W., & Kaushal, R. (2004). Overcoming barriers to adopting and implementing computerized physician order entry systems in U.S. hospitals. *Health Affairs*, *23*(4), 184–190. doi:10.1377/hlthaff.23.4.184 PMID:15318579

Post, R. E., Mainous, A. G., King, D. E., & Simpson, K. N. (2012). Dietary fiber for the treatment of type 2 diabetes mellitus: A meta-analysis. *Journal of the American Board of Family Medicine*, *25*(1), 16–23. doi:10.3122/jabfm.2012.01.110148 PMID:22218620

Priester, R. (1992). A values framework for health system reform. *Health Affairs*, *11*(1), 84–107. doi:10.1377/hlthaff.11.1.84 PMID:1577390

Protti, D., Edworthy, S., & Johansen, I. (2007). Adoption of information technology in primary care physician offices in Alberta and Denmark, Part 1: Historical, technical and cultural forces. *Healthcare Quarterly*, *10*(3), 95–102. PMID:17626551

Pugnetti, L., Mendozzi, L., Attree, E. A., Barbieri, E., Brooks, B. M., Cazzullo, C. L., ... Rose, F. D. (1998). Probing memory and executive functions with virtual reality: Past and present studies. *Cyberpsychology & Behavior*, *1*(2), 151–161. doi:10.1089/cpb.1998.1.151

Raben, A., Christensen, N. J., Madsen, J., Holst, J. J., & Astrup, A. (1994). Decreased postprandial thermogenesis and fat oxidation but increased fullness after a high-fiber meal compared with a low-fiber meal. *The American Journal of Clinical Nutrition*, *59*(6), 1386–1394. doi:10.1093/ajcn/59.6.1386 PMID:8198065

Radloff, L. S. (1977). The CES-D Scale: A Self-Report Depression Scale for Research in the General Population. *Applied Psychological Measurement*, *1*(3), 385–401. doi:10.1177/014662167700100306

Ramsey, G. W., & Bapna, S. (2014). A Technique to Exploit Free-Form Notes to Predict Customer Churn. *International Journal of Computational Models and Algorithms in Medicine*, *4*(1), 1–16. doi:10.4018/ijcmam.2014010101

Ranade, P., Londhe, S., & Mishra, A. (2015). Smart villages through information technology – need for emerging India. *International Journal of Information Technology, 3*(7), 1–7.

Raspelli, S., Pallavicini, F., Carelli, L., Morganti, F., Poletti, B., & ... Riva, G. (2011). Validation of a neuro virtual reality –based version of the multiple errands test for the assessment of executive functions. *Studies in Health Technology and Informatics, 167*, 92–97. PMID:21685648

Reichheld, F. F., Teal, T., & Smith, D. K. (1996). The loyalty effect: Vol. 1. *No. 3* (pp. 78–84). Boston, MA: Harvard Business School Press.

Rentz, D. M. (2016). Validating Use of Technology for Cognitive Test Assessment. *EBioMedicine, 11*, 23–24. doi:10.1016/j.ebiom.2016.08.002 PMID:27498366

Richter, Y., Yom-Tov, E., & Slonim, N. (2010, April). Predicting customer churn in mobile networks through analysis of social groups. In *Proceedings of the 2010 SIAM international conference on data mining* (pp. 732-741). Society for Industrial and Applied Mathematics. 10.1137/1.9781611972801.64

Riese, H., Van Doornen, L. J., Houtman, I. L., & De Geus, E. J. (2004). Job strain in relation to ambulatory blood pressure, heart rate, and heart rate variability among female nurses. *Scandinavian Journal of Work, Environment & Health, 30*(6), 477–485. doi:10.5271jweh.837 PMID:15635758

Rosa, P. J., Gamito, P., Oliveira, J., Morais, D., Pavlovic, M., & Smyth, O. (2015). Show me your eyes! The combined use of eye tracking and virtual reality applications for cognitive assessment. In *Proceedings of the 3rd 2015 Workshop on ICTs for improving Patients Rehabilitation Research Techniques (REHAB '15)* (pp. 135-138). New York, NY: ACM. 10.1145/2838944.2838977

Roumani, Y. F., May, J. H., Strum, D. P., & Vargas, L. G. (2013). Classifying highly imbalanced ICU data. *Health Care Management Science, 16*(2), 119–128. doi:10.100710729-012-9216-9 PMID:23132123

Ryan, A. M., Bishop, T. F., Shih, S., & Casalino, L. P. (2013). Small physician practices in New York needed sustained help to realize gains in quality from use of electronic health records. *Health Affairs, 32*(1), 53–62. doi:10.1377/hlthaff.2012.0742 PMID:23297271

Sackett, D., Rosenberg, W. M. C., Gray, M. J. A., Haynes, B. R., & Richardson, W. S. (1996). Evidence based medicine: What it is and what it isn't. *BMJ (Clinical Research Ed.)*, *312*(7023), 71–72. doi:10.1136/bmj.312.7023.71 PMID:8555924

Saha, A., & Sindhwani, V. (2012). Learning evolving and emerging topics in social media: A dynamic NMF approach with temporal regularization. *Paper presented at the Proceedings of the 5th International Conference on Web Search and Data Mining (WSDM)*. 10.1145/2124295.2124376

Sahu, A. (2017). Feasibility of using tablet-based cognitive screening tools in India: A short review. *International Journal of Computers in Clinical Practice*, *2*(1), 34–44. doi:10.4018/IJCCP.2017010103

Sánchez, D., & Batet, M. (2011). Semantic similarity estimation in the biomedical domain: An ontology-based information-theoretic perspective. *Journal of Biomedical Informatics*, *44*(5), 749–759. doi:10.1016/j.jbi.2011.03.013 PMID:21463704

Sayers, B. M. (1973). Analysis of heart rate variability. *Ergonomics*, *16*(1), 17–32. doi:10.1080/00140137308924479 PMID:4702060

Schaffer, S. K., Messner, D., Mestre-Ferrandiz, J., Tambor, E., & Towse, A. (2018). Paying for Cures: Perspectives on Solutions to the "Affordability Issue." *Value in Health*, *21*(3), 276–279. doi:10.1016/j.jval.2017.12.013 PMID:29566833

Scheurer, D., McKean, S., Miller, J., & Wetterneck, T. (2009). U.S. physician satisfaction: A systematic review. *Journal of Hospital Medicine*, *177*(8), 883–888. PMID:20013859

Schriml, L. M., Arze, C., Nadendla, S., Chang, Y. W. W., Mazaitis, M., Felix, V., ... Kibbe, W. A. (2012). Disease ontology: A backbone for disease semantic integration. *Nucleic Acids Research*, *40*(D1), D940–D946. doi:10.1093/nar/gkr972 PMID:22080554

Schultheis, M., Himelstein, J., & Rizzo, A. A. (2002). Virtual reality and neuropsychology: Upgrading the current tools. *The Journal of Head Trauma Rehabilitation*, *17*(5), 378–394. doi:10.1097/00001199-200210000-00002 PMID:12802250

Schwab, K. (2016). The Fourth Industrial Revolution. World Economic Forum, Geneva, Switzerland.

Schwab, K., & Davis, N. (2018). Shaping the Fourth Industrial Revolution. World Economic Forum, Geneva, Switzerland.

Scotch, M., Duggal, M., Brandt, C., Lin, Z., & Schiffman, R. (2010). Use of statistical analysis in the biomedical informatics literature. *Journal of the American Medical Informatics Association*, *17*(1), 3–5. doi:10.1197/jamia.M2853 PMID:20064794

Sempionatto, J. R., Nakagawa, T., Pavinatto, A., Mensah, S. T., Imani, S., Mercier, P., & Wang, J. (2017). Eyeglasses based wireless electrolyte and metabolite sensor platform. *Lab on a Chip*, *17*(10), 1834–1842. doi:10.1039/C7LC00192D PMID:28470263

Senders, J. T., Harary, M., Stopa, B. M., Staples, P., Broekman, M. L. D., Smith, T. R., ... Arnaout, O. (2018). Information-based medicine in glioma patients: A clinical perspective. *Computational and Mathematical Methods in Medicine*, *2018*, 8572058. doi:10.1155/2018/8572058 PMID:30008798

Serino, S., Pedroli, E., Cipresso, P., Pallavicini, F., Albani, G., ... Riva, G. (2014). The role of virtual reality in neuropsychology: The virtual multiple errands test (VMET) for the assessment of executive functions in Parkinson's disease. *Intelligent Systems. The Reference Librarian*, *68*, 257–274. doi:10.1007/978-3-642-54816-1_14

Shabi, I. S., Shabi, O. M., Akewukereke, M. A., & Udofia, E. P. (2011). Physicians utilisation of internet medical databases at the tertiary health institutions in Soun state, south west Nigeria. *Health Information and Libraries Journal*, *28*(4), 313–320. doi:10.1111/j.1471-1842.2011.00962.x PMID:22051130

Shadbolt, N., Hall, W., & Berners-Lee, T. (2006). The semantic web revisited. *IEEE Intelligent Systems*, *21*(3), 96–101. doi:10.1109/MIS.2006.62

Shahnaz, F., Berry, M. W., Pauca, V. P., & Plemmons, R. J. (2006). Document clustering using nonnegative matrix factorization. *Information Processing & Management*, *42*(2), 373–386. doi:10.1016/j.ipm.2004.11.005

Shallice, T., & Burgess, P. (1991). Deficits in strategy application following frontal lobe damage in man. *Brain*, *114*(2), 727–741. doi:10.1093/brain/114.2.727 PMID:2043945

Shanafelt, T. D., Dyrbye, L. N., Sinsky, C., Hasan, O., Satele, D., Sloan, J., & West, C. P. (2016, July). Relationship between clerical burden and characteristics of the electronic environment with physician burnout and professional satisfaction. *Mayo Clinic Proceedings, 91*(7), 836–848. doi:10.1016/j.mayocp.2016.05.007 PMID:27313121

Shanafelt, T. D., Sloan, J. A., & Habermann, T. M.Association of Professors of Medicine. (2003). The well-being of physicians. *The American Journal of Medicine, 114*(6), 513–519. doi:10.1016/S0002-9343(03)00117-7 PMID:12727590

Shimono, F., Ohsuga, M., & Terashita, H. (1998). Method for assessment of mental stress during high-tension and monotonous tasks using heart rate. respiration and blood pressure. Japan Ergonomics Society, 34(3), 107-115.

Shittu, A., Ajayi, A., and Garba, S. (2008). Information and Communication Technologies (ICT) Knowledge and Utilization for Healthcare Delivery among Zaria Medical Doctors. *The Nigerian Journal of Communication, 6*(1 & 2), 28-43.

Shvaiko, P., & Euzenat, J. (2013). Ontology Matching: State of the Art and Future Challenges. *IEEE Transactions on Knowledge and Data Engineering, 25*(1), 158–176. doi:10.1109/TKDE.2011.253

Siadat, M. R., Soltanian-Zadeh, H., Fotouhi, F., & Elisevich, K. (2005). Content-based image database system for epilepsy. *Computer Methods and Programs in Biomedicine, 79*(3), 209–226. doi:10.1016/j.cmpb.2005.03.012 PMID:15955590

Siegrist, J., Peter, R., Junge, A., Cremer, P., & Seidel, D. (1990). Low status control, high effort at work and ischemic heart disease: Prospective evidence from bluecollar men. *Social Science & Medicine, 31*(10), 1127–1134. doi:10.1016/0277-9536(90)90234-J PMID:2274801

Singh, B. (2007). Psyllium as therapeutic and drug delivery agent. *International Journal of Pharmaceutics, 334*(1-2), 1–14. doi:10.1016/j.ijpharm.2007.01.028 PMID:17329047

Sinha, N., Dauwels, J., Kaiser, M., Cash, S. S., Brandon Westover, M., Wang, Y., & Taylor, P. N. (2016). Predicting neurosurgical outcomes in focal epilepsy patients using computational modelling. *Brain, 140*(2), 319–332. doi:10.1093/brain/aww299 PMID:28011454

Sinsky, C., Colligan, L., Li, L., Prgomet, M., Reynolds, S., Goeders, L., ... Blike, G. (2016). Allocation of physician time in ambulatory practice: A time and motion study in 4 specialties. *Annals of Internal Medicine*, *165*(11), 753–760. doi:10.7326/M16-0961 PMID:27595430

Sirois, F. M., Molnar, D. S., & Hirsch, J. K. (2015). Self-compassion, stress, and coping in the context of chronic illness. *Self and Identity*, *3*(3), 334–347. doi:10.1080/15298868.2014.996249

Slade, M. (2017). Implementing shared decision making in routine mental health care. *World Psychiatry; Official Journal of the World Psychiatric Association (WPA)*, *16*(2), 146–153. doi:10.1002/wps.20412 PMID:28498575

Smith, B., Ashburner, M., Rosse, C., Bard, J., Bug, W., & Ceusters, W. … Lewis, S. (2007). The OBO Foundry: Coordinated evolution of ontologies to support biomedical data integration. *Nature Biotechnology*. doi:10.1038/nbt1346

Søreide, K., & Wijnhoven, B. P. L. (2016). Surgery for an ageing population. *British Journal of Surgery*, *103*(2), e7–e9. doi:10.1002/bjs.10071 PMID:26771471

Sowmya, R. R., DesRoches, C. M., Donelan, K., Campbell, E. G., Miralles, P. D., & Jha, A. K. (2011). Electronic health records in small physician practices: Availability, use, and perceived benefits. *Journal of the American Medical Informatics Association*, *18*(3), 271–275. doi:10.1136/amiajnl-2010-000010 PMID:21486885

Spasić, I., & Ananiadou, S. (2005). A flexible measure of contextual similarity for biomedical terms. In *Pacific Symposium on Biocomputing. Pacific Symposium on Biocomputing*.

Spencer, S. S., Berg, A. T., Vickrey, B. G., Sperling, M. R., Bazil, C. W., Shinnar, S., ... Pacia, S. V. (2005). Predicting long-term seizure outcome after resective epilepsy surgery: The multicenter study. *Neurology*, *65*(6), 912–918. doi:10.1212/01.wnl.0000176055.45774.71 PMID:16186534

Srinivas, K., Rani, B. K., & Govrdhan, A. (2010). Applications of Data Mining Techniques in Healthcare and Prediction of Heart Attacks. *International Journal on Computer Science and Engineering*, *2*(02), 250–255.

Srivastava, A. (2005). *Accelerating Delivery of Health Services*. New Delhi: UN World Food Programme.

Stansfeld, S. A., Fuhrer, R., Shipley, M. J., & Marmot, M. G. (1999). Work characteristics predict psychiatric disorder: Prospective results from the Whitehall II study. *Occupational and Environmental Medicine*, *56*(5), 302–307. doi:10.1136/oem.56.5.302 PMID:10472303

Statista. (2018). Forecast of mobile phone users in India. Retrieved from https://www.statista.com/statistics/274658/forecast-of-mobile-phone-users-in-india/

Stein, M. B., & Smoller, J. W. (2018). Precision psychiatry– Will genomic medicine lead the way? *JAMA Psychiatry*, *75*(7), 663–664. doi:10.1001/jamapsychiatry.2018.0375 PMID:29800947

Stern, D. T. (2006). *Measuring medical professionalism*. Oxford University Press.

Stewart, R., & Davis, K. (2016). 'Big Data' in mental health research: Current status and emerging possibilities. *Social Psychiatry and Psychiatric Epidemiology*, *51*(8), 1055–1072. doi:10.100700127-016-1266-8 PMID:27465245

Straus, S. E., Glasziou, P., Richardson, W. S., & Haynes, R. B. (2019). *Evidence-based medicine: How to practice and teach EBM* (5th ed.). Edinburgh: Elsevier.

Strauss, C., Lever Taylor, B., Gu, J., Kuyken, W., Baer, R., Jones, F., & Cavanagh, K. (2016). What is compassion and how can we measure it? A review of definitions and measures. *Clinical Psychology Review*, *47*, 15–27. doi:10.1016/j.cpr.2016.05.004 PMID:27267346

Sun, W., Rumshisky, A., & Uzuner, O. (2013). Evaluating temporal relations in clinical text: 2012 i2b2 challenge. *Journal of the American Medical Informatics Association*, *20*(5), 806–813. doi:10.1136/amiajnl-2013-001628 PMID:23564629

Svensson, E., Baggesen, L. M., Johnsen, S. P., Pedersen, L., Nørrelund, H., Buhl, E. S., ... Thomsen, R. W. (2017). Early glycemic control and magnitude of HbA1c reduction predict cardiovascular events and mortality: Population-based cohort study of 24,752 metformin initiators. *Diabetes Care*. PMID:28404659

Tabe, N., Tkara, T., & Hoshino, K. (1996). Pupillary diameter and heart rate under active and passive stress. *IEICE*, *96*(116), 75–79.

Takatsu, H., Murnakata, M., Ozeki, O., Yokoyama, K., Watanabe, Y., & Takata, K. (2000). An Evaluation of the Quantitative Relationship between the Subjective Stress Value and Heart Rate Variability. *The trans. of the Institute of Electrical Engineers of Japan*, *120*(1), 104-110.

Tam, C. S., Xie, W., Johnson, W. D., Cefalu, W. T., Redman, L. M., & Ravussin, E. (2012). Defining insulin resistance from hyperinsulinemic-euglycemic clamps. *Diabetes Care*, *35*(7), 1605–1610. doi:10.2337/dc11-2339 PMID:22511259

Tanaka, T., & Sugiyama, Y. (2015). Improvement effect of positive affect on aggravation of burnout tendency in university athletes: Focusing on negative affect. *Japan J. Phys. Educ. Hlth. Sport Sci.*, *60*(2), 479–488. doi:10.5432/jjpehss.15016

Taneja, A., Bhat, C., Arora, A., & Kaur, A. (1989). Effect of incorporation of isabgol husk in a low fibre diet on faecal excretion and serum levels of lipids in adolescent girls. *European Journal of Clinical Nutrition*, *43*, 197. PMID:2543555

Tang, B., Shepherd, M., Milios, E., & Heywood, M. I. (2008). Comparing and combining dimension reduction techniques for efficient text clustering.

Tang, Z., Wang, S., Zhang, X., Wei, W., & Zhao, Y. (2011). Lexicographical framework for image hashing with implementation based on DCT and NMF. *Multimedia Tools and Applications*, *52*(2-3), 325–345. doi:10.100711042-009-0437-y

Tapscott, D. (1998). *Growing up digital: The rise of the next generation*. New York: McGraw-Hill.

Tarnanas, I., Schlee, W., Tsolaki, M., Müri, R., Mosimann, U., & Nef, T. (2013). Ecological validity of virtual reality daily living activities screening for early dementia: longitudinal study. *JMIR Serious Games, 1*(1), 1-14.

Terwisscha van Scheltinga, A. F., Bakker, S. C., van Haren, N. E., Derks, E. M., Buizer-Voskamp, J. E., Cahn, W., & Ripke, S.Psychiatric Genome-Wide Association Study (GWAS) Consortium. (2013). Schizophrenia genetic variants are not associated with intelligence. *Psychological Medicine*, *43*(12), 2563–2570. doi:10.1017/S003329171300196 PMID:23410598

The Physician Foundation. (2016). 2016 Survey of America's Physicians; Practice Patterns & Perspectives. Retrieved from https://www.merritthawkins.com/uploadedFiles/Physicians%20Foundation%202016%20Survey%20of%20Americas%20Physicians.pdf

Thornton, T. (2013). *Clinical judgment, tacit knowledge, and recognition in psychiatric diagnosis*. Oxford: Oxford Handbooks Online.

Tierney, M. J., Tamada, J. A., Potts, R. O., Jovanovic, L., & Garg, S. (2001). Clinical evaluation of the GlucoWatch® biographer: A continual, non-invasive glucose monitor for patients with diabetes. *Biosensors & Bioelectronics*, *16*(9-12), 621–629. doi:10.1016/S0956-5663(01)00189-0 PMID:11679237

Tkachenko, P., Kriukova, G., Aleksandrova, M., Chertov, O., Renard, E., & Pereverzyev, S. V. (2016). Prediction of nocturnal hypoglycemia by an aggregation of previously known prediction approaches: Proof of concept for clinical application. *Computer Methods and Programs in Biomedicine*, *134*, 179–186. doi:10.1016/j.cmpb.2016.07.003 PMID:27480742

Tonini, C., Beghi, E., Berg, A. T., Bogliun, G., Giordano, L., Newton, R. W., ... Wiebe, S. (2004). Predictors of epilepsy surgery outcome: A meta-analysis. *Epilepsy Research*, *62*(1), 75–87. doi:10.1016/j.eplepsyres.2004.08.006 PMID:15519134

Tornatore, J. B., Hill, E., Laboff, J. A., & McGann, M. E. (2005). Self-administered screening for mild cognitive impairment: Initial validation of a computerized test battery. *The Journal of Neuropsychiatry and Clinical Neurosciences*, *17*(1), 98–105. doi:10.1176/jnp.17.1.98 PMID:15746489

Toyo, O. D. (2016). Information and Communication Technology (ICT): A catalyst for promoting primary healthcare delivery services in rural communities in Nigeria. *International Journal of Sustainable Development, 11*(1), 49-57. Retrieved from www.africarsearchcorps.com

Trotman, B. W., Bernstein, S. E., Bove, K. E., & Wirth, G. D. (1980). Studies on the pathogenesis of pigment gallstones in hemolytic anemia. Description and characteristics of a mouse model. *The Journal of Clinical Investigation*, *65*(6), 1301–1308. doi:10.1172/JCI109793 PMID:7410545

Trumbo, P., Schlicker, S., Yates, A. A., & Poos, M. (2002). Dietary reference intakes for energy, carbohydrate, fiber, fat, fatty acids, cholesterol, protein and amino acids. *Journal of the American Dietetic Association*, *102*(11), 1621–1630. doi:10.1016/S0002-8223(02)90346-9 PMID:12449285

Tsarkov, D., Riazanov, A., Bechhofer, S., & Horrocks, I. (2004, November). Using Vampire to reason with OWL. In International Semantic Web Conference (pp. 471-485). Springer. doi:10.1007/978-3-540-30475-3_33

Turgeon, M. L. (2015). *Linne & Ringsrud's Clinical Laboratory Science: The Basics and Routine Techniques*. Retrieved from https://books.google.com/books?id=D1umBgAAQBAJ&pgis=1

Tuzhilin, A. (2012). Customer relationship management and Web mining: The next frontier. *Data Mining and Knowledge Discovery*, 1–29.

Udousoro, N.W. (2014). Use and gratification of ICTs by Health Care Personnel in Nigerian South-South Tertiary Hospitals. *Asian Journal of Social Sciences and Humanities, 3*(4), 226-235.

Uijl, S. G., Leijten, F. S., Arends, J. B., Parra, J., van Huffelen, A. C., & Moons, K. G. (2008). Prognosis after temporal lobe epilepsy surgery: The value of combining predictors. *Epilepsia, 49*(8), 1317–1323. doi:10.1111/j.1528-1167.2008.01695.x PMID:18557776

Underhill, D. G. (2007). Exploring Dimensionality Reduction for Text Mining: DTIC Document.

Unertl, K. M., Johnson, K. B., & Lorenzi, N. M. (2012). Health information exchange technology on the front lines of healthcare: Workflow factors and patterns of use. *Journal of the American Medical Informatics Association, 19*(3), 392–400. doi:10.1136/amiajnl-2011-000432 PMID:22003156

Unruh, L. Y., & Fottler, M. D. (2006). Patient turnover and nursing staff adequacy. *Health Services Research, 41*(2), 599–612. doi:10.1111/j.1475-6773.2005.00496.x PMID:16584467

Vafeiadis, T., Diamantaras, K. I., Sarigiannidis, G., & Chatzisavvas, K. C. (2015). A comparison of machine learning techniques for customer churn prediction. *Simulation Modelling Practice and Theory, 55*, 1–9. doi:10.1016/j.simpat.2015.03.003

VanFosson, C. A., Yoder, L. H., & Jones, T. L. (2017). Patient turnover: A concept analysis. *Advances in Nursing Science, 40*(3), 300–312. doi:10.1097/ANS.0000000000000171 PMID:28266962

Verbeke, W., Martens, D., Mues, C., & Baesens, B. (2011). Building comprehensible customer churn prediction models with advanced rule induction techniques. *Expert Systems with Applications, 38*(3), 2354–2364. doi:10.1016/j.eswa.2010.08.023

Vrijkotte, T. G., van Doornen, L. J., & de Geus, E. J. (2000). Effects of work stress on ambulatory blood pressure, heart rate, and heart rate variability. *Hypertension, 35*(4), 880–886. doi:10.1161/01.HYP.35.4.880 PMID:10775555

Vydra, T.P., Cuaresma, E., Kretovics, M., & Bose-Brill, S. (2015). Diffusion and use of tethered personal health records in primary care. *Perspective in Health Information Management,* (Spring), 1-16.

W3C. (2014). RDF Schema 1.1. World Wide Web Consortium.

Wallace, T. M., Levy, J. C., & Matthews, D. R. (2004). Use and abuse of HOMA modeling. *Diabetes Care, 27*(6), 1487–1495. doi:10.2337/diacare.27.6.1487 PMID:15161807

Wang, H. C., & Lee, A. R. (2015). Recent developments in blood glucose sensors. *Journal of Food and Drug Analysis, 23*(2), 191–200. doi:10.1016/j.jfda.2014.12.001 PMID:28911373

Watkins, J., Kitner, K. R., & Mehta, D. (2012). Mobile and smartphone use in urban and rural India. *Journal of Media & Cultural Studies, 26*(5), 685–697. doi:10.1080/10304312.2012.706458

Wears, R. L., & Berg, M. (2005). Computer technology and clinical work: Still waiting for Godot. *Journal of the American Medical Association, 293*(10), 1261–1263. doi:10.1001/jama.293.10.1261 PMID:15755949

Weickert, M. O., & Pfeiffer, A. F. (2008). Metabolic effects of dietary fiber consumption and prevention of diabetes. *The Journal of Nutrition, 138*(3), 439–442. doi:10.1093/jn/138.3.439 PMID:18287346

Weniger, G., Ruhleder, M., Lange, C., Wolf, S., & Irle, E. (2011). Egocentric and allocentric memory as assessed by virtual reality in individuals with amnestic mild cognitive impairments. *Neuropsychologia, 49*(3), 518–527. doi:10.1016/j.neuropsychologia.2010.12.031 PMID:21185847

West, M., & Spendlove, M. (2006). The impact of culture and climate in healthcare organizations. In J. Cox, J. King, A. Hutchinson, & P. McAvoy (Eds.), *Understanding doctors' performance* (pp. 91–105). Oxford: Radcliffe Publishing.

William, J. A., & Murugesh, R. (2016). Cognitive modeling in human computer interaction: Understanding technology usage in elderly people. In *2016 IEEE International Conference on Advances in Computer Applications (ICACA)* (pp. 115-120). 10.1109/ICACA.2016.7887934

Wilson, K. B., Tete-Mensah, I., & Boateng, K.A. (2014). Information and Communication Technology Use in Higher Education: Perspectives from Students. *European Scientific Journal, 10*(19), 161–171.

Witten, I. H., & Frank, E. (2005). *Data Mining: Practical machine learning tools and techniques* (2nd ed.). San Francisco, CA: Morgan Kaufmann.

Witt, J.-A., Alpherts, W., & Helmstaedter, C. (2013). Computerized neuropsychological testing in epilepsy: Overview of available tools. *Seizure, 22*(6), 416–423. doi:10.1016/j.seizure.2013.04.004 PMID:23628168

World Health Organization. (2016). Global report on diabetes.

Wu, C., Steinbauer, J. R., & Kuo, G. M. (2005). EM Clustering Analysis of Diabetes Patients Basic Diagnosis Index. *Paper presented at the AMIA Annual Symposium Proceedings.*

Wu, R. C., Abrams, H., Baker, M., & Rossos, P. G. (2006). Implementation of a computerized physician order entry system of medications at the University Health Network – Physicians' perspectives on the critical issues. *Healthcare Quarterly, 9*, 106–109. PMID:16548441

Xie, Y., & Li, X. (2008). Churn prediction with Linear Discriminant Boosting algorithm. *Paper presented at the 2008 International Conference on Machine Learning and Cybernetics.*

Xierali, I. M., Phillips, R. L., Green, L. A., Bazemore, A. W., & Puffer, J. C. (2013). Factors influencing family physician adoption of electronic health records (EHRs). *Journal of the American Board of Family Medicine, 26*(4), 399–393. doi:10.3122/jabfm.2013.04.120351 PMID:23833153

Yang, N., & Hing, E. (2017). Table of Electronic Health Record Adoption and Use among Office-based Physicians in the U.S., by Specialty: 2015 National Electronic Health Records Survey. *CDC*. Retrieved from https://www.cdc.gov/nchs/data/ahcd/nehrs/2015_nehrs_ehr_by_specialty.pdf

Yun, C. H., Lee, S. K., Lee, S. Y., Kim, K. K., Jeong, S. W., & Chung, C. K. (2006). Prognostic factors in neocortical epilepsy surgery: Multivariate analysis. *Epilepsia, 47*(3), 574–579. doi:10.1111/j.1528-1167.2006.00470.x PMID:16529624

Yu, X., Rashid, M., Feng, J., Hobbs, N., Hajizadeh, I., Samadi, S., ... Quinn, L. (2018). Online Glucose Prediction Using Computationally Efficient Sparse Kernel Filtering Algorithms in Type-1 Diabetes. *IEEE Transactions on Control Systems Technology, 99*, 1–13.

Zanstra, Y. J., Schellekens, J. M., Schaap, C., & Kooistra, L. (2006). Vagal and sympathetic activity in burnouts during a mentally demanding workday. *Psychosomatic Medicine, 68*(4), 583–590. doi:10.1097/01.psy.0000228012.38884.49 PMID:16868268

Zecchin, C., Facchinetti, A., Sparacino, G., & Cobelli, C. (2013). Reduction of number and duration of hypoglycemic events by glucose prediction methods: A proof-of-concept in silico study. *Diabetes Technology & Therapeutics*, *15*(1), 66–77. doi:10.1089/dia.2012.0208 PMID:23297671

Zecchin, C., Facchinetti, A., Sparacino, G., & Cobelli, C. (2016). How much is short-term glucose prediction in type 1 diabetes improved by adding insulin delivery and meal content information to CGM data? A proof-of-concept study. *Journal of Diabetes Science and Technology*, *10*(5), 1149–1160. doi:10.1177/1932296816654161 PMID:27381030

Zhao, M., Zhang, S., Li, W., & Chen, G. (2018). Matching biomedical ontologies based on formal concept analysis. *Journal of Biomedical Semantics*, *9*(1), 11. doi:10.118613326-018-0178-9 PMID:29554977

Zitner, D. (2006). Physicians will happily adopt information technology. *Canadian Medical Association Journal*, *174*(11), 1583–1584. doi:10.1503/cmaj.060470 PMID:16717267

Zuger, A. (2004). Dissatisfaction with medical practice. *The New England Journal of Medicine*, *350*(1), 69–75. doi:10.1056/NEJMsr031703 PMID:14702431

Zvárová, J., & Zvára, K. (2011). e3Health: Three main features of modern healthcare. In A. Moumtzoglou & A. Kastania (Eds.), E-health systems quality and reliability. Models and standards (pp. 18-27). Hershey, PA: IGI Global.

Zvárová, J. (2014). Information-based holistic electronic healthcare. *International Journal of Biomedicine and Healthcare*, *2*(2), 2–7.

Related References

To continue our tradition of advancing information science and technology research, we have compiled a list of recommended IGI Global readings. These references will provide additional information and guidance to further enrich your knowledge and assist you with your own research and future publications.

Abu Seman, S. A., & Ramayah, T. (2017). Are We Ready to App?: A Study on mHealth Apps, Its Future, and Trends in Malaysia Context. In J. Pelet (Ed.), *Mobile Platforms, Design, and Apps for Social Commerce* (pp. 69–83). Hershey, PA: IGI Global. doi:10.4018/978-1-5225-2469-4.ch005

Aggarwal, S., & Azad, V. (2017). A Hybrid System Based on FMM and MLP to Diagnose Heart Disease. In S. Bhattacharyya, S. De, I. Pan, & P. Dutta (Eds.), *Intelligent Multidimensional Data Clustering and Analysis* (pp. 293–325). Hershey, PA: IGI Global. doi:10.4018/978-1-5225-1776-4.ch011

Akaichi, J., & Mhadhbi, L. (2016). A Clinical Decision Support System: Ontology-Driven Approach for Effective Emergency Management. In J. Moon & M. Galea (Eds.), *Improving Health Management through Clinical Decision Support Systems* (pp. 270–294). Hershey, PA: IGI Global. doi:10.4018/978-1-4666-9432-3.ch013

Akerkar, R. (2016). Towards an Intelligent Integrated Approach for Clinical Decision Support. In A. Aggarwal (Ed.), *Managing Big Data Integration in the Public Sector* (pp. 187–205). Hershey, PA: IGI Global. doi:10.4018/978-1-4666-9649-5.ch011

Al-Busaidi, S. S. (2018). Interdisciplinary Relationships Between Medicine and Social Sciences. In M. Al-Suqri, A. Al-Kindi, S. AlKindi, & N. Saleem (Eds.), *Promoting Interdisciplinarity in Knowledge Generation and Problem Solving* (pp. 124–137). Hershey, PA: IGI Global. doi:10.4018/978-1-5225-3878-3.ch009

Al Kareh, T., & Thoumy, M. (2018). The Impact of Health Information Digitization on the Physiotherapist-Patient Relationship: A Pilot Study of the Lebanese Community. *International Journal of Healthcare Information Systems and Informatics, 13*(2), 29–53. doi:10.4018/IJHISI.2018040103

Alenzuela, R. (2017). Research, Leadership, and Resource-Sharing Initiatives: The Role of Local Library Consortia in Access to Medical Information. In S. Ram (Ed.), *Library and Information Services for Bioinformatics Education and Research* (pp. 199–211). Hershey, PA: IGI Global. doi:10.4018/978-1-5225-1871-6.ch012

Ameri, H., Alizadeh, S., & Noughabi, E. A. (2017). Application of Data Mining Techniques in Clinical Decision Making: A Literature Review and Classification. In E. Noughabi, B. Raahemi, A. Albadvi, & B. Far (Eds.), *Handbook of Research on Data Science for Effective Healthcare Practice and Administration* (pp. 257–295). Hershey, PA: IGI Global. doi:10.4018/978-1-5225-2515-8.ch012

Anand, S. (2017). Medical Image Enhancement Using Edge Information-Based Methods. In B. Singh (Ed.), *Computational Tools and Techniques for Biomedical Signal Processing* (pp. 123–148). Hershey, PA: IGI Global. doi:10.4018/978-1-5225-0660-7.ch006

Angjellari-Dajci, F., Sapienza, C., Lawless, W. F., & Kavanagh, K. (2016). Human Capital Accumulation in Medical Simulated Learning Environments: A Framework for Economic Evaluation. In M. Russ (Ed.), *Quantitative Multidisciplinary Approaches in Human Capital and Asset Management* (pp. 65–88). Hershey, PA: IGI Global. doi:10.4018/978-1-4666-9652-5.ch004

Anil, M., Ayyildiz-Tamis, D., Tasdemir, S., Sendemir-Urkmez, A., & Gulce-Iz, S. (2016). Bioinspired Materials and Biocompatibility. In M. Bououdina (Ed.), *Emerging Research on Bioinspired Materials Engineering* (pp. 294–322). Hershey, PA: IGI Global. doi:10.4018/978-1-4666-9811-6.ch011

Anton, J. L., Soriano, J. V., Martinez, M. I., & Garcia, F. B. (2018). Comprehensive E-Learning Appraisal System. In M. Khosrow-Pour, D.B.A. (Ed.), Encyclopedia of Information Science and Technology, Fourth Edition (pp. 5787-5799). Hershey, PA: IGI Global. doi:10.4018/978-1-5225-2255-3.ch503

Arabi, M. (2016). Redesigning the Organizational Structure to Reach Efficiency: The Case of Ministry of Health and Medical Education of Iran. In R. Gholipour & K. Rouzbehani (Eds.), *Social, Economic, and Political Perspectives on Public Health Policy-Making* (pp. 257–294). Hershey, PA: IGI Global. doi:10.4018/978-1-4666-9944-1.ch012

Assis-Hassid, S., Heart, T., Reychav, I., & Pliskin, J. S. (2016). Modelling Factors Affecting Patient-Doctor-Computer Communication in Primary Care. *International Journal of Reliable and Quality E-Healthcare*, *5*(1), 1–17. doi:10.4018/IJRQEH.2016010101

Atzori, B., Hoffman, H. G., Vagnoli, L., Messeri, A., & Grotto, R. L. (2018). Virtual Reality as Distraction Technique for Pain Management in Children and Adolescents. In M. Khosrow-Pour, D.B.A. (Ed.), Encyclopedia of Information Science and Technology, Fourth Edition (pp. 5955-5965). Hershey, PA: IGI Global. doi:10.4018/978-1-5225-2255-3.ch518

Audibert, M., Mathonnat, J., Pélissier, A., & Huang, X. X. (2018). The Impact of the New Rural Cooperative Medical Scheme on Township Hospitals' Utilization and Income Structure in Weifang Prefecture, China. In I. Management Association (Ed.), Health Economics and Healthcare Reform: Breakthroughs in Research and Practice (pp. 109-121). Hershey, PA: IGI Global. doi:10.4018/978-1-5225-3168-5.ch007

Ayyachamy, S. (2016). Analysis and Comparison of Developed 2D Medical Image Database Design using Registration Scheme, Retrieval Scheme, and Bag-of-Visual-Words. In N. Dey & A. Ashour (Eds.), *Classification and Clustering in Biomedical Signal Processing* (pp. 149–168). Hershey, PA: IGI Global. doi:10.4018/978-1-5225-0140-4.ch007

Babalola, A. C. (2016). Literacy and Decision Making on Health Issues among Married Women in Southwest Nigeria. In V. Wang (Ed.), *Handbook of Research on Advancing Health Education through Technology* (pp. 191–212). Hershey, PA: IGI Global. doi:10.4018/978-1-4666-9494-1.ch009

Babu, A., & Ayyappan, S. (2017). A Methodological Evaluation of Crypto-Watermarking System for Medical Images. In C. Bhatt & S. Peddoju (Eds.), *Cloud Computing Systems and Applications in Healthcare* (pp. 189–217). Hershey, PA: IGI Global. doi:10.4018/978-1-5225-1002-4.ch010

Bakke, A. (2017). Ethos in E-Health: From Informational to Interactive Websites. In M. Folk & S. Apostel (Eds.), *Establishing and Evaluating Digital Ethos and Online Credibility* (pp. 85–103). Hershey, PA: IGI Global. doi:10.4018/978-1-5225-1072-7.ch005

Bali, S. (2018). Enhancing the Reach of Health Care Through Telemedicine: Status and New Possibilities in Developing Countries. In U. Pandey & V. Indrakanti (Eds.), *Open and Distance Learning Initiatives for Sustainable Development* (pp. 339–354). Hershey, PA: IGI Global. doi:10.4018/978-1-5225-2621-6.ch019

Barrett, T. E. (2018). Essentials for Education and Training for Tomorrow's Physicians. In C. Smith (Ed.), *Exploring the Pressures of Medical Education From a Mental Health and Wellness Perspective* (pp. 230–252). Hershey, PA: IGI Global. doi:10.4018/978-1-5225-2811-1.ch010

Barrett, T. J. (2016). Knowledge in Action: Fostering Health Education through Technology. In V. Wang (Ed.), *Handbook of Research on Advancing Health Education through Technology* (pp. 39–62). Hershey, PA: IGI Global. doi:10.4018/978-1-4666-9494-1.ch003

Berrahal, S., & Boudriga, N. (2017). The Risks of Wearable Technologies to Individuals and Organizations. In A. Marrington, D. Kerr, & J. Gammack (Eds.), *Managing Security Issues and the Hidden Dangers of Wearable Technologies* (pp. 18–46). Hershey, PA: IGI Global. doi:10.4018/978-1-5225-1016-1.ch002

Bhagat, A. P., & Atique, M. (2016). Medical Image Mining Using Fuzzy Connectedness Image Segmentation: Efficient Retrieval of Patients' Stored Images. In W. Karâa & N. Dey (Eds.), *Biomedical Image Analysis and Mining Techniques for Improved Health Outcomes* (pp. 184–209). Hershey, PA: IGI Global. doi:10.4018/978-1-4666-8811-7.ch009

Bhargava, P. (2018). Blended Learning: An Effective Application to Clinical Teaching. In S. Tang & C. Lim (Eds.), *Preparing the Next Generation of Teachers for 21st Century Education* (pp. 302–320). Hershey, PA: IGI Global. doi:10.4018/978-1-5225-4080-9.ch018

Binh, N. T., & Tuyet, V. T. (2016). The Combination of Adaptive Filters to Improve the Quality of Medical Images in New Wavelet Domain. In N. Dey & A. Ashour (Eds.), *Classification and Clustering in Biomedical Signal Processing* (pp. 46–76). Hershey, PA: IGI Global. doi:10.4018/978-1-5225-0140-4.ch003

Bird, J. L. (2017). Writing Healing Narratives. In V. Bryan & J. Bird (Eds.), *Healthcare Community Synergism between Patients, Practitioners, and Researchers* (pp. 1–28). Hershey, PA: IGI Global. doi:10.4018/978-1-5225-0640-9.ch001

Bottrighi, A., Leonardi, G., Piovesan, L., & Terenziani, P. (2016). Knowledge-Based Support to the Treatment of Exceptions in Computer Interpretable Clinical Guidelines. *International Journal of Knowledge-Based Organizations*, *6*(3), 1–27. doi:10.4018/IJKBO.2016070101

Bougoulias, K., Kouris, I., Prasinos, M., Giokas, K., & Koutsouris, D. (2017). Ob/Gyn EMR Software: A Solution for Obstetricians and Gynecologists. In A. Moumtzoglou (Ed.), *Design, Development, and Integration of Reliable Electronic Healthcare Platforms* (pp. 101–111). Hershey, PA: IGI Global. doi:10.4018/978-1-5225-1724-5.ch006

Bouslimi, R., Ayadi, M. G., & Akaichi, J. (2018). Medical Image Retrieval in Healthcare Social Networks. *International Journal of Healthcare Information Systems and Informatics, 13*(2), 13–28. doi:10.4018/IJHISI.2018040102

Bouzaabia, O., Bouzaabia, R., & Mejri, K. (2017). Role of Internet in the Development of Medical Tourism Service in Tunisia. In A. Capatina & E. Rancati (Eds.), *Key Challenges and Opportunities in Web Entrepreneurship* (pp. 211–241). Hershey, PA: IGI Global. doi:10.4018/978-1-5225-2466-3.ch009

Briz-Ponce, L., Juanes-Méndez, J. A., & García-Peñalvo, F. J. (2016). The Role of Gender in Technology Acceptance for Medical Education. In M. Cruz-Cunha, I. Miranda, R. Martinho, & R. Rijo (Eds.), *Encyclopedia of E-Health and Telemedicine* (pp. 1013–1027). Hershey, PA: IGI Global. doi:10.4018/978-1-4666-9978-6.ch079

Briz-Ponce, L., Juanes-Méndez, J. A., & García-Peñalvo, F. J. (2016). A Research Contribution to the Analysis of Mobile Devices in Higher Education from Medical Students' Point of View. In L. Briz-Ponce, J. Juanes-Méndez, & F. García-Peñalvo (Eds.), *Handbook of Research on Mobile Devices and Applications in Higher Education Settings* (pp. 196–221). Hershey, PA: IGI Global. doi:10.4018/978-1-5225-0256-2.ch009

Brown-Jackson, K. L. (2018). Telemedicine and Telehealth: Academics Engaging the Community in a Call to Action. In S. Burton (Ed.), *Engaged Scholarship and Civic Responsibility in Higher Education* (pp. 166–193). Hershey, PA: IGI Global. doi:10.4018/978-1-5225-3649-9.ch008

Bwalya, K. J. (2017). Next Wave of Tele-Medicine: Virtual Presence of Medical Personnel. In K. Moahi, K. Bwalya, & P. Sebina (Eds.), *Health Information Systems and the Advancement of Medical Practice in Developing Countries* (pp. 168–180). Hershey, PA: IGI Global. doi:10.4018/978-1-5225-2262-1.ch010

Carlton, E. L., Holsinger, J. W. Jr, & Anunobi, N. (2016). Physician Engagement with Health Information Technology: Implications for Practice and Professionalism. *International Journal of Computers in Clinical Practice, 1*(2), 51–73. doi:10.4018/IJCCP.2016070103

Castillo-Page, L., Eliason, J., Conrad, S. S., & Nivet, M. A. (2016). Diversity in Undergraduate Medical Education: An Examination of Organizational Culture and Climate in Medical Schools. In C. Scott & J. Sims (Eds.), *Developing Workforce Diversity Programs, Curriculum, and Degrees in Higher Education* (pp. 304–326). Hershey, PA: IGI Global. doi:10.4018/978-1-5225-0209-8.ch016

Cebeci, H. I., & Hiziroglu, A. (2016). Review of Business Intelligence and Intelligent Systems in Healthcare Domain. In N. Celebi (Ed.), *Intelligent Techniques for Data Analysis in Diverse Settings* (pp. 192–206). Hershey, PA: IGI Global. doi:10.4018/978-1-5225-0075-9.ch009

Celik, G. (2018). Determining Headache Diseases With Genetic Algorithm. In U. Kose, G. Guraksin, & O. Deperlioglu (Eds.), *Nature-Inspired Intelligent Techniques for Solving Biomedical Engineering Problems* (pp. 249–262). Hershey, PA: IGI Global. doi:10.4018/978-1-5225-4769-3.ch012

Chakraborty, C., Gupta, B., & Ghosh, S. K. (2016). Mobile Telemedicine Systems for Remote Patient's Chronic Wound Monitoring. In A. Moumtzoglou (Ed.), *M-Health Innovations for Patient-Centered Care* (pp. 213–239). Hershey, PA: IGI Global. doi:10.4018/978-1-4666-9861-1.ch011

Chakraborty, S., Chatterjee, S., Ashour, A. S., Mali, K., & Dey, N. (2018). Intelligent Computing in Medical Imaging: A Study. In N. Dey (Ed.), *Advancements in Applied Metaheuristic Computing* (pp. 143–163). Hershey, PA: IGI Global. doi:10.4018/978-1-5225-4151-6.ch006

Chavez, A., & Kovarik, C. (2017). Open Source Technology for Medical Practice in Developing Countries. In K. Moahi, K. Bwalya, & P. Sebina (Eds.), *Health Information Systems and the Advancement of Medical Practice in Developing Countries* (pp. 33–59). Hershey, PA: IGI Global. doi:10.4018/978-1-5225-2262-1.ch003

Chen, E. T. (2016). Examining the Influence of Information Technology on Modern Health Care. In P. Manolitzas, E. Grigoroudis, N. Matsatsinis, & D. Yannacopoulos (Eds.), *Effective Methods for Modern Healthcare Service Quality and Evaluation* (pp. 110–136). Hershey, PA: IGI Global. doi:10.4018/978-1-4666-9961-8.ch006

Chin, S. (2016). Surviving Sandy: Recovering Collections after a Natural Disaster. In E. Decker & J. Townes (Eds.), *Handbook of Research on Disaster Management and Contingency Planning in Modern Libraries* (pp. 366–388). Hershey, PA: IGI Global. doi:10.4018/978-1-4666-8624-3.ch016

Chojnacki, M., & Wójcik, A. (2016). Security and the Role of New Technologies and Innovation in Medical Ethics. In A. Rosiek & K. Leksowski (Eds.), *Organizational Culture and Ethics in Modern Medicine* (pp. 52–77). Hershey, PA: IGI Global. doi:10.4018/978-1-4666-9658-7.ch003

Cılız, N., Yıldırım, H., & Temizel, Ş. (2016). Structure Development for Effective Medical Waste and Hazardous Waste Management System. In U. Akkucuk (Ed.), *Handbook of Research on Waste Management Techniques for Sustainability* (pp. 303–327). Hershey, PA: IGI Global. doi:10.4018/978-1-4666-9723-2.ch016

Ciufudean, C. (2018). Innovative Formalism for Biological Data Analysis. In M. Khosrow-Pour, D.B.A. (Ed.), Encyclopedia of Information Science and Technology, Fourth Edition (pp. 1814-1824). Hershey, PA: IGI Global. doi:10.4018/978-1-5225-2255-3.ch158

Ciufudean, C., & Ciufudean, O. (2016). Tele-Monitoring for Medical Diagnosis Availability. In M. Cruz-Cunha, I. Miranda, R. Martinho, & R. Rijo (Eds.), *Encyclopedia of E-Health and Telemedicine* (pp. 401–411). Hershey, PA: IGI Global. doi:10.4018/978-1-4666-9978-6.ch032

Colaguori, R., & Danesi, M. (2017). Medical Semiotics: A Revisitation and an Exhortation. *International Journal of Semiotics and Visual Rhetoric*, *1*(1), 11–18. doi:10.4018/IJSVR.2017010102

Cole, A. W., & Salek, T. A. (2017). Adopting a Parasocial Connection to Overcome Professional Kakoethos in Online Health Information. In M. Folk & S. Apostel (Eds.), *Establishing and Evaluating Digital Ethos and Online Credibility* (pp. 104–120). Hershey, PA: IGI Global. doi:10.4018/978-1-5225-1072-7.ch006

Contreras, E. C., & Puente, G. J. (2016). How to Identify Rheumatic Diseases by General Physicians. In T. Gasmelseid (Ed.), *Advancing Pharmaceutical Processes and Tools for Improved Health Outcomes* (pp. 136–166). Hershey, PA: IGI Global. doi:10.4018/978-1-5225-0248-7.ch006

D'Andrea, A., Ferri, F., & Grifoni, P. (2016). RFID Technologies in Healthcare Setting: Applications and Future Perspectives. *International Journal of Computers in Clinical Practice*, *1*(1), 15–27. doi:10.4018/IJCCP.2016010102

Damianakis, A., Kallonis, P., Loudos, G., Tsatsos, D., & Tsoukalis, A. (2016). Exploiting 3D Medical Equipment Simulations to Support Biomedical Engineering Academic Courses: Design Methodology and Implementation in a Small Scale National Project. In B. Khan (Ed.), *Revolutionizing Modern Education through Meaningful E-Learning Implementation* (pp. 277–295). Hershey, PA: IGI Global. doi:10.4018/978-1-5225-0466-5.ch015

Demiroz, E. (2016). Principles of Instructional Design for E-Learning and Online Learning Practices: Implications for Medical Education. In V. Wang (Ed.), *Handbook of Research on Advancing Health Education through Technology* (pp. 419–451). Hershey, PA: IGI Global. doi:10.4018/978-1-4666-9494-1.ch018

Deperlioglu, O. (2018). Intelligent Techniques Inspired by Nature and Used in Biomedical Engineering. In U. Kose, G. Guraksin, & O. Deperlioglu (Eds.), *Nature-Inspired Intelligent Techniques for Solving Biomedical Engineering Problems* (pp. 51–77). Hershey, PA: IGI Global. doi:10.4018/978-1-5225-4769-3.ch003

Dey, N., & Ashour, A. S. (2018). Meta-Heuristic Algorithms in Medical Image Segmentation: A Review. In N. Dey (Ed.), *Advancements in Applied Metaheuristic Computing* (pp. 185–203). Hershey, PA: IGI Global. doi:10.4018/978-1-5225-4151-6.ch008

Dey, N., Ashour, A. S., & Althoupety, A. S. (2017). Thermal Imaging in Medical Science. In V. Santhi (Ed.), *Recent Advances in Applied Thermal Imaging for Industrial Applications* (pp. 87–117). Hershey, PA: IGI Global. doi:10.4018/978-1-5225-2423-6.ch004

Di Virgilio, F., Camillo, A. A., & Camillo, I. C. (2017). The Impact of Social Network on Italian Users' Behavioural Intention for the Choice of a Medical Tourist Destination. *International Journal of Tourism and Hospitality Management in the Digital Age, 1*(1), 36–49. doi:10.4018/IJTHMDA.2017010103

Dias, C. M., Ribeiro, A. G., & Furtado, S. F. (2016). An Overview about the Use of Healthcare Applications on Mobile Devices. In M. Cruz-Cunha, I. Miranda, R. Martinho, & R. Rijo (Eds.), *Encyclopedia of E-Health and Telemedicine* (pp. 285–298). Hershey, PA: IGI Global. doi:10.4018/978-1-4666-9978-6.ch024

Dogra, A. K., & Dogra, P. (2017). The Medical Tourism Industry in the BRIC Nations: An Indian Analysis. In M. Dhiman (Ed.), *Opportunities and Challenges for Tourism and Hospitality in the BRIC Nations* (pp. 320–336). Hershey, PA: IGI Global. doi:10.4018/978-1-5225-0708-6.ch020

Drowos, J. L., & Wood, S. K. (2017). Preparing Future Physicians to Adapt to the Changing Health Care System: Promoting Humanism through Curricular Design. In V. Bryan & J. Bird (Eds.), *Healthcare Community Synergism between Patients, Practitioners, and Researchers* (pp. 106–125). Hershey, PA: IGI Global. doi:10.4018/978-1-5225-0640-9.ch006

Dulam, K. (2017). Medical Patents and Impact on Availability and Affordability of Essential Medicines in India. In R. Aggarwal & R. Kaur (Eds.), *Patent Law and Intellectual Property in the Medical Field* (pp. 41–57). Hershey, PA: IGI Global. doi:10.4018/978-1-5225-2414-4.ch003

Dutta, P. (2017). Decision Making in Medical Diagnosis via Distance Measures on Interval Valued Fuzzy Sets. *International Journal of System Dynamics Applications*, *6*(4), 63–83. doi:10.4018/IJSDA.2017100104

Edoh, T. O., Pawar, P. A., Brügge, B., & Teege, G. (2016). A Multidisciplinary Remote Healthcare Delivery System to Increase Health Care Access, Pathology Screening, and Treatment in Developing Countries: The Case of Benin. *International Journal of Healthcare Information Systems and Informatics*, *11*(4), 1–31. doi:10.4018/IJHISI.2016100101

El Guemhioui, K., & Demurjian, S. A. (2017). Semantic Reconciliation of Electronic Health Records Using Semantic Web Technologies. *International Journal of Information Technology and Web Engineering*, *12*(2), 26–48. doi:10.4018/IJITWE.2017040102

Ellouze, N., Rekhis, S., & Boudriga, N. (2016). Forensic Investigation of Digital Crimes in Healthcare Applications. In O. Isafiade & A. Bagula (Eds.), *Data Mining Trends and Applications in Criminal Science and Investigations* (pp. 169–210). Hershey, PA: IGI Global. doi:10.4018/978-1-5225-0463-4.ch007

Eneanya, A. N. (2016). Health Policy Implementation and Its Barriers: The Case Study of US Health System. In R. Gholipour & K. Rouzbehani (Eds.), *Social, Economic, and Political Perspectives on Public Health Policy-Making* (pp. 42–63). Hershey, PA: IGI Global. doi:10.4018/978-1-4666-9944-1.ch003

Entico, G. J. (2016). Knowledge Management and the Medical Health Librarians: A Perception Study. In J. Yap, M. Perez, M. Ayson, & G. Entico (Eds.), *Special Library Administration, Standardization and Technological Integration* (pp. 52–77). Hershey, PA: IGI Global. doi:10.4018/978-1-4666-9542-9.ch003

Ferradji, M. A., & Zidani, A. (2016). Collaborative Environment for Remote Clinical Reasoning Learning. *International Journal of E-Health and Medical Communications*, *7*(4), 62–81. doi:10.4018/IJEHMC.2016100104

Fisher, J. (2018). Sociological Perspectives on Improving Medical Diagnosis Emphasizing CAD. In M. Khosrow-Pour, D.B.A. (Ed.), Encyclopedia of Information Science and Technology, Fourth Edition (pp. 1017-1024). Hershey, PA: IGI Global. doi:10.4018/978-1-5225-2255-3.ch088

Flores, C. D., Respício, A., Coelho, H., Bez, M. R., & Fonseca, J. M. (2016). Simulation for Medical Training. In M. Cruz-Cunha, I. Miranda, R. Martinho, & R. Rijo (Eds.), *Encyclopedia of E-Health and Telemedicine* (pp. 827–842). Hershey, PA: IGI Global. doi:10.4018/978-1-4666-9978-6.ch064

Frank, E. M. (2018). Healthcare Education: Integrating Simulation Technologies. In V. Bryan, A. Musgrove, & J. Powers (Eds.), *Handbook of Research on Human Development in the Digital Age* (pp. 163–182). Hershey, PA: IGI Global. doi:10.4018/978-1-5225-2838-8.ch008

Garner, G. (2018). Foundations for Yoga Practice in Rehabilitation. In S. Telles & N. Singh (Eds.), *Research-Based Perspectives on the Psychophysiology of Yoga* (pp. 263–307). Hershey, PA: IGI Global. doi:10.4018/978-1-5225-2788-6.ch015

Gasmelseid, T. M. (2016). Improving Pharmaceutical Care through the Use of Intelligent Pharmacoinformatics. In T. Gasmelseid (Ed.), *Advancing Pharmaceutical Processes and Tools for Improved Health Outcomes* (pp. 167–188). Hershey, PA: IGI Global. doi:10.4018/978-1-5225-0248-7.ch007

Gavurová, B., Kováč, V., & Šoltés, M. (2018). Medical Equipment and Economic Determinants of Its Structure and Regulation in the Slovak Republic. In M. Khosrow-Pour, D.B.A. (Ed.), Encyclopedia of Information Science and Technology, Fourth Edition (pp. 5841-5852). Hershey, PA: IGI Global. doi:10.4018/978-1-5225-2255-3.ch508

Ge, X., Wang, Q., Huang, K., Law, V., & Thomas, D. C. (2017). Designing Simulated Learning Environments and Facilitating Authentic Learning Experiences in Medical Education. In J. Stefaniak (Ed.), *Advancing Medical Education Through Strategic Instructional Design* (pp. 77–100). Hershey, PA: IGI Global. doi:10.4018/978-1-5225-2098-6.ch004

Gewald, H., & Gewald, C. (2018). Inhibitors of Physicians' Use of Mandatory Hospital Information Systems (HIS). *International Journal of Healthcare Information Systems and Informatics, 13*(1), 29–44. doi:10.4018/IJHISI.2018010103

Ghosh, D., & Dinda, S. (2017). Health Infrastructure and Economic Development in India. In R. Das (Ed.), *Social, Health, and Environmental Infrastructures for Economic Growth* (pp. 99–119). Hershey, PA: IGI Global. doi:10.4018/978-1-5225-2364-2.ch006

Ghosh, K., & Sen, K. C. (2017). The Potential of Crowdsourcing in the Health Care Industry. In N. Wickramasinghe (Ed.), *Handbook of Research on Healthcare Administration and Management* (pp. 418–427). Hershey, PA: IGI Global. doi:10.4018/978-1-5225-0920-2.ch024

Ghrab, S., & Saad, I. (2016). Identifying Crucial Know-How and Knowing-That for Medical Decision Support. *International Journal of Decision Support System Technology, 8*(4), 14–33. doi:10.4018/IJDSST.2016100102

Giokas, K., Tsirmpas, C., Anastasiou, A., Iliopoulou, D., Costarides, V., & Koutsouris, D. (2016). Contemporary Heart Failure Treatment Based on Improved Knowledge and Personalized Care of Comorbidities. In D. Fotiadis (Ed.), *Handbook of Research on Trends in the Diagnosis and Treatment of Chronic Conditions* (pp. 301–314). Hershey, PA: IGI Global. doi:10.4018/978-1-4666-8828-5.ch014

Gopalan, V., Chan, E., & Ho, D. T. (2018). Deliberate Self-Harm and Suicide Ideology in Medical Students. In C. Smith (Ed.), *Exploring the Pressures of Medical Education From a Mental Health and Wellness Perspective* (pp. 122–143). Hershey, PA: IGI Global. doi:10.4018/978-1-5225-2811-1.ch005

Goswami, S., Dey, U., Roy, P., Ashour, A., & Dey, N. (2017). Medical Video Processing: Concept and Applications. In N. Dey, A. Ashour, & P. Patra (Eds.), *Feature Detectors and Motion Detection in Video Processing* (pp. 1–17). Hershey, PA: IGI Global. doi:10.4018/978-1-5225-1025-3.ch001

Goswami, S., Mahanta, K., Goswami, S., Jigdung, T., & Devi, T. P. (2018). Ageing and Cancer: The Epigenetic Basis, Alternative Treatment, and Care. In B. Prasad & S. Akbar (Eds.), *Handbook of Research on Geriatric Health, Treatment, and Care* (pp. 206–235). Hershey, PA: IGI Global. doi:10.4018/978-1-5225-3480-8.ch012

Gouva, M. I. (2017). The Psychological Impact of Medical Error on Patients, Family Members, and Health Professionals. In M. Riga (Ed.), *Impact of Medical Errors and Malpractice on Health Economics, Quality, and Patient Safety* (pp. 171–196). Hershey, PA: IGI Global. doi:10.4018/978-1-5225-2337-6.ch007

Gürcü, M., & Tengilimoğlu, D. (2017). Health Tourism-Based Destination Marketing. In A. Bayraktar & C. Uslay (Eds.), *Strategic Place Branding Methodologies and Theory for Tourist Attraction* (pp. 308–331). Hershey, PA: IGI Global. doi:10.4018/978-1-5225-0579-2.ch015

Gürsel, G. (2016). Mobility in Healthcare: M-Health. In A. Panagopoulos (Ed.), *Handbook of Research on Next Generation Mobile Communication Systems* (pp. 485–511). Hershey, PA: IGI Global. doi:10.4018/978-1-4666-8732-5.ch019

Gürsel, G. (2017). For Better Healthcare Mining Health Data. In S. Bhattacharyya, S. De, I. Pan, & P. Dutta (Eds.), *Intelligent Multidimensional Data Clustering and Analysis* (pp. 135–158). Hershey, PA: IGI Global. doi:10.4018/978-1-5225-1776-4.ch006

Guzman-Lugo, G., Lopez-Martinez, M., Lopez-Ramirez, B., & Avila-Vazquez, D. (2016). City-Driven Approach to Determine Health Services Based on Current User Location and Collaborative Information. *International Journal of Knowledge Society Research, 7*(1), 53–62. doi:10.4018/IJKSR.2016010104

Gyaase, P. O., Darko-Lartey, R., William, H., & Borkloe, F. (2017). Towards an Integrated Electronic Medical Records System for Quality Healthcare in Ghana: An Exploratory Factor Analysis. *International Journal of Computers in Clinical Practice, 2*(2), 38–55. doi:10.4018/IJCCP.2017070103

Handayani, P. W., Sandhyaduhita, P. I., Hidayanto, A. N., Pinem, A. A., Fajrina, H. R., Junus, K. M., ... Ayuningtyas, D. (2016). Integrated Hospital Information System Architecture Design in Indonesia. In T. Iyamu & A. Tatnall (Eds.), *Maximizing Healthcare Delivery and Management through Technology Integration* (pp. 207–236). Hershey, PA: IGI Global. doi:10.4018/978-1-4666-9446-0.ch013

Hanel, P. (2017). Is China Catching Up?: Health-Related Applications of Biotechnology. In T. Bas & J. Zhao (Eds.), *Comparative Approaches to Biotechnology Development and Use in Developed and Emerging Nations* (pp. 465–520). Hershey, PA: IGI Global. doi:10.4018/978-1-5225-1040-6.ch016

Harmsen, C. A., & Royle, R. N. (2016). St. Stephen's Hospital Hervey Bay: Study of Developing a Digital Hospital. In J. Moon & M. Galea (Eds.), *Improving Health Management through Clinical Decision Support Systems* (pp. 127–153). Hershey, PA: IGI Global. doi:10.4018/978-1-4666-9432-3.ch006

Harp, D., Shim, R. S., Johnson, J., Harp, J. A., Wilcox, W. C., & Wilcox, J. K. (2016). Race and Gender Inequalities in Medicine and Biomedical Research. In U. Thomas & J. Drake (Eds.), *Critical Research on Sexism and Racism in STEM Fields* (pp. 115–134). Hershey, PA: IGI Global. doi:10.4018/978-1-5225-0174-9.ch006

Hartman, A., & Brown, S. (2017). Synergism through Therapeutic Visual Arts. In V. Bryan & J. Bird (Eds.), *Healthcare Community Synergism between Patients, Practitioners, and Researchers* (pp. 29–48). Hershey, PA: IGI Global. doi:10.4018/978-1-5225-0640-9.ch002

Hazra, J., Chowdhury, A. R., & Dutta, P. (2016). Cluster Based Medical Image Registration Using Optimized Neural Network. In S. Bhattacharyya, P. Banerjee, D. Majumdar, & P. Dutta (Eds.), *Handbook of Research on Advanced Hybrid Intelligent Techniques and Applications* (pp. 551–581). Hershey, PA: IGI Global. doi:10.4018/978-1-4666-9474-3.ch018

Hung, S., Huang, W., Yen, D. C., Chang, S., & Lu, C. (2016). Effect of Information Service Competence and Contextual Factors on the Effectiveness of Strategic Information Systems Planning in Hospitals. *Journal of Global Information Management, 24*(1), 14–36. doi:10.4018/JGIM.2016010102

Iltchev, P., Śliwczyński, A., Szynkiewicz, P., & Marczak, M. (2016). Mobile Health Applications Assisting Patients with Chronic Diseases: Examples from Asthma Care. In A. Moumtzoglou (Ed.), *M-Health Innovations for Patient-Centered Care* (pp. 170–196). Hershey, PA: IGI Global. doi:10.4018/978-1-4666-9861-1.ch009

Iqbal, S., Ahmad, S., & Willis, I. (2017). Influencing Factors for Adopting Technology Enhanced Learning in the Medical Schools of Punjab, Pakistan. *International Journal of Information and Communication Technology Education, 13*(3), 27–39. doi:10.4018/IJICTE.2017070103

Jagan, J., Dalkiliç, Y., & Samui, P. (2016). Utilization of SVM, LSSVM and GP for Predicting the Medical Waste Generation. In G. Hua (Ed.), *Smart Cities as a Solution for Reducing Urban Waste and Pollution* (pp. 224–251). Hershey, PA: IGI Global. doi:10.4018/978-1-5225-0302-6.ch008

Jagiello, K., Sosnowska, A., Mikolajczyk, A., & Puzyn, T. (2017). Nanomaterials in Medical Devices: Regulations' Review and Future Perspectives. *Journal of Nanotoxicology and Nanomedicine*, *2*(2), 1–11. doi:10.4018/JNN.2017070101

Jena, T. K. (2018). Skill Training Process in Medicine Through Distance Mode. In U. Pandey & V. Indrakanti (Eds.), *Optimizing Open and Distance Learning in Higher Education Institutions* (pp. 228–243). Hershey, PA: IGI Global. doi:10.4018/978-1-5225-2624-7.ch010

Jesus, Â., & Gomes, M. J. (2016). Web 2.0 Tools in Biomedical and Pharmaceutical Education: Updated Review and Commentary. In T. Gasmelseid (Ed.), *Advancing Pharmaceutical Processes and Tools for Improved Health Outcomes* (pp. 52–78). Hershey, PA: IGI Global. doi:10.4018/978-1-5225-0248-7.ch003

Joseph, V., & Miller, J. M. (2018). Medical Students' Perceived Stigma in Seeking Care: A Cultural Perspective. In C. Smith (Ed.), *Exploring the Pressures of Medical Education From a Mental Health and Wellness Perspective* (pp. 44–67). Hershey, PA: IGI Global. doi:10.4018/978-1-5225-2811-1.ch002

Joyce, B. L., & Swanberg, S. M. (2017). Using Backward Design for Competency-Based Undergraduate Medical Education. In J. Stefaniak (Ed.), *Advancing Medical Education Through Strategic Instructional Design* (pp. 53–76). Hershey, PA: IGI Global. doi:10.4018/978-1-5225-2098-6.ch003

Kaljo, K., & Jacques, L. (2018). Flipping the Medical School Classroom. In M. Khosrow-Pour, D.B.A. (Ed.), Encyclopedia of Information Science and Technology, Fourth Edition (pp. 5800-5809). Hershey, PA: IGI Global. doi:10.4018/978-1-5225-2255-3.ch504

Karon, R. (2016). Utilisation of Health Information Systems for Service Delivery in the Namibian Environment. In T. Iyamu & A. Tatnall (Eds.), *Maximizing Healthcare Delivery and Management through Technology Integration* (pp. 169–183). Hershey, PA: IGI Global. doi:10.4018/978-1-4666-9446-0.ch011

Kasina, H., Bahubalendruni, M. V., & Botcha, R. (2017). Robots in Medicine: Past, Present and Future. *International Journal of Manufacturing, Materials, and Mechanical Engineering*, *7*(4), 44–64. doi:10.4018/IJMMME.2017100104

Katehakis, D. G. (2018). Electronic Medical Record Implementation Challenges for the National Health System in Greece. *International Journal of Reliable and Quality E-Healthcare*, *7*(1), 16–30. doi:10.4018/IJRQEH.2018010102

Katz, A., & Shtub, A. (2016). Design and Build a Wizard of Oz (WOZ) Telemedicine Simulator Platform. In M. Cruz-Cunha, I. Miranda, R. Martinho, & R. Rijo (Eds.), *Encyclopedia of E-Health and Telemedicine* (pp. 128–141). Hershey, PA: IGI Global. doi:10.4018/978-1-4666-9978-6.ch011

Kaur, P. D., & Sharma, P. (2017). Success Dimensions of ICTs in Healthcare. In B. Singh (Ed.), *Computational Tools and Techniques for Biomedical Signal Processing* (pp. 149–173). Hershey, PA: IGI Global. doi:10.4018/978-1-5225-0660-7.ch007

Kaushik, P. (2018). Comorbidity of Medical and Psychiatric Disorders in Geriatric Population: Treatment and Care. In B. Prasad & S. Akbar (Eds.), *Handbook of Research on Geriatric Health, Treatment, and Care* (pp. 448–474). Hershey, PA: IGI Global. doi:10.4018/978-1-5225-3480-8.ch025

Khachane, M. Y. (2017). Organ-Based Medical Image Classification Using Support Vector Machine. *International Journal of Synthetic Emotions*, *8*(1), 18–30. doi:10.4018/IJSE.2017010102

Kirci, P. (2018). Intelligent Techniques for Analysis of Big Data About Healthcare and Medical Records. In N. Shah & M. Mittal (Eds.), *Handbook of Research on Promoting Business Process Improvement Through Inventory Control Techniques* (pp. 559–582). Hershey, PA: IGI Global. doi:10.4018/978-1-5225-3232-3.ch029

Kldiashvili, E. (2016). Cloud Computing as the Useful Resource for Application of the Medical Information System for Quality Assurance Purposes. *International Journal of Computers in Clinical Practice*, *1*(2), 1–23. doi:10.4018/IJCCP.2016070101

Kldiashvili, E. (2018). Cloud Approach for the Medical Information System: MIS on Cloud. In M. Khosrow-Pour (Ed.), *Incorporating Nature-Inspired Paradigms in Computational Applications* (pp. 238–261). Hershey, PA: IGI Global. doi:10.4018/978-1-5225-5020-4.ch008

Kldiashvili, E., Burduli, A., Ghortlishvili, G., & Sheklashvili, I. (2016). Georgian Experience in Telecytology. In M. Cruz-Cunha, I. Miranda, R. Martinho, & R. Rijo (Eds.), *Encyclopedia of E-Health and Telemedicine* (pp. 62–71). Hershey, PA: IGI Global. doi:10.4018/978-1-4666-9978-6.ch006

Ko, H., Mesicek, L., Choi, J., Choi, J., & Hwang, S. (2018). A Study on Secure Contents Strategies for Applications With DRM on Cloud Computing. *International Journal of Cloud Applications and Computing*, *8*(1), 143–153. doi:10.4018/IJCAC.2018010107

Komendziński, T., Dreszer-Drogorób, J., Mikołajewska, E., Mikołajewski, D., & Bałaj, B. (2016). Interdisciplinary Education for Research and Everyday Clinical Practice: Lessons Learned from InteRDoCTor Project. In A. Rosiek & K. Leksowski (Eds.), *Organizational Culture and Ethics in Modern Medicine* (pp. 78–110). Hershey, PA: IGI Global. doi:10.4018/978-1-4666-9658-7.ch004

Komendziński, T., Mikołajewska, E., & Mikołajewski, D. (2018). Cross-Cultural Decision-Making in Healthcare: Theory and Practical Application in Real Clinical Conditions. In A. Rosiek-Kryszewska & K. Leksowski (Eds.), *Healthcare Administration for Patient Safety and Engagement* (pp. 276–298). Hershey, PA: IGI Global. doi:10.4018/978-1-5225-3946-9.ch015

Konecny, L. T. (2018). Medical School Wellness Initiatives. In C. Smith (Ed.), *Exploring the Pressures of Medical Education From a Mental Health and Wellness Perspective* (pp. 209–228). Hershey, PA: IGI Global. doi:10.4018/978-1-5225-2811-1.ch009

Konieczna, A., & Słomkowski, P. (2016). Confrontation of Human Rights in Daily Clinical Situations. In A. Rosiek & K. Leksowski (Eds.), *Organizational Culture and Ethics in Modern Medicine* (pp. 255–281). Hershey, PA: IGI Global. doi:10.4018/978-1-4666-9658-7.ch011

Kromrei, H., Solomonson, W. L., & Juzych, M. S. (2017). Teaching Residents How to Teach. In J. Stefaniak (Ed.), *Advancing Medical Education Through Strategic Instructional Design* (pp. 164–185). Hershey, PA: IGI Global. doi:10.4018/978-1-5225-2098-6.ch008

Kulkarni, S., Savyanavar, A., Kulkarni, P., Stranieri, A., & Ghorpade, V. (2018). Framework for Integration of Medical Image and Text-Based Report Retrieval to Support Radiological Diagnosis. In M. Kolekar & V. Kumar (Eds.), *Biomedical Signal and Image Processing in Patient Care* (pp. 86–122). Hershey, PA: IGI Global. doi:10.4018/978-1-5225-2829-6.ch006

Kumar, A., & Sarkar, B. K. (2018). Performance Analysis of Nature-Inspired Algorithms-Based Bayesian Prediction Models for Medical Data Sets. In U. Singh, A. Tiwari, & R. Singh (Eds.), *Soft-Computing-Based Nonlinear Control Systems Design* (pp. 134–155). Hershey, PA: IGI Global. doi:10.4018/978-1-5225-3531-7.ch007

Kurtz, R. S. (2016). Fortitude: A Study of African Americans in Surgery in New York City. In U. Thomas & J. Drake (Eds.), *Critical Research on Sexism and Racism in STEM Fields* (pp. 153–169). Hershey, PA: IGI Global. doi:10.4018/978-1-5225-0174-9.ch009

Labbadi, W., & Akaichi, J. (2017). Efficient Algorithm for Answering Fuzzy Medical Requests in Pervasive Healthcare Information Systems. *International Journal of Healthcare Information Systems and Informatics, 12*(2), 46–64. doi:10.4018/IJHISI.2017040103

Lagumdzija, A., & Swing, V. K. (2017). Health, Digitalization, and Individual Empowerment. In F. Topor (Ed.), *Handbook of Research on Individualism and Identity in the Globalized Digital Age* (pp. 380–402). Hershey, PA: IGI Global. doi:10.4018/978-1-5225-0522-8.ch017

Lamey, T. W., & Davidson-Shivers, G. V. (2017). Instructional Strategies and Sequencing. In J. Stefaniak (Ed.), *Advancing Medical Education Through Strategic Instructional Design* (pp. 30–52). Hershey, PA: IGI Global. doi:10.4018/978-1-5225-2098-6.ch002

Leon, G. (2017). The Role of Forensic Medicine in Medical Errors. In M. Riga (Ed.), *Impact of Medical Errors and Malpractice on Health Economics, Quality, and Patient Safety* (pp. 144–170). Hershey, PA: IGI Global. doi:10.4018/978-1-5225-2337-6.ch006

Lidia, B., Federica, G., & Maria, V. E. (2016). The Patient-Centered Medicine as the Theoretical Framework for Patient Engagement. In G. Graffigna (Ed.), *Promoting Patient Engagement and Participation for Effective Healthcare Reform* (pp. 25–39). Hershey, PA: IGI Global. doi:10.4018/978-1-4666-9992-2.ch002

Love, L., & McDowelle, D. (2018). Developing a Comprehensive Wellness Program for Medical Students. In C. Smith (Ed.), *Exploring the Pressures of Medical Education From a Mental Health and Wellness Perspective* (pp. 190–208). Hershey, PA: IGI Global. doi:10.4018/978-1-5225-2811-1.ch008

Lovell, K. L. (2017). Development and Evaluation of Neuroscience Computer-Based Modules for Medical Students: Instructional Design Principles and Effectiveness. In J. Stefaniak (Ed.), *Advancing Medical Education Through Strategic Instructional Design* (pp. 262–276). Hershey, PA: IGI Global. doi:10.4018/978-1-5225-2098-6.ch013

Lubin, R., & Hamlin, M. D. (2018). Medical Student Burnout: A Social Cognitive Learning Perspective on Medical Student Mental Health and Wellness. In C. Smith (Ed.), *Exploring the Pressures of Medical Education From a Mental Health and Wellness Perspective* (pp. 92–121). Hershey, PA: IGI Global. doi:10.4018/978-1-5225-2811-1.ch004

Luk, C. Y. (2018). Moving Towards Universal Health Coverage: Challenges for the Present and Future in China. In B. Fong, A. Ng, & P. Yuen (Eds.), *Sustainable Health and Long-Term Care Solutions for an Aging Population* (pp. 19–45). Hershey, PA: IGI Global. doi:10.4018/978-1-5225-2633-9.ch002

Mahat, M., & Pettigrew, A. (2017). The Regulatory Environment of Non-Profit Higher Education and Research Institutions and Its Implications for Managerial Strategy: The Case of Medical Education and Research. In L. West & A. Worthington (Eds.), *Handbook of Research on Emerging Business Models and Managerial Strategies in the Nonprofit Sector* (pp. 336–351). Hershey, PA: IGI Global. doi:10.4018/978-1-5225-2537-0.ch017

Maitra, I. K., & Bandhyopadhyaay, S. K. (2017). Adaptive Edge Detection Method towards Features Extraction from Diverse Medical Imaging Technologies. In S. Bhattacharyya, S. De, I. Pan, & P. Dutta (Eds.), *Intelligent Multidimensional Data Clustering and Analysis* (pp. 159–192). Hershey, PA: IGI Global. doi:10.4018/978-1-5225-1776-4.ch007

Mangu, V. P. (2017). Mobile Health Care: A Technology View. In C. Bhatt & S. Peddoju (Eds.), *Cloud Computing Systems and Applications in Healthcare* (pp. 1–18). Hershey, PA: IGI Global. doi:10.4018/978-1-5225-1002-4.ch001

Manirabona, A., Fourati, L. C., & Boudjit, S. (2017). Investigation on Healthcare Monitoring Systems: Innovative Services and Applications. *International Journal of E-Health and Medical Communications*, *8*(1), 1–18. doi:10.4018/IJEHMC.2017010101

Mannai, M. M., & Karâa, W. B. (2016). Biomedical Image Processing Overview. In W. Karâa & N. Dey (Eds.), *Biomedical Image Analysis and Mining Techniques for Improved Health Outcomes* (pp. 1–12). Hershey, PA: IGI Global. doi:10.4018/978-1-4666-8811-7.ch001

Manzoor, A. (2016). RFID in Health Care-Building Smart Hospitals for Quality Healthcare. *International Journal of User-Driven Healthcare*, *6*(2), 21–45. doi:10.4018/IJUDH.2016070102

Marwan, M., Kartit, A., & Ouahmane, H. (2018). A Framework to Secure Medical Image Storage in Cloud Computing Environment. *Journal of Electronic Commerce in Organizations*, *16*(1), 1–16. doi:10.4018/JECO.2018010101

Masoud, M. P., Nejad, M. K., Darebaghi, H., Chavoshi, M., & Farahani, M. (2018). The Decision Support System and Conventional Method of Telephone Triage by Nurses in Emergency Medical Services: A Comparative Investigation. *International Journal of E-Business Research, 14*(1), 77–88. doi:10.4018/IJEBR.2018010105

McDonald, W. G., Martin, M., & Salzberg, L. D. (2018). From Medical Student to Medical Resident: Graduate Medical Education and Mental Health in the United States. In C. Smith (Ed.), *Exploring the Pressures of Medical Education From a Mental Health and Wellness Perspective* (pp. 145–169). Hershey, PA: IGI Global. doi:10.4018/978-1-5225-2811-1.ch006

Medhekar, A. (2017). The Role of Social Media for Knowledge Dissemination in Medical Tourism: A Case of India. In R. Chugh (Ed.), *Harnessing Social Media as a Knowledge Management Tool* (pp. 25–54). Hershey, PA: IGI Global. doi:10.4018/978-1-5225-0495-5.ch002

Medhekar, A., & Haq, F. (2018). Urbanization and New Jobs Creation in Healthcare Services in India: Challenges and Opportunities. In U. Benna & I. Benna (Eds.), *Urbanization and Its Impact on Socio-Economic Growth in Developing Regions* (pp. 198–218). Hershey, PA: IGI Global. doi:10.4018/978-1-5225-2659-9.ch010

Mehta, G., Dutta, M. K., & Kim, P. S. (2016). An Efficient and Lossless Cryptosystem for Security in Tele-Ophthalmology Applications Using Chaotic Theory. *International Journal of E-Health and Medical Communications, 7*(4), 28–47. doi:10.4018/IJEHMC.2016100102

Mehta, P. (2017). Framework of Indian Healthcare System and its Challenges: An Insight. In V. Bryan & J. Bird (Eds.), *Healthcare Community Synergism between Patients, Practitioners, and Researchers* (pp. 247–271). Hershey, PA: IGI Global. doi:10.4018/978-1-5225-0640-9.ch011

Metelmann, B., & Metelmann, C. (2016). M-Health in Prehospital Emergency Medicine: Experiences from the EU funded Project LiveCity. In A. Moumtzoglou (Ed.), *M-Health Innovations for Patient-Centered Care* (pp. 197–212). Hershey, PA: IGI Global. doi:10.4018/978-1-4666-9861-1.ch010

Mi, M. (2017). Informal Learning in Medical Education. In J. Stefaniak (Ed.), *Advancing Medical Education Through Strategic Instructional Design* (pp. 225–244). Hershey, PA: IGI Global. doi:10.4018/978-1-5225-2098-6.ch011

Miglioretti, M., Mariani, F., & Vecchio, L. (2016). Could Patient Engagement Promote a Health System Free From Malpractice Litigation Risk? In G. Graffigna (Ed.), *Promoting Patient Engagement and Participation for Effective Healthcare Reform* (pp. 240–264). Hershey, PA: IGI Global. doi:10.4018/978-1-4666-9992-2.ch012

Misra, S. C., & Bisui, S. (2016). Feasibility of Large Scale Implementation of Personalized Medicine in the Current Scenario. *International Journal of E-Health and Medical Communications*, *7*(2), 30–49. doi:10.4018/IJEHMC.2016040103

Misra, S. C., Bisui, S., & Fantazy, K. (2016). Identifying Critical Changes in Adoption of Personalized Medicine (PM) in Healthcare Management. *International Journal of E-Health and Medical Communications*, *7*(3), 1–15. doi:10.4018/IJEHMC.2016070101

Mohammadian, M., Hatzinakos, D., Spachos, P., & Jentzsh, R. (2016). An Intelligent and Secure Framework for Wireless Information Technology in Healthcare for User and Data Classification in Hospitals. In V. Wang (Ed.), *Handbook of Research on Advancing Health Education through Technology* (pp. 452–479). Hershey, PA: IGI Global. doi:10.4018/978-1-4666-9494-1.ch019

Mokeddem, S., & Atmani, B. (2016). Assessment of Clinical Decision Support Systems for Predicting Coronary Heart Disease. *International Journal of Operations Research and Information Systems*, *7*(3), 57–73. doi:10.4018/IJORIS.2016070104

Mokrzycka, A., & Kowalska-Bobko, I. (2016). Public Health Legislation and Patient's Rights: Health2020 Strategy, European Perspective. In A. Rosiek & K. Leksowski (Eds.), *Organizational Culture and Ethics in Modern Medicine* (pp. 298–322). Hershey, PA: IGI Global. doi:10.4018/978-1-4666-9658-7.ch013

Moon, J. D., & Galea, M. P. (2016). Overview of Clinical Decision Support Systems in Healthcare. In J. Moon & M. Galea (Eds.), *Improving Health Management through Clinical Decision Support Systems* (pp. 1–27). Hershey, PA: IGI Global. doi:10.4018/978-1-4666-9432-3.ch001

Mosadeghrad, A. M., & Woldemichael, A. (2017). Application of Quality Management in Promoting Patient Safety and Preventing Medical Errors. In M. Riga (Ed.), *Impact of Medical Errors and Malpractice on Health Economics, Quality, and Patient Safety* (pp. 91–112). Hershey, PA: IGI Global. doi:10.4018/978-1-5225-2337-6.ch004

Moumtzoglou, A. (2017). Digital Medicine: The Quality Standpoint. In A. Moumtzoglou (Ed.), *Design, Development, and Integration of Reliable Electronic Healthcare Platforms* (pp. 179–195). Hershey, PA: IGI Global. doi:10.4018/978-1-5225-1724-5.ch011

Moumtzoglou, A., & Pouliakis, A. (2018). Population Health Management and the Science of Individuality. *International Journal of Reliable and Quality E-Healthcare, 7*(2), 1–26. doi:10.4018/IJRQEH.2018040101

Mpofu, C. (2016). International Medical Experiences Outbound New Zealand: An Economic and Medical Workforce Strategy. In D. Velliaris & D. Coleman-George (Eds.), *Handbook of Research on Study Abroad Programs and Outbound Mobility* (pp. 446–469). Hershey, PA: IGI Global. doi:10.4018/978-1-5225-0169-5.ch018

Mukhtar, W. F., & Abuelyaman, E. S. (2017). Opportunities and Challenges of Big Data in Healthcare. In N. Wickramasinghe (Ed.), *Handbook of Research on Healthcare Administration and Management* (pp. 47–58). Hershey, PA: IGI Global. doi:10.4018/978-1-5225-0920-2.ch004

Munugala, S., Brar, G. K., Syed, A., Mohammad, A., & Halgamuge, M. N. (2018). The Much Needed Security and Data Reforms of Cloud Computing in Medical Data Storage. In M. Lytras & P. Papadopoulou (Eds.), *Applying Big Data Analytics in Bioinformatics and Medicine* (pp. 99–113). Hershey, PA: IGI Global. doi:10.4018/978-1-5225-2607-0.ch005

Narasimhamurthy, A. (2016). An Overview of Machine Learning in Medical Image Analysis: Trends in Health Informatics. In N. Dey & A. Ashour (Eds.), *Classification and Clustering in Biomedical Signal Processing* (pp. 23–45). Hershey, PA: IGI Global. doi:10.4018/978-1-5225-0140-4.ch002

Ngara, R. (2017). Multiple Voices, Multiple Paths: Towards Dialogue between Western and Indigenous Medical Knowledge Systems. In P. Ngulube (Ed.), *Handbook of Research on Theoretical Perspectives on Indigenous Knowledge Systems in Developing Countries* (pp. 332–358). Hershey, PA: IGI Global. doi:10.4018/978-1-5225-0833-5.ch015

O'Connor, Y., & Heavin, C. (2018). Defining and Characterising the Landscape of eHealth. In M. Khosrow-Pour, D.B.A. (Ed.), Encyclopedia of Information Science and Technology, Fourth Edition (pp. 5864-5875). Hershey, PA: IGI Global. doi:10.4018/978-1-5225-2255-3.ch510

Ochonogor, W. C., & Okite-Amughoro, F. A. (2018). Building an Effective Digital Library in a University Teaching Hospital (UTH) in Nigeria. In A. Tella & T. Kwanya (Eds.), *Handbook of Research on Managing Intellectual Property in Digital Libraries* (pp. 184–204). Hershey, PA: IGI Global. doi:10.4018/978-1-5225-3093-0.ch010

Olaniran, B. A. (2016). ICTs, E-health, and Multidisciplinary Healthcare Teams: Promises and Challenges. *International Journal of Privacy and Health Information Management, 4*(2), 62–75. doi:10.4018/IJPHIM.2016070105

Olaniran, B. A. (2016). ICT Use and Multidisciplinary Healthcare Teams in the Age of e-Health. *International Journal of Reliable and Quality E-Healthcare, 5*(1), 18–31. doi:10.4018/IJRQEH.2016010102

Olivares, S. L., Cruz, A. G., Cabrera, M. V., Regalado, A. I., & García, J. E. (2017). An Assessment Study of Quality Model for Medical Schools in Mexico. In S. Mukerji & P. Tripathi (Eds.), *Handbook of Research on Administration, Policy, and Leadership in Higher Education* (pp. 404–439). Hershey, PA: IGI Global. doi:10.4018/978-1-5225-0672-0.ch016

Omidoyin, E. O., Opeke, R. O., & Osagbemi, G. K. (2016). Utilization Pattern and Privacy Issues in the use of Health Records for Research Practice by Doctors: Selected Nigerian Teaching Hospitals as Case Study. *International Journal of Privacy and Health Information Management, 4*(1), 1–11. doi:10.4018/IJPHIM.2016010101

Omoruyi, E. A., & Omidele, F. (2018). Resident Physician and Medical Academic Faculty Burnout: A Review of Current Literature. In C. Smith (Ed.), *Exploring the Pressures of Medical Education From a Mental Health and Wellness Perspective* (pp. 171–189). Hershey, PA: IGI Global. doi:10.4018/978-1-5225-2811-1.ch007

Osop, H., & Sahama, T. (2016). Data-Driven and Practice-Based Evidence: Design and Development of Efficient and Effective Clinical Decision Support System. In J. Moon & M. Galea (Eds.), *Improving Health Management through Clinical Decision Support Systems* (pp. 295–328). Hershey, PA: IGI Global. doi:10.4018/978-1-4666-9432-3.ch014

Ossowski, R., & Izdebski, P. (2016). Ethical Aspects of Talking to a Patient. In A. Rosiek & K. Leksowski (Eds.), *Organizational Culture and Ethics in Modern Medicine* (pp. 203–235). Hershey, PA: IGI Global. doi:10.4018/978-1-4666-9658-7.ch009

Pandian, P. S. (2016). An Overview of Telemedicine Technologies for Healthcare Applications. *International Journal of Biomedical and Clinical Engineering, 5*(2), 29–52. doi:10.4018/IJBCE.2016070103

Papadopoulou, P., Lytras, M., & Marouli, C. (2018). Bioinformatics as Applied to Medicine: Challenges Faced Moving from Big Data to Smart Data to Wise Data. In M. Lytras & P. Papadopoulou (Eds.), *Applying Big Data Analytics in Bioinformatics and Medicine* (pp. 1–25). Hershey, PA: IGI Global. doi:10.4018/978-1-5225-2607-0.ch001

Paraskou, A., & George, B. P. (2018). An Overview of Reproductive Tourism. In *Legal and Economic Considerations Surrounding Reproductive Tourism: Emerging Research and Opportunities* (pp. 1–17). Hershey, PA: IGI Global. doi:10.4018/978-1-5225-2694-0.ch001

Park, S., & Moon, J. (2016). Strategic Approach towards Clinical Information Security. In J. Moon & M. Galea (Eds.), *Improving Health Management through Clinical Decision Support Systems* (pp. 329–359). Hershey, PA: IGI Global. doi:10.4018/978-1-4666-9432-3.ch015

Pereira, D., Castro, A., Gomes, P., Areias, J. C., Reis, Z. S., Coimbra, M. T., & Cruz-Correia, R. (2016). Digital Auscultation: Challenges and Perspectives. In M. Cruz-Cunha, I. Miranda, R. Martinho, & R. Rijo (Eds.), *Encyclopedia of E-Health and Telemedicine* (pp. 910–927). Hershey, PA: IGI Global. doi:10.4018/978-1-4666-9978-6.ch070

Peters, R. A., & Cruz, M. (2016). The States as Generators of Incremental Change in American Health Care Policy: 1935 to 1965. In R. Gholipour & K. Rouzbehani (Eds.), *Social, Economic, and Political Perspectives on Public Health Policy-Making* (pp. 86–114). Hershey, PA: IGI Global. doi:10.4018/978-1-4666-9944-1.ch005

Phuritsabam, B., & Devi, A. B. (2017). Information Seeking Behavior of Medical Scientists at Jawaharlal Nehru Institute of Medical Science: A Study. In S. Ram (Ed.), *Library and Information Services for Bioinformatics Education and Research* (pp. 177–187). Hershey, PA: IGI Global. doi:10.4018/978-1-5225-1871-6.ch010

Pieczka, B. (2018). Management of Risk and Adverse Events in Medical Entities. In A. Rosiek-Kryszewska & K. Leksowski (Eds.), *Healthcare Administration for Patient Safety and Engagement* (pp. 31–46). Hershey, PA: IGI Global. doi:10.4018/978-1-5225-3946-9.ch003

Poduval, J. (2016). Curriculum Development. In *Optimizing Medicine Residency Training Programs* (pp. 45–102). Hershey, PA: IGI Global. doi:10.4018/978-1-4666-9527-6.ch003

Poduval, J. (2016). Ethics and Professionalism. In *Optimizing Medicine Residency Training Programs* (pp. 103–133). Hershey, PA: IGI Global. doi:10.4018/978-1-4666-9527-6.ch004

Poduval, J. (2016). Management Skills and Leadership. In *Optimizing Medicine Residency Training Programs* (pp. 182–205). Hershey, PA: IGI Global. doi:10.4018/978-1-4666-9527-6.ch008

Poduval, J. (2016). Medicine Residency Training. In *Optimizing Medicine Residency Training Programs* (pp. 1–27). Hershey, PA: IGI Global. doi:10.4018/978-1-4666-9527-6.ch001

Poduval, J. (2016). Personal Issues. In *Optimizing Medicine Residency Training Programs* (pp. 206–221). Hershey, PA: IGI Global. doi:10.4018/978-1-4666-9527-6.ch009

Poduval, J. (2017). Medical Errors: Impact on Health Care Quality. In M. Riga (Ed.), *Impact of Medical Errors and Malpractice on Health Economics, Quality, and Patient Safety* (pp. 33–60). Hershey, PA: IGI Global. doi:10.4018/978-1-5225-2337-6.ch002

Politis, D., Stagiopoulos, P., Aidona, S., Kyriafinis, G., & Constantinidis, I. (2018). Autonomous Learning and Skill Accreditation: A Paradigm for Medical Studies. In A. Kumar (Ed.), *Optimizing Student Engagement in Online Learning Environments* (pp. 266–296). Hershey, PA: IGI Global. doi:10.4018/978-1-5225-3634-5.ch012

Pomares-Quimbaya, A., Gonzalez, R. A., Quintero, S., Muñoz, O. M., Bohórquez, W. R., García, O. M., & Londoño, D. (2016). A Review of Existing Applications and Techniques for Narrative Text Analysis in Electronic Medical Records. In M. Cruz-Cunha, I. Miranda, R. Martinho, & R. Rijo (Eds.), *Encyclopedia of E-Health and Telemedicine* (pp. 796–811). Hershey, PA: IGI Global. doi:10.4018/978-1-4666-9978-6.ch062

Pomares-Quimbaya, A., González, R. A., Sierra, A., Daza, J. C., Muñoz, O., García, A., ... Bohórquez, W. R. (2017). ICT for Enabling the Quality Evaluation of Health Care Services: A Case Study in a General Hospital. In A. Moumtzoglou (Ed.), *Design, Development, and Integration of Reliable Electronic Healthcare Platforms* (pp. 196–210). Hershey, PA: IGI Global. doi:10.4018/978-1-5225-1724-5.ch012

Pouliakis, A., Margari, N., Karakitsou, E., Archondakis, S., & Karakitsos, P. (2018). Emerging Technologies Serving Cytopathology: Big Data, the Cloud, and Mobile Computing. In I. El Naqa (Ed.), *Emerging Developments and Practices in Oncology* (pp. 114–152). Hershey, PA: IGI Global. doi:10.4018/978-1-5225-3085-5.ch005

Queirós, A., Silva, A. G., Ferreira, A., Caravau, H., Cerqueira, M., & Rocha, N. P. (2016). Assessing Mobile Applications Considered Medical Devices. In M. Cruz-Cunha, I. Miranda, R. Martinho, & R. Rijo (Eds.), *Encyclopedia of E-Health and Telemedicine* (pp. 111–127). Hershey, PA: IGI Global. doi:10.4018/978-1-4666-9978-6.ch010

Raffaeli, L., Spinsante, S., & Gambi, E. (2016). Integrated Smart TV-Based Personal e-Health System. *International Journal of E-Health and Medical Communications, 7*(1), 48–64. doi:10.4018/IJEHMC.2016010103

Rai, A., Kothari, R., & Singh, D. P. (2017). Assessment of Available Technologies for Hospital Waste Management: A Need for Society. In R. Singh, A. Singh, & V. Srivastava (Eds.), *Environmental Issues Surrounding Human Overpopulation* (pp. 172–188). Hershey, PA: IGI Global. doi:10.4018/978-1-5225-1683-5.ch010

Ramamoorthy, S., & Sivasubramaniam, R. (2018). Image Processing Including Medical Liver Imaging: Medical Image Processing from Big Data Perspective, Ultrasound Liver Images, Challenges. In M. Lytras & P. Papadopoulou (Eds.), *Applying Big Data Analytics in Bioinformatics and Medicine* (pp. 380–392). Hershey, PA: IGI Global. doi:10.4018/978-1-5225-2607-0.ch016

Rathor, G. P., & Gupta, S. K. (2017). Improving Multimodality Image Fusion through Integrate AFL and Wavelet Transform. In V. Tiwari, B. Tiwari, R. Thakur, & S. Gupta (Eds.), *Pattern and Data Analysis in Healthcare Settings* (pp. 143–157). Hershey, PA: IGI Global. doi:10.4018/978-1-5225-0536-5.ch008

Rawat, D. B., & Bhattacharya, S. (2016). Wireless Body Area Network for Healthcare Applications. In N. Meghanathan (Ed.), *Advanced Methods for Complex Network Analysis* (pp. 343–358). Hershey, PA: IGI Global. doi:10.4018/978-1-4666-9964-9.ch014

Rea, P. M. (2016). Advances in Anatomical and Medical Visualisation. In M. Pinheiro & D. Simões (Eds.), *Handbook of Research on Engaging Digital Natives in Higher Education Settings* (pp. 244–264). Hershey, PA: IGI Global. doi:10.4018/978-1-5225-0039-1.ch011

Rexhepi, H., & Persson, A. (2017). Challenges to Implementing IT Support for Evidence Based Practice Among Nurses and Assistant Nurses: A Qualitative Study. *Journal of Electronic Commerce in Organizations, 15*(2), 61–76. doi:10.4018/JECO.2017040105

Reychav, I., & Azuri, J. (2016). Including Elderly Patients in Decision Making via Electronic Health Literacy. In M. Cruz-Cunha, I. Miranda, R. Martinho, & R. Rijo (Eds.), *Encyclopedia of E-Health and Telemedicine* (pp. 241–249). Hershey, PA: IGI Global. doi:10.4018/978-1-4666-9978-6.ch020

Richards, D., & Caldwell, P. H. (2016). Gamification to Improve Adherence to Clinical Treatment Advice: Improving Adherence to Clinical Treatment. In D. Novák, B. Tulu, & H. Brendryen (Eds.), *Handbook of Research on Holistic Perspectives in Gamification for Clinical Practice* (pp. 47–77). Hershey, PA: IGI Global. doi:10.4018/978-1-4666-9522-1.ch004

Rissman, B. (2016). Medical Conditions Associated with NLD. In B. Rissman (Ed.), *Medical and Educational Perspectives on Nonverbal Learning Disability in Children and Young Adults* (pp. 27–66). Hershey, PA: IGI Global. doi:10.4018/978-1-4666-9539-9.ch002

Rosiek, A. (2018). The Assessment of Actions of the Environment and the Impact of Preventive Medicine for Public Health in Poland. In A. Rosiek-Kryszewska & K. Leksowski (Eds.), *Healthcare Administration for Patient Safety and Engagement* (pp. 106–119). Hershey, PA: IGI Global. doi:10.4018/978-1-5225-3946-9.ch006

Rosiek, A., Leksowski, K., Goch, A., Rosiek-Kryszewska, A., & Leksowski, Ł. (2016). Medical Treatment and Difficult Ethical Decisions in Interdisciplinary Hospital Teams. In A. Rosiek & K. Leksowski (Eds.), *Organizational Culture and Ethics in Modern Medicine* (pp. 121–153). Hershey, PA: IGI Global. doi:10.4018/978-1-4666-9658-7.ch006

Rosiek, A., & Rosiek-Kryszewska, A. (2018). Managed Healthcare: Doctor Life Satisfaction and Its Impact on the Process of Communicating With the Patient. In A. Rosiek-Kryszewska & K. Leksowski (Eds.), *Healthcare Administration for Patient Safety and Engagement* (pp. 244–261). Hershey, PA: IGI Global. doi:10.4018/978-1-5225-3946-9.ch013

Rosiek-Kryszewska, A., Leksowski, Ł., Rosiek, A., Leksowski, K., & Goch, A. (2016). Clinical Communication in the Aspect of Development of New Technologies and E-Health in the Doctor-Patient Relationship. In A. Rosiek & K. Leksowski (Eds.), *Organizational Culture and Ethics in Modern Medicine* (pp. 18–51). Hershey, PA: IGI Global. doi:10.4018/978-1-4666-9658-7.ch002

Rosiek-Kryszewska, A., & Rosiek, A. (2018). The Involvement of the Patient and his Perspective Evaluation of the Quality of Healthcare. In A. Rosiek-Kryszewska & K. Leksowski (Eds.), *Healthcare Administration for Patient Safety and Engagement* (pp. 121–144). Hershey, PA: IGI Global. doi:10.4018/978-1-5225-3946-9.ch007

Rosiek-Kryszewska, A., & Rosiek, A. (2018). The Impact of Management and Leadership Roles in Building Competitive Healthcare Units. In A. Rosiek-Kryszewska & K. Leksowski (Eds.), *Healthcare Administration for Patient Safety and Engagement* (pp. 13–30). Hershey, PA: IGI Global. doi:10.4018/978-1-5225-3946-9.ch002

Roşu, S. M., Păvăloiu, I. B., Dragoi, G., Apostol, C. G., & Munteanu, D. (2016). Telemedicine Based on LMDS in the Urban/Metropolitan Area: A Romanian Case Study. In M. Cruz-Cunha, I. Miranda, R. Martinho, & R. Rijo (Eds.), *Encyclopedia of E-Health and Telemedicine* (pp. 96–109). Hershey, PA: IGI Global. doi:10.4018/978-1-4666-9978-6.ch009

Rouzbehani, K. (2017). Health Policy Implementation: Moving Beyond Its Barriers in United States. In N. Wickramasinghe (Ed.), *Handbook of Research on Healthcare Administration and Management* (pp. 541–552). Hershey, PA: IGI Global. doi:10.4018/978-1-5225-0920-2.ch032

Ruiz, I. M., Cohen, D. S., & Marco, Á. M. (2016). ISO/IEEE11073 Family of Standards: Trends and Applications on E-Health Monitoring. In M. Cruz-Cunha, I. Miranda, R. Martinho, & R. Rijo (Eds.), *Encyclopedia of E-Health and Telemedicine* (pp. 646–660). Hershey, PA: IGI Global. doi:10.4018/978-1-4666-9978-6.ch050

Sam, S. (2017). Mobile Phones and Expanding Human Capabilities in Plural Health Systems. In K. Moahi, K. Bwalya, & P. Sebina (Eds.), *Health Information Systems and the Advancement of Medical Practice in Developing Countries* (pp. 93–114). Hershey, PA: IGI Global. doi:10.4018/978-1-5225-2262-1.ch006

Sankaranarayanan, S., & Ganesan, S. (2016). Applications of Intelligent Agents in Health Sector-A Review. *International Journal of E-Health and Medical Communications*, *7*(1), 1–30. doi:10.4018/IJEHMC.2016010101

Santos-Trigo, M., Suaste, E., & Figuerola, P. (2018). Technology Design and Routes for Tool Appropriation in Medical Practices. In M. Khosrow-Pour, D.B.A. (Ed.), Encyclopedia of Information Science and Technology, Fourth Edition (pp. 3794-3804). Hershey, PA: IGI Global. doi:10.4018/978-1-5225-2255-3.ch329

Sarivougioukas, J., Vagelatos, A., Parsopoulos, K. E., & Lagaris, I. E. (2018). Home UbiHealth. In M. Khosrow-Pour, D.B.A. (Ed.), Encyclopedia of Information Science and Technology, Fourth Edition (pp. 7765-7774). Hershey, PA: IGI Global. doi:10.4018/978-1-5225-2255-3.ch675

Sarkar, B. K. (2017). Big Data and Healthcare Data: A Survey. *International Journal of Knowledge-Based Organizations*, *7*(4), 50–77. doi:10.4018/IJKBO.2017100104

Saxena, K., & Banodha, U. (2017). An Essence of the SOA on Healthcare. In R. Bhadoria, N. Chaudhari, G. Tomar, & S. Singh (Eds.), *Exploring Enterprise Service Bus in the Service-Oriented Architecture Paradigm* (pp. 283–304). Hershey, PA: IGI Global. doi:10.4018/978-1-5225-2157-0.ch018

Schmeida, M., & McNeal, R. (2016). Consulting Online Healthcare Information: E-Caregivers as Knowledgeable Decision Makers. *International Journal of Computers in Clinical Practice*, *1*(1), 42–52. doi:10.4018/IJCCP.2016010104

Sen, K., & Ghosh, K. (2018). Incorporating Global Medical Knowledge to Solve Healthcare Problems: A Framework for a Crowdsourcing System. *International Journal of Healthcare Information Systems and Informatics*, *13*(1), 1–14. doi:10.4018/IJHISI.2018010101

Shakdher, A., & Pandey, K. (2017). REDAlert+: Medical/Fire Emergency and Warning System using Android Devices. *International Journal of E-Health and Medical Communications*, *8*(1), 37–51. doi:10.4018/IJEHMC.2017010103

Shekarian, E., Abdul-Rashid, S. H., & Olugu, E. U. (2017). An Integrated Fuzzy VIKOR Method for Performance Management in Healthcare. In M. Tavana, K. Szabat, & K. Puranam (Eds.), *Organizational Productivity and Performance Measurements Using Predictive Modeling and Analytics* (pp. 40–61). Hershey, PA: IGI Global. doi:10.4018/978-1-5225-0654-6.ch003

Shi, J., Erdem, E., & Liu, H. (2016). Expanding Role of Telephone Systems in Healthcare: Developments and Opportunities. In A. Dwivedi (Ed.), *Reshaping Medical Practice and Care with Health Information Systems* (pp. 87–131). Hershey, PA: IGI Global. doi:10.4018/978-1-4666-9870-3.ch004

Shijina, V., & John, S. J. (2017). Multiple Relations and its Application in Medical Diagnosis. *International Journal of Fuzzy System Applications, 6*(4), 47–62. doi:10.4018/IJFSA.2017100104

Shipley, N., & Chakraborty, J. (2018). Big Data and mHealth: Increasing the Usability of Healthcare Through the Customization of Pinterest – Literary Perspective. In J. Machado, A. Abelha, M. Santos, & F. Portela (Eds.), *Next-Generation Mobile and Pervasive Healthcare Solutions* (pp. 46–66). Hershey, PA: IGI Global. doi:10.4018/978-1-5225-2851-7.ch004

Singh, A., & Dutta, M. K. (2017). A Reversible Data Hiding Scheme for Efficient Management of Tele-Ophthalmological Data. *International Journal of E-Health and Medical Communications, 8*(3), 38–54. doi:10.4018/IJEHMC.2017070103

Sivaji, A., Radjo, H. K., Amin, M., & Abu Hashim, M. A. (2016). Design of a Hospital Interactive Wayfinding System: Designing for Malaysian Users. In N. Mohamed, T. Mantoro, M. Ayu, & M. Mahmud (Eds.), *Critical Socio-Technical Issues Surrounding Mobile Computing* (pp. 88–123). Hershey, PA: IGI Global. doi:10.4018/978-1-4666-9438-5.ch005

Skourti, P. K., & Pavlakis, A. (2017). The Second Victim Phenomenon: The Way Out. In M. Riga (Ed.), *Impact of Medical Errors and Malpractice on Health Economics, Quality, and Patient Safety* (pp. 197–222). Hershey, PA: IGI Global. doi:10.4018/978-1-5225-2337-6.ch008

Smith, C. R. (2018). Medical Students' Quest Towards the Long White Coat: Impact on Mental Health and Well-Being. In C. Smith (Ed.), *Exploring the Pressures of Medical Education From a Mental Health and Wellness Perspective* (pp. 1–42). Hershey, PA: IGI Global. doi:10.4018/978-1-5225-2811-1.ch001

Smith, S. I., & Dandignac, M. (2018). Perfectionism: Addressing Lofty Expectations in Medical School. In C. Smith (Ed.), *Exploring the Pressures of Medical Education From a Mental Health and Wellness Perspective* (pp. 68–91). Hershey, PA: IGI Global. doi:10.4018/978-1-5225-2811-1.ch003

Sobrinho, Á. A., Dias da Silva, L., Perkusich, A., Cunha, P., Pinheiro, M. E., & Melo de Medeiros, L. (2016). Towards Medical Systems to Aid the Detection and Treatment of Chronic Diseases. In D. Fotiadis (Ed.), *Handbook of Research on Trends in the Diagnosis and Treatment of Chronic Conditions* (pp. 50–69). Hershey, PA: IGI Global. doi:10.4018/978-1-4666-8828-5.ch003

Soczywko, J., & Rutkowska, D. (2018). The Patient/Provider Relationship in Emergency Medicine: Organization, Communication, and Understanding. In A. Rosiek-Kryszewska & K. Leksowski (Eds.), *Healthcare Administration for Patient Safety and Engagement* (pp. 74–105). Hershey, PA: IGI Global. doi:10.4018/978-1-5225-3946-9.ch005

Sołtysik-Piorunkiewicz, A., Furmankiewicz, M., & Ziuziański, P. (2016). Web Healthcare Applications in Poland: Trends, Standards, Barriers and Possibilities of Implementation and Usage of E-Health Systems. In I. Deliyannis, P. Kostagiolas, & C. Banou (Eds.), *Experimental Multimedia Systems for Interactivity and Strategic Innovation* (pp. 258–283). Hershey, PA: IGI Global. doi:10.4018/978-1-4666-8659-5.ch013

Soni, P. (2018). Implications of HIPAA and Subsequent Regulations on Information Technology. In M. Gupta, R. Sharman, J. Walp, & P. Mulgund (Eds.), *Information Technology Risk Management and Compliance in Modern Organizations* (pp. 71–98). Hershey, PA: IGI Global. doi:10.4018/978-1-5225-2604-9.ch004

Spinelli, R., & Benevolo, C. (2016). From Healthcare Services to E-Health Applications: A Delivery System-Based Taxonomy. In A. Dwivedi (Ed.), *Reshaping Medical Practice and Care with Health Information Systems* (pp. 205–245). Hershey, PA: IGI Global. doi:10.4018/978-1-4666-9870-3.ch007

Srivastava, A., & Aggarwal, A. K. (2018). Medical Image Fusion in Spatial and Transform Domain: A Comparative Analysis. In M. Anwar, A. Khosla, & R. Kapoor (Eds.), *Handbook of Research on Advanced Concepts in Real-Time Image and Video Processing* (pp. 281–300). Hershey, PA: IGI Global. doi:10.4018/978-1-5225-2848-7.ch011

Srivastava, S. K., & Roy, S. N. (2018). Recommendation System: A Potential Tool for Achieving Pervasive Health Care. In J. Machado, A. Abelha, M. Santos, & F. Portela (Eds.), *Next-Generation Mobile and Pervasive Healthcare Solutions* (pp. 111–127). Hershey, PA: IGI Global. doi:10.4018/978-1-5225-2851-7.ch008

Stancu, A. (2016). Correlations and Patterns of Food and Health Consumer Expenditure. In A. Jean-Vasile (Ed.), *Food Science, Production, and Engineering in Contemporary Economies* (pp. 44–101). Hershey, PA: IGI Global. doi:10.4018/978-1-5225-0341-5.ch003

Stanimirovic, D. (2017). Digitalization of Death Certification Model: Transformation Issues and Implementation Concerns. In S. Saeed, Y. Bamarouf, T. Ramayah, & S. Iqbal (Eds.), *Design Solutions for User-Centric Information Systems* (pp. 22–43). Hershey, PA: IGI Global. doi:10.4018/978-1-5225-1944-7.ch002

Stavros, A., Vavoulidis, E., & Nasioutziki, M. (2016). The Use of Mobile Health Applications for Quality Control and Accreditational Purposes in a Cytopathology Laboratory. In A. Moumtzoglou (Ed.), *M-Health Innovations for Patient-Centered Care* (pp. 262–283). Hershey, PA: IGI Global. doi:10.4018/978-1-4666-9861-1.ch013

Sukkird, V., & Shirahada, K. (2018). E-Health Service Model for Asian Developing Countries: A Case of Emergency Medical Service for Elderly People in Thailand. In M. Khosrow-Pour (Ed.), *Optimizing Current Practices in E-Services and Mobile Applications* (pp. 214–232). Hershey, PA: IGI Global. doi:10.4018/978-1-5225-5026-6.ch011

Sygit, B., & Wąsik, D. (2016). Patients' Rights and Medical Personnel Duties in the Field of Hospital Care. In A. Rosiek & K. Leksowski (Eds.), *Organizational Culture and Ethics in Modern Medicine* (pp. 282–297). Hershey, PA: IGI Global. doi:10.4018/978-1-4666-9658-7.ch012

Sygit, B., & Wąsik, D. (2016). The Idea of Human Rights in Conditions of Hospital Treatment. In A. Rosiek & K. Leksowski (Eds.), *Organizational Culture and Ethics in Modern Medicine* (pp. 236–254). Hershey, PA: IGI Global. doi:10.4018/978-1-4666-9658-7.ch010

Talbot, T. B. (2017). Making Lifelike Medical Games in the Age of Virtual Reality: An Update on "Playing Games with Biology" from 2013. In B. Dubbels (Ed.), *Transforming Gaming and Computer Simulation Technologies across Industries* (pp. 103–119). Hershey, PA: IGI Global. doi:10.4018/978-1-5225-1817-4.ch006

Tamposis, I., Pouliakis, A., Fezoulidis, I., & Karakitsos, P. (2016). Mobile Platforms Supporting Health Professionals: Need, Technical Requirements, and Applications. In A. Moumtzoglou (Ed.), *M-Health Innovations for Patient-Centered Care* (pp. 91–114). Hershey, PA: IGI Global. doi:10.4018/978-1-4666-9861-1.ch005

Tiago, M. T., Tiago, F., Amaral, F. E., & Silva, S. (2016). Healthy 3.0: Healthcare Digital Dimensions. In A. Dwivedi (Ed.), *Reshaping Medical Practice and Care with Health Information Systems* (pp. 287–322). Hershey, PA: IGI Global. doi:10.4018/978-1-4666-9870-3.ch010

Tripathy, B. (2016). Application of Rough Set Based Models in Medical Diagnosis. In S. Dash & B. Subudhi (Eds.), *Handbook of Research on Computational Intelligence Applications in Bioinformatics* (pp. 144–168). Hershey, PA: IGI Global. doi:10.4018/978-1-5225-0427-6.ch008

Turcu, C. E., & Turcu, C. O. (2017). Social Internet of Things in Healthcare: From Things to Social Things in Internet of Things. In C. Reis & M. Maximiano (Eds.), *Internet of Things and Advanced Application in Healthcare* (pp. 266–295). Hershey, PA: IGI Global. doi:10.4018/978-1-5225-1820-4.ch010

Unwin, D. W., Sanzogni, L., & Sandhu, K. (2017). Developing and Measuring the Business Case for Health Information Technology. In K. Moahi, K. Bwalya, & P. Sebina (Eds.), *Health Information Systems and the Advancement of Medical Practice in Developing Countries* (pp. 262–290). Hershey, PA: IGI Global. doi:10.4018/978-1-5225-2262-1.ch015

Urooj, S., & Singh, S. P. (2016). Wavelet Transform-Based Soft Computational Techniques and Applications in Medical Imaging. In P. Saxena, D. Singh, & M. Pant (Eds.), *Problem Solving and Uncertainty Modeling through Optimization and Soft Computing Applications* (pp. 339–363). Hershey, PA: IGI Global. doi:10.4018/978-1-4666-9885-7.ch016

Vasant, P. (2018). A General Medical Diagnosis System Formed by Artificial Neural Networks and Swarm Intelligence Techniques. In U. Kose, G. Guraksin, & O. Deperlioglu (Eds.), *Nature-Inspired Intelligent Techniques for Solving Biomedical Engineering Problems* (pp. 130–145). Hershey, PA: IGI Global. doi:10.4018/978-1-5225-4769-3.ch006

Waegemann, C. P. (2016). mHealth: History, Analysis, and Implementation. In A. Moumtzoglou (Ed.), M-Health Innovations for Patient-Centered Care (pp. 1-19). Hershey, PA: IGI Global. doi:10.4018/978-1-4666-9861-1.ch001

Watfa, M. K., Majeed, H., & Salahuddin, T. (2016). Computer Based E-Healthcare Clinical Systems: A Comprehensive Survey. *International Journal of Privacy and Health Information Management, 4*(1), 50–69. doi:10.4018/IJPHIM.2016010104

Wietholter, J. P., Coetzee, R., Nardella, B., Kincaid, S. E., & Slain, D. (2016). International Healthcare Experiences: Caring While Learning and Learning While Caring. In D. Velliaris & D. Coleman-George (Eds.), *Handbook of Research on Study Abroad Programs and Outbound Mobility* (pp. 470–496). Hershey, PA: IGI Global. doi:10.4018/978-1-5225-0169-5.ch019

Witzke, K., & Specht, O. (2017). M-Health Telemedicine and Telepresence in Oral and Maxillofacial Surgery: An Innovative Prehospital Healthcare Concept in Structurally Weak Areas. *International Journal of Reliable and Quality E-Healthcare*, *6*(4), 37–48. doi:10.4018/IJRQEH.2017100105

Wójcik, A., & Chojnacki, M. (2016). Behavior and Ethical Problems in the Functioning of the Operating Theater (Case Study). In A. Rosiek & K. Leksowski (Eds.), *Organizational Culture and Ethics in Modern Medicine* (pp. 154–179). Hershey, PA: IGI Global. doi:10.4018/978-1-4666-9658-7.ch007

Wolk, K., & Marasek, K. P. (2016). Translation of Medical Texts using Neural Networks. *International Journal of Reliable and Quality E-Healthcare*, *5*(4), 51–66. doi:10.4018/IJRQEH.2016100104

Wong, A. K., & Lo, M. F. (2018). Using Pervasive Computing for Sustainable Healthcare in an Aging Population. In B. Fong, A. Ng, & P. Yuen (Eds.), *Sustainable Health and Long-Term Care Solutions for an Aging Population* (pp. 187–202). Hershey, PA: IGI Global. doi:10.4018/978-1-5225-2633-9.ch010

Wu, W., Martin, B. C., & Ni, C. (2017). A Systematic Review of Competency-Based Education Effort in the Health Professions: Seeking Order Out of Chaos. In K. Rasmussen, P. Northrup, & R. Colson (Eds.), *Handbook of Research on Competency-Based Education in University Settings* (pp. 352–378). Hershey, PA: IGI Global. doi:10.4018/978-1-5225-0932-5.ch018

Yadav, N., Aliasgari, M., & Poellabauer, C. (2016). Mobile Healthcare in an Increasingly Connected Developing World. *International Journal of Privacy and Health Information Management*, *4*(2), 76–97. doi:10.4018/IJPHIM.2016070106

Yadav, S., Ekbal, A., Saha, S., Pathak, P. S., & Bhattacharyya, P. (2017). Patient Data De-Identification: A Conditional Random-Field-Based Supervised Approach. In S. Saha, A. Mandal, A. Narasimhamurthy, S. V, & S. Sangam (Eds.), Handbook of Research on Applied Cybernetics and Systems Science (pp. 234-253). Hershey, PA: IGI Global. doi:10.4018/978-1-5225-2498-4.ch011

Yu, B., Wijesekera, D., & Costa, P. C. (2017). Informed Consent in Healthcare: A Study Case of Genetic Services. In A. Moumtzoglou (Ed.), *Design, Development, and Integration of Reliable Electronic Healthcare Platforms* (pp. 211–242). Hershey, PA: IGI Global. doi:10.4018/978-1-5225-1724-5.ch013

Yu, B., Wijesekera, D., & Costa, P. C. (2017). Informed Consent in Electronic Medical Record Systems. In I. Management Association (Ed.), Healthcare Ethics and Training: Concepts, Methodologies, Tools, and Applications (pp. 1029-1049). Hershey, PA: IGI Global. doi:10.4018/978-1-5225-2237-9.ch049

Yu, M., Li, J., & Wang, W. (2017). Creative Life Experience among Students in Medical Education. In C. Zhou (Ed.), *Handbook of Research on Creative Problem-Solving Skill Development in Higher Education* (pp. 158–184). Hershey, PA: IGI Global. doi:10.4018/978-1-5225-0643-0.ch008

Zarour, K. (2017). Towards a Telehomecare in Algeria: Case of Diabetes Measurement and Remote Monitoring. *International Journal of E-Health and Medical Communications*, *8*(4), 61–80. doi:10.4018/IJEHMC.2017100104

Zavyalova, Y. V., Korzun, D. G., Meigal, A. Y., & Borodin, A. V. (2017). Towards the Development of Smart Spaces-Based Socio-Cyber-Medicine Systems. *International Journal of Embedded and Real-Time Communication Systems*, *8*(1), 45–63. doi:10.4018/IJERTCS.2017010104

Zeinali, A. A. (2018). Word Formation Study in Developing Naming Guidelines in the Translation of English Medical Terms Into Persian. In M. Khosrow-Pour, D.B.A. (Ed.), Encyclopedia of Information Science and Technology, Fourth Edition (pp. 5136-5147). Hershey, PA: IGI Global. doi:10.4018/978-1-5225-2255-3.ch446

Ziminski, T. B., Demurjian, S. A., Sanzi, E., & Agresta, T. (2016). Toward Integrating Healthcare Data and Systems: A Study of Architectural Alternatives. In T. Iyamu & A. Tatnall (Eds.), *Maximizing Healthcare Delivery and Management through Technology Integration* (pp. 270–304). Hershey, PA: IGI Global. doi:10.4018/978-1-4666-9446-0.ch016

Ziminski, T. B., Demurjian, S. A., Sanzi, E., Baihan, M., & Agresta, T. (2016). An Architectural Solution for Health Information Exchange. *International Journal of User-Driven Healthcare*, *6*(1), 65–103. doi:10.4018/IJUDH.2016010104

Zineldin, M., & Vasicheva, V. (2018). Reducing Medical Errors and Increasing Patient Safety: TRM and 5 Q's Approaches for Better Quality of Life. In *Technological Tools for Value-Based Sustainable Relationships in Health: Emerging Research and Opportunities* (pp. 87–115). Hershey, PA: IGI Global. doi:10.4018/978-1-5225-4091-5.ch005

About the Contributors

Kwok Tai Chui, Dr., received his B.Eng. degree in electronic and communication engineering - business intelligence minor from and a Ph.D. degree from the City University of Hong Kong in 2013 and 2017, respectively. His research interests include artificial intelligence, data analytics, wireless communication, pattern recognition, healthcare, machine learning algorithms and optimization. He was the recipient of the 2nd Prize Award (Postgraduate Category) at the 2014 IEEE Region 10 Student Paper Contest. Also, he received the Best Paper Award from the IEEE International Conference on Consumer Electronics-China, in both 2014 and 2015. He has around 30 research publications, journal papers, conference papers and book chapters. His research interests include complex network, wireless communication, pattern recognition, healthcare, machine learning algorithms and optimization. He has served as various editorial positions and guest editors in referred international journals and conferences.

Miltiadis D. Lytras, Dr., is a Research Professor at Deree- ACG with a research focus on the semantic web, knowledge management, and e-learning, with more than 200 publications. He has co-edited more than 45 special issues in international journals (IEEE Transaction on Knowledge and Data Engineering, IEEE Internet Computing, IEEE Transactions on Education, Computers in Human Behaviour, Interactive Learning Environments, Journal of Knowledge Management, Journal of Computer Assisted Learning) and has authored/(co-)edited 42 books (e.g. Open Source for Knowledge and Learning Management, Ubiquitous and Pervasive Knowledge Management, Intelligent Learning Infrastructures for Knowledge Intensive Organizations, Semantic Web Based Information Systems, China Information Technology Handbook, Real World Applications of Semantic Web and Ontologies, Web 2.0: The Business Model, etc.). He has served as the (Co)Editor in Chief of 8 international journals (e.g. International Journal on Semantic Web and Information Systems, International Journal of Knowledge Society Research, International Journal of Knowledge and Learning, International Journal of Technology Enhanced Learning).

* * *

Said Abdelmaged received the M.S. degree in Computer Science from Alexandria University, Alexandria, Egypt, in 2013. In 2007-2016 he has been working as Assistant Lecturer at Department of Mathematics and Computer Science, Faculty of Science, Alexandria University, Alexandria, Egypt. He is currently pursuing a Ph.D. degree in Computer Science at Smart Data Analytics (SDA), University of Bonn, Bonn, Germany. His research focus in semantic web technologies, scholarly communication, knowledge graph construction, semantic reasoning, and natural language processing. He has several conference and journal publications in the semantic web, text classification, Bioinformatics, scholarly communication, and knowledge engineering. He participated in the program committee of several conferences.

Jeremiah Ademola Balogun is a graduate research assistant in the Department of Computer Science and Engineering, Obafemi Awolowo University, Nigeria. His focus is in the area of applied computing that is application of computing theories to address and solve health related problems in Sub Saharan Africa. He has published in journals and has presented papers at conferences within Nigeria. He is currently researching into Cancer and environmental-related diseases in Nigeria. His research interest includes health informatics, data mining, machine learning, software engineering and geographical information systems. He enjoys reading and brainstorming sessions.

Sanjay Bapna is a Professor and Chair of the Department of Information Science and Systems at Morgan State University. His background is in the field of cyber-security, business intelligence, econometrics, blockchain, data mining, and evaluations. Dr. Bapna is the recipient of the best paper from National Decision Sciences Institute Conference in 2009 and 2011. Another of his papers was awarded the Best Paper from the International Association of Computer Information Systems. He has been awarded numerous grants from the state of Maryland in the area of Intelligent Transportation Systems. He has published extensively in quality journals including Decision Sciences, the Journal of Strategic Information Systems, and Decision Support Systems.

Erik L. Carlton, Dr. PH, MS is Associate Dean of Professional Programs and Associate Professor of Health Policy, Management and Leadership at the West Virginia University School of Public Health. Prior to joining WVU, Dr. Carlton spent six years on the faculty at the University of Memphis School of Public Health and the University of Tennessee Health Sciences Center Colleges of Medicine and Nursing. Dr. Carlton has nearly two decades of managerial and leadership experience in both private and public sector organizations. He is the founder and principal of Elevation Consulting Group, a healthcare consulting firm focused on leadership development, team building, and delivery innovation strategies. His research focuses on healthcare leadership development and the integration of healthcare and public health systems. Having lived internationally in both France and China, and through his work with St. Jude Global, Dr. Carlton has a strong presence in global healthcare leadership development. He has trained clinical and administrative leaders from 28 countries. Dr. Carlton has published and presented his scholarly work nationally and internationally, and is the author of three books.

Kost Elisevich, MD, PhD, is Chair of the Department of Clinical Neurosciences at Spectrum Health in Grand Rapids, Michigan, USA and Professor at the College of Human Medicine of Michigan State University. He obtained his medical degree from the University of Western Ontario in London, Canada in 1978, and completed his neurosurgery training with McGill University at the Montreal Neurological Institute and affiliated hospitals in 1986. Doctoral studies in the Department of Anatomy and Cell Biology at the University of Western Ontario were also completed in the interim. Dr. Elisevich is a Fellow of the Royal College of Physicians and Surgeons of Canada and the American College of Surgeons. His particular interests include the surgical management of epilepsy, studies in epileptogenesis and both electrographic and imaging features of focal epileptogenicity in humans. He has over 150 publications including a book entitled, Case Studies and Commentaries in Epilepsy.

Hidehiko Hayashi, Dr., is currently a professor at Hokusei Gakuen University, Hokkaido, Japan. He received his M.S in Information Science and a PhD degree in Knowledge Science from the Japan Advanced Institute of Science and Technology (JAIST) in 2000 and 2003, respectively. His research interests are information and knowledge science, human sensing technology, brain computer interface, medical information, mathematical analysis of innovation system and ecosystem, and entrepreneurship education.

James W. Holsinger Jr., MD, PhD, currently serves as Chancellor Emeritus and the Charles T. Wethington Jr. Endowed Chair in the Health Sciences Emeritus at the University of Kentucky. His faculty appointments include Preventive Medicine and Environmental Health and Health Management and Policy in the College of Public Health; and Internal Medicine, Surgery, and Anatomy in the College of Medicine. He served for 26 years in the Department of Veterans Affairs and was nominated by President George H. W. Bush and confirmed by the United States Senate as the first presidentially appointed Chief Medical Director of the Veterans Health Administration.

Peter Adebayo Idowu is a Senior Researcher in the Department of Computer Science and Engineering, Obafemi Awolowo University, Nigeria. His research focus is on applied computing that is application of computing to address and solve health related problems in Sub Saharan Africa. He has over 60 publications to his credit in local journals, international journals and referred conference proceedings. He is currently researching into HIV/AIDS, disease modelling, and cloud computing in health care delivery. He is also a Member of the British Computer Society, Internet Society Nigeria Chapter, Nigerian Computer Society, Computer Professional Registration Council of Nigeria, Nigerian Young Academy, International Geospatial Society, International Association of Engineers and International Federation of Information Processing WG 9.4. His research interest includes health informatics, data modelling, software engineering, GIS, and informatics. Within the last five years, Dr Idowu has successively trained over 15 graduate students (both master's and doctoral students). He is blessed with three research associates; Praise, Vicky and Peter. He enjoys reading and driving.

Jan Kalina is a researcher at the boundary between informatics and statistics. He studied mathematical statistics at the Faculty of Mathematics and Physics of the Charles University in Prague and then obtained his Ph.D. from the University of Duisburg-Essen in Germany in 2007. His Ph.D. thesis was devoted to image analysis with medical motivation. He works at the Institute of Computer Science of the Czech Academy of Sciences since 2010, where he has experienced both mathematical and cross-disciplinary applied research and served as a head of Department of Medical Informatics and Biostatistics in 2013-2017. Currently, he serves as associate editor of Sequential Analysis and editorial board member of Applications of Mathematics. He supervises a Ph.D. student working on improving reference charts for fetal biometry at the First Faculty of Medicine of Charles University in Prague. He is passionate about popularization of science and won a gold medal at FameLab Olympics in Dublin in 2012.

Yaman Kannot was born in Hama City, Syrian Arab Republic in 1989. He received a B.S degree in Computer Engineering from the Arab Academy for Science, Technology & Maritime Transport (AAST), Latakia, in 2012 and the M.S. degree in Computer Engineering from the Arab Academy for Science, Technology & Maritime Transport (AAST), Alexandria, in 2016.

Masoud Latifi-Navid, PhD, was born in Ardebil, Iran in 1982. He received his BS degree in Mechanical Engineering in 2007 and then continued his academic education in Mechatronics and received his MS degree from Sharif University of

Technology, Iran in 2009. Mr. Latifinavid received his Ph.D. degree in Mechanical Engineering from Middle East Technical University, Turkey in 2017. He worked as a researcher in the School of Cognitive Sciences at the Institute for Research in Fundamental Sciences (IPM) in Tehran, Iran, from 2008 to 2009. Mr. Latifinavid is currently an assistant professor in Mechatronic Engineering Department of University of Turkish Aeronautical Association in Ankara/Turkey.

Asos Q. Mahmood, MD, MPH, is a doctoral candidate and currently pursuing his degree in Health Systems and Policy doctoral program at the University of Memphis School of Public Health. Mr. Mahmood's research interest areas include chronic medical conditions, ageing populations, and home health care services.

Akinori Minazuki is currently a professor, Kushiro Public University, Hokkaido, Japan. He received his PhD degree in Knowledge Science from Japan Advanced Institute of Science and Technology, Japan (JAIST) in 2003. His research interests are information and knowledge science, information technology for social systems, information education, emergency medical services and medical information.

Heba Mohamed is a Ph.D. candidate in the Smart Data Analytics (SDA) research group at the University of Bonn, Bonn, Germany. She received her master's degree in Computer Science in 2012 from Alexandria University, Egypt. In 2007-2016 she has been working as Assistant Lecturer at Mathematics and Computer Science Department, Faculty of Science, Alexandria, Egypt. Her research interests include Semantic Web, Big Data, Machine Learning.

Sally Shuk Han Pang received her B.Sc. degree in Food & Nutritional Science - Biology Minor with First Class Honor, from The University of Hong Kong in 2014. Her research interests include food and nutritional science, bioinformatics, healthcare, and patient monitoring.

Gregory Ramsey is an associate professor of Information Science and Systems at the Earl G. Graves School of Business and Management at Morgan State University. His research centers on human decision making, data analytics, sources of errors in decision-making processes, process characterization, and health informatics. He earned a BS in Electrical Engineering from Duke University, an MS in Electrical Engineering from the Georgia Institute of Technology, an MSIA from the Tepper School at Carnegie Mellon University, and a PhD. in Information and Decision Sciences from the Carlson School at the University of Minnesota. Additionally, he is a member of the KPMG PhD Project.

Aparna Sahu currently serves as a consultant at Turiyan Psyneuronics Private Limited, a company she co-founded that holds a vision to create computer aided/ tablet assisted neurocognitive assessments and cognitive remediation modules. She received her MA and PhD in Experimental -Cognitive Psychology from the University of Toledo, USA, following which she was a visiting post-doctoral trainee and researcher at the Cognitive Neuropsychology Centre, Department of Experimental Psychology, University of Oxford, UK. She recently served as an Assistant Professor in the Psychology Department at CHRIST (Deemed to be University), Bangalore, India. She has in recent times provided consultation to start-up companies in India that aspire to integrate digital technologies with cognitive psychology for areas such as education and talent management.

Hamid Soltanian-Zadeh, PhD, received his BS/MS degrees in electrical engineering: electronics (with honors) from the University of Tehran, Tehran, Iran in 1986 and MSE/PhD degrees in electrical engineering: systems and bioelectrical sciences from the University of Michigan, Ann Arbor, Michigan, USA, in 1992. Since 1988, he has been with Henry Ford Health System, Detroit, Michigan, USA, where he is currently the director of the Medical Image Analysis Laboratory. Since 1994, he has also been with University of Tehran, Tehran, Iran, where he is currently a Full Professor. Prof. Soltanian-Zadeh has co-authored over 850 papers in journals and conference records and delivered numerous invited lectures nationally and internationally. He has served on the review boards of over 60 scientific journals and study sections of National Institutes of Health (NIH), National Science Foundation (NSF), American Institute of Biological Sciences (AIBS), and international funding agencies.

Index

P

R

S

T

U

V

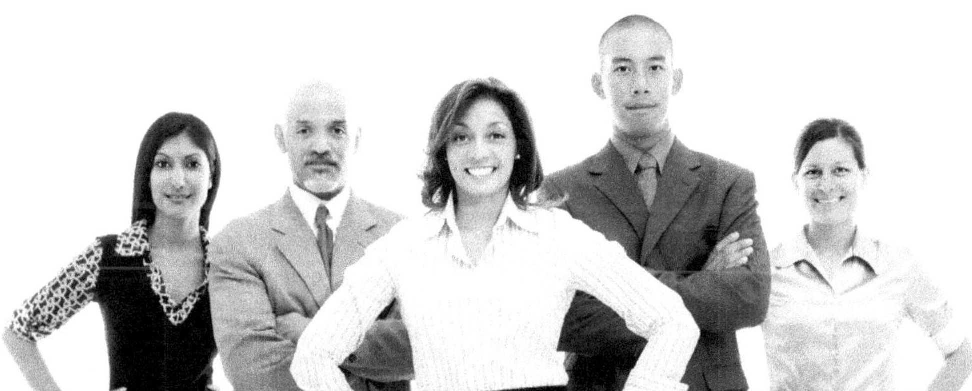

www.ingramcontent.com/pod-product-compliance
Lightning Source LLC
LaVergne TN
LVHW081331021026
849161LV00008BA/1932